CHRONIC RHONCHOPATHY

CHRONIC RHONCHOPATHY

Proceedings of the 1st International
Congress on Chronic Rhonchopathy
Paris, 6-8 July 1987

Editor C.H. Chouard

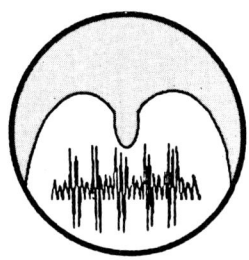

PARIS - 1987

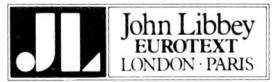

British Library Cataloguing in Publication Data

International Congress on Chronic
  Rhonchopathy. *(1st : 1987 : Paris)*
  chronic rhonchopathy
  1. Snoring
  I. Title II. Chouard, C.H.
  616.2   RF470

ISBN 0-86196-157-9

First published in 1988 by
John Libbey & Company Ltd
80/84 Bondway, London SW8 1SF, England. (01) 582 5266
John Libbey Eurotext Ltd
6 rue Blanche, 92120 Montrouge, France. (1) 47 35 85 52

© John Libbey & Company Ltd, 1988. All rights reserved
Unauthorized duplication contravenes applicable laws

Typesetting in Helvetica by
Gwynne Printers, Hurstpierpoint, Sussex

Printed in Great Britain by
Whitstable Litho, Whitstable, Kent

FIRST INTERNATIONAL CONGRESS ON CHRONIC RHONCHOPATHY

An international congress
held in Paris, 6-8 July 1987
under the patronage of
Mme le Ministre délégué
chargé de la Santé et de la Famille

Collège Français d'ORL et de Chirurgie Cervico-Faciale

and

Société Française de Cardiologie
Société Française de Chirurgie Plastique et Reconstructive
Société d'Electroencéphalographie de Langue Française
Société Française de Neurologie
Société Française de Pneumologie

PARIS
6-8 July 1987

The Organizing Committee would like to thank the
following companies for their generous grants:

ALVAR ELECTRONIC (F)
AUDIT LABORATORIES (F)
BARCLAYS BANK (F)
BOUCHARA LABORATORIES (F)
CENTRE DE CORRECTION AUDITIVE WAGRAM – NATION (F)
EUROTHERAPIE (F)
INAVA LABORATORIES (F)
LAFON LABORATORIES (F)
Ets. POURET (F)
SEFAM (F)
SYNTHEX – LAROCHE NAVARRON LABORATORIES (F)

HONORARY PRESIDENT
T. IKEMATSU (J)

PRESIDENT
C. H. CHOUARD (F)

VICE-PRESIDENTS
H. P. CATHALA (F)
Y. DEJEAN (F)
J. Ph. DERENNE (F)
J. VALTY (F)

SCIENTIFIC ADVISORY BOARD
M. BILLIARD (F)
E. DOUEK (UK)
B. DURON (F)
C. GUILLEMINAULT (USA)
E. LUGARESI (I)
J. M. PIEYRE (CH)
J. E. REMMERS (CAN)

SCIENTIFIC SECRETARIAT
B. MEYER (F)
F. CHABOLLE (F)
B. FLEURY (F)

ORGANISING COMMITTEE
SIR SYMPOSIUM
6 rue Blanche – 92120 MONTROUGE
(1) 46 57 38 38

Contents

INTRODUCTION   1   C.H. Chouard (Editor)

CHRONIC RHONCHOPATHY GENERAL FEATURES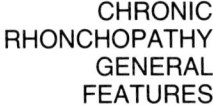

Chairman: F. Chabolle

- 5   Clinical study of snoring for the past 30 years
  Takenosuke Ikematsu
- 15   Anatomic mechanism of snoring
  F. Chabolle
- 20   Eléments de physiologie du sommeil
  M. Minz
- 30   Correlation of structure and mechanics in pharyngeal obstruction during sleep
  J.E. Remmers, T. Feroah, J.R. Perez-Padilla and W.A. Whitelaw
- 36   Epidemiology of snoring and obstructive sleep apnea syndrome
  E. Lugaresi, F. Cirignotta and P. Montagna

CHRONIC RHONCHOPATHY GENERAL FEATURES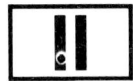

Chairman: B. Fleury

- 45   Detection of the partial upper airway obstruction by the SCSB-method
  O. Polo, M. Tafti and P. Vaara
- 50   Cinematographic X-ray study on snoring
  C. Hannig, A. Wuttge-Hannig and H.W. Mahlo
- 53   Videoradiography of obstructive sleep apnea, OSAS: technical description with a case report
  Birgitta Hillarp
- 59   Respiratory muscles activity in children with sleep obstructive apnea syndrome
  J.P. Praud, J.P. Monrigal, M.F. Delaperche, A.M. d'Allest, H. Nedelco and C.H. Gaultier
- 64   Prognostic value of magnetic resonnance imaging cephalometric study in snorers with or without sleep apnea syndrome
  F. Chabolle, B. Fleury, M.I. Ibazizen and A.E. Cabanis

CHRONIC
RHONCHOPATHY
GENERAL
FEATURES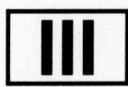

Chairman: J.F. DERENNE

73 Computerized analysis of snoring
ALBERTO LEIBERMAN AND ARNON COHEN

78 Upper respiratory tract resistance and snoring in dogs
J.G. WIDDICOMBE AND A. DAVIES

82 Upper airway anatomic abnormality of chronic snorers with obstructive sleep apnea (methods of evaluation and classification)
SHIRO FUJITA, EUGENE POTESTA AND JACK L. CLARK

85 Combined video endoscopy and frequency spectrum analysis of snoring sounds in heavy snorers. A video demonstration
J.W. SCHÄFER AND W. PIRSIG

88 Polysomnographic study of obstructive sleep dyspnea and snoring
S. MIYAZAKI, K. TOGAWA, K. YAMAKAWA, Y. ITASAKA AND M. OKAWA

93 Do people know about their snoring?
M. PARTINEN, T. TELAKIVI, M. KOSHENVUO AND J. KAPRIO

97 The "common" snorer in front of his doctor
F. LANGRAF-FAVRE

CHRONIC
RHONCHOPATHY
AND
NEUROLOGICAL
DISEASES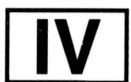

Chairman: H.P. CATHALA

105 Snoring and occurrence in brain infarction
H. PALOMÄKI, M. PARTINEN, S. JUVELA AND M. KASTE

109 Snoring as a risk factor for nocturnal sudden death in spinocerebellar degeneration
SOICHI KATAYAMA, YOSHIRO HIRANO, SEISHI YOKOYAMA, SEIICHI TADA AND MARI KATAYAMA

114 Brainstem dysfunction in sleep apneics as assessed by electrophysiological methods
R.M. KOUTLIDIS, B. FLEURY, M.C.L. ROUSSEAU AND F. CHABOLLE

120 Brainstem structure and function in patients with sleep apnea syndrome
B. FLEURY, R. MORIZOT-KOUTLIDIS, M.C. LAVALLARD-ROUSSEAU, F. CHABOLLE, E. CABANIS AND J. PH. DERENNE

125 Etude du sommeil chez les patients améliorés après uvulopalatopharyngoplastie (UPPP)
F. LAFFON, M.O. JOSSE, M. MINZ, P. WAISBORD, B. FLEURY AND F. CHABOLLE

CHRONIC RHONCHOPATHY AND CARDIO VASCULAR DISEASES V

Chairman: P. VALTY

135 Prevalence and correlates of snoring in an adult population
W.W. SCHMIDT-NOWARA, D.B. COULTAS, C. WIGGINS, B.E. SKIPPER AND J.M. SAMET

141 Apport de l'enregistrement holter au diagnostic du syndrome d'apnées du sommeil
J.Y. LE HEUZEY, P. ROMEJKO, B. FLEURY, J. PH. DERENNE, C.H. CHOUARD AND J. VALTY

144 Snoring and cardiovascular diseases
JEAN VALTY, CLAUDE HENRI CHOUARD, JEAN YVES LE HEUZEY AND ANTOINE BUONCUORE

149 A battery-operated device for home monitoring of oximetry, heart rate, respiration, eye movements, sleeping position, and body movement in patients with snoring and sleep apnea
LAUGHTON E. MILES

152 Sleep apnea syndrome without apnea
G. AUBREY-TULKENS, D.O. RODENSTEIN, C. CULÉE AND D.C. STANESCU

157 The effects of alcohol on snoring-induced hypoxic events in males during the first 3 hours of sleep
P.G. HARTMAN, L. SCRIMA, D. STEDMAN AND F.C. HILLER

158 Effects of alcohol on snoring in men ages 30-50
L. SCRIMA, P. HARTMAN, F. JOHNSON, D. STEDMAN AND F.C. HILLIER

160 The velo-impedancemetry – a new technique for dynamic study of soft palate
C.H. CHOUARD, B. MEYER AND F. CHABOLLE

177 Snoring of nasal origin by vibrations of the salpingoseptal fold
VINCENT BOUTON

181 The endoscopic examination of voluntary snoring
E. TRUFFER

185 Studies of snoring disease by videofiberscope, X-rays and xerography – 23 cases
JEAN ABITOL AND P. KATZ

CLINICAL ASPECTS OF SLEEP APNEAS SYNDROME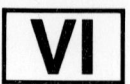

Chairman: J.F. DERENNE

193 Cardio-respiratory investigations during sleep in subjects with chronic rhonchopathy: the use of the static charge sensitive bed method
M. BILLIARD, L. BRISSAUD, B. SALES AND O. POLO

197 Sleep apnea syndrome (SAS) and respiration
B. FLEURY AND J. PH. DERENNE

203 Sleep apnea syndrome: ENT features
Y. DEJEAN AND L CRAMPETTE

CHRONIC RHONCHOPATHY IN CHILDREN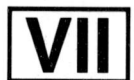

Chairman: A. GRIMFIELD

211 Gradual childhood development of obstructive sleep apnea and behavioral sequelae treated with adenoidectomy
L. SCRIMA, S. SKAKICH-SCRIMA AND N. SNYDERMAN

213 Noisy snoring during sleep in infants with pulmonary disease. Isn't pathologic?
E.N. GARABEDIAN, M. BOULE, M. EISENFIZ AND A. GRIMFIELD

218 Heavy snorers disease in children
M. ZUCCONI, F. CIRIGNOTTA, E. SFORZA, S. MONDINI, A. RINALDI CERONI, F. TARTARI AND E. LUGARESI

227 Treatment of sleep apnea in children with adenotonsillar hypertrophy by adenotonsillectomy
V. WOOTEN, G. PETERS AND JUDY HUBBARD

232 Apnées obstructives du sommeil chez l'enfant: à propos de 28 observations
S. BOBIN, C. LE PAJOLEC, P. ATTAL AND C. GAULTIER

TREATMENTS OF CHRONIC RHONCHOPATHY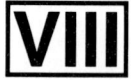

Chairman: Y. DEJEAN

241 Social problems relating to snoring
ELLIS DOUEK

244 The positional treatment of snoring
JEAN MICHEL PIEYRE

250 Prosthetic treatments of chronic rhoncopathy
BERNARD MEYER

TREATMENTS OF CHRONIC RHONCHOPATHY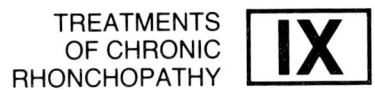

Chairman: E. DOUEK

263 Did Napoleon suffer from sleep apneas syndrome?
C.H. CHOUARD, B. MEYER AND F. CHABOLLE

273 Objective monitoring of therapeutical success in heavy snorers: a new technique
T. PENZEL, G. AMEND, J.H. PETER, T. PODSZUS, P. VON WICHERT AND M. ZAHORKA

279 Polysomnographic evaluation of the effect of uvulopalatopharyngoplasty (UPPP) on obstructive sleep dyspneas
K. TOGAWA, S. MIYAZAKI, K. YAMAKAWA, Y. ITASAKA AND M. OKAWA

284 Effect of nasal application of asonor on snoring
POUL JENNUM

289 Elimination of snoring by means of nasal continuous positive airway pressure reduces airway resistance and respiratory work in obstructive sleep apnea patients
J. KRIEGER AND D. KURTZ

294 Efficiency of continue positive airway pressure (CPAP) after uvulopalatopharyngoplasty (UPPP) failure for obstructive sleep apnea syndrome (OSAS)
B. FLEURY, F. LAFFONT, F. CHABOLLE AND J. PH. DERENNE

300 Surgical management of chronic snoring with obstructive sleep apnea and polysomnographic evaluation
SHIRO FUJITA, ROBERT WITTIG, FRANK ZORICK AND THOMAS ROTH

305 Effectiveness of uvulopalatopharyngoplasty in snorers with sleep apnea syndrome
F. CHABOLLE, B. FLEURY, M. MEYER AND J.P. DERENNE

311 The relative importance of cranio-mandibular abnormalities in obstructive sleep apnea syndrome
M. PARTINEN AND C. GUILLEMINAULT

320 Maxillo-mandibular surgery as a treatment for obstructive sleep apnea
CHRISTIAN GUILLEMINAULT, MARIA ANTONIA QUERA-SALVA, NELSON B. POWELL AND ROBERT W. RILEY

328 Multidisciplinary approach to the diagnosis and treatment of snoring and obstructive sleep apnea
J.M. TRIGLIA, F. PHILIP-JOET, M. REY, M. CANNONI AND A. PECH

TREATMENTS OF CHRONIC RHONCHOPATHY — X

Chairman: E. LUGARESI

- **335** Veloplastics in simple rhonchopathy
  A.H. MORGON AND F. DISANT

- **338** Nocturnal respiratory obstruction and modified technique of uvulo-pharyngoplasty
  JACQUES PICHÉ

- **349** Snoring revealing hypothyroidism
  J. SOUDANT, J.M. ZIZA, G. LAMAS, K. BOUSSEN, B. WECHSLER, M. CHIC AND C. CHAPELON

- **354** Five year follow-up of daytime sleepiness and snoring after tracheostomy in patients with obstructive sleep apnea
  P.S. LEDEREICH, M.J. THORPY, P.B. GLOVINSKY, B. BURACK, P. MCGREGOR, D.L. ROZYCKI AND A.E. SHER

TREATMENTS OF CHRONIC RHONCHOPATHY — XI

Chairman: J.P. PIEYRE

- **361** Assessment and surgical considerations of snoring and OSA
  H.B. HOLDEN, A.D. CHEESMAN AND B.H. PICKARD

- **363** Surgical concepts in uvulo-palato-pharyngoplasty. Complications and sequelae
  Y. ZOHAR, Y. FINKELSTEIN AND Y. TALMI

- **368** Uvulopalatopharyngoplasty sequelae and velopharyngeal valve mechanism
  Y. FINKELSTEIN, Y. TALMI AND Y. ZOHAR

- **373** Results of uvulopalatopharyngoplasty: an evaluation emphasizing preoperative selection criteria and tailoring technique of the procedure
  PH VAN DE HEYNING, J. CLAES, H. VALCKE, J. DE ROECK, E. KOEKELKOREN AND J. BRU

- **379** Clinical results in 790 cases of operated chronic rhonchopathy
  C.H. CHOUARD, B. MEYER AND F. CHABOLLE

- **385** Partial rejection of palate (PRP) as surgical treatment of OSAS
  E. PERELLÓ, P. QUESADA, J. PEDRO-BOTET AND A. ROCA

- **387** Anesthesia for snoring surgery: methods and techniques, problems and risk factors
  J.M. DE LARMINAT, C. BOUCHEREZ, P. BRARD, L. NACCACHE AND S. BOUCLIER

Foreword

C.H. Chouard

Hôpital Saint-Antoine, Service ORL, 184 rue du Faubourg Saint-Antoine, 75012 Paris, France.

It was a pleasure and a great honour to welcome the participants to Paris for the 3 days of the Symposium to study the symptom of chronic snoring and its consequences. The delegates were drawn from so many diverse specialities that it would be almost easier to list those that were absent. Pneumologists, cardiologists, neurologists, sleep specialists, radiologists, epidemiologists, otorhinolaryngologists, all are interested in chronic rhonchopathy: totally unknown a few years ago, today it seems to afflict a large part of the population. Young children, old people, male or female, everyone may start to snore, and this will usually affect them for the rest of their lives, except if proper treatment is given.

The First International Congress on Chronic Rhonchopathy had several goals: (1) to assess the epidemiology and risk factors of the disease; (2) to determine its mechanisms; (3) to study the repercussions of chronic nocturnal hypoxia in various fields of pathology; (4) to describe the various clinical aspects of the disease (from the mild and latent form with only social and personal consequences to severe and dangerous forms which are sometimes responsible for sudden death during sleep), and (5) to expose the various therapeutic possibilities, postural treatment, prosthetic treatment, surgical treatment, and to objectively assess the advantages, the efficacy and the inconveniences of each.

The best incentive to our attempts is to know that our efforts are appreciated by the official bodies responsible for our various specialities. It is a great honour and a great encouragement for us to know that the First International Congress on Chronic Rhonchopathy has received the official support of the French Society of ENT and Cervico-Facial Surgery, the French Society of Cardiology, the French Society of Neurology, the French Society of Pneumology, the French Society of Plastic and Reconstructive Surgery and the French Society of Electro-encephalography. I thank them, their members and their presidents.

Despite the extensive tasks we have to achieve, the facilities provided by SIR Symposium have greatly assisted us. I thank them for the excellent organization of the Congress.

I CHRONIC RHONCHOPATHY GENERAL FEATURES
Chairman: F. Chabolle

Clinical study of snoring for the past 30 years

Takenosuke Ikematsu

Ikematsu Clinic of Otorhinolaryngology, 226 Nakanodai, Noda City, Chiba Prefecture, Japan

ABSTRACT

This paper presents the author's clinical experience in evaluation and treatment of more than 4,000 habitual snorers in Japan during the past 30 years. The data in this study are based on 1,979 patients seen in my clinic from 1970 through 1983.

In 1952, a 23 years old woman came to my clinic with a complaint of her loud snoring which subsequently caused a divorce. She was desperately asking for medical help to eliminate her obnoxious snoring.

On examination, she had no enlarged adenoid, tonsils or nasal obstruction that would be a frequent cause for heavy snoring. The only unusual finding in this examination was the presence of an extremely redundant soft palate, a webbing of the posterior pillar mucosa. After serious thinking, I raised a question whether the removal of these excessive tissues of the soft palate could improve her snoring. With the consent of the patient and her family, I finally decided to go ahead with an operation, a resection of the redundant posterior pillar mucosa and partial excision of elongated uvula under local anesthesia. Since this was my first trial of this procedure, I was naturally a little apprehensive about the outcome, particularly concerning possible complications, in relation to functional disturbance of speech or deglutition. One week after the surgery, she returned to my office with a big smile. She was literally delighted to report that her loud snoring had nearly gone without complications. This was the day I decided to pursue my life long investigation of snoring which is reported here.

METHOD OF INVESTIGATION

The author's initial approach in this endeavor was to study tape recorded snorings of 300 cases collected in 5 years between 1952 and 1956. These were correlated to oropharyngeal anatomy, facial appearance, or any other contributing factors such as sex difference, physical condition, sleeping posture, etc.

Secondly, I conducted an epidemiological study of snoring, its incidence, age distribution and relation to general health.

Questionnaires of snoring were sent to 20,000 residents, including all age groups (0-70 years of age) in Noda City, Chiba-Prefecture. 12,700 individuals responded to the questionnaires for study.

INCIDENCE OF SNORING

In this survey, 92% (excluding infants) indicated that they snored either habitually or non-habitually. 62% were habitual snorers, including heavy snorers 10% and light snorers 52% while 30% were non-habitual snorers and 8% had hardly any snore. 72% of snorers reported their habit of sleeping with mouth open while 60% would snore on sleeping in a supine position (Table 1).

AGE AND SEX DISTRIBUTION

The incidence of snoring increases with age showing the highest among the age group between 50 and 60. There is a tendency of higher incidence of snoring among younger children under age 10. The incidence of habitual snoring tends to decline after age 10 until age 30 in males and 15 in females. Thereafter, it increases with age. (Fig. 1(B)). The males snore slightly more than the females throughout the entire age group. (Fig. 1(A)).

INCIDENCE OF SNORING AMONG THE OLDEST AGE GROUP ABOVE 80

In 1957, the author visited Shirahama Village in Chiba-Prefecture to interview 47 elderly residents ranging from 80 through 108 years of age in order to obtain epidemiological data of snoring among this age group. Shirahama is noted to have the highest longevity among residents in the nation. 76% of this group were found to be non-habitual snorers or non-snorers. They were generally in good health.

HEAVY HABITUAL SNORERS AND GENERAL HEALTH

Among 130 heavy habitual snorers, 65% were found to have significant upper airway obstructive disease or systemic disorder such as obesity, Pickwick disease, obstructive sleep apnea syndrome, hypertension, heart disease, etc.

CONTRIBUTING FACTORS AND/OR PHYSICAL SIGNS ASSOCIATED WITH HABITUAL SNORING

The following is a list of underlying conditions, contributing factors or physical signs frequently seen in heavy habitual snorers.
1. Obesity
2. Upper airway abnormality or obstruction
   (a) Nasal obstruction - sleeping with mouth open
   (b) Excessive secretion or dryness in the upper airway tract
   (c) Oro- or hypopharyngeal mass (enlarged tonsils, lingual tonsils, cyst)
   (d) Nasopharyngeal mass or stenosis
3. Upper airway anatomical deviation
   (a) Enlarged or elongated uvula
   (b) Redundant pillar mucosa (soft palatal arch)
   (c) Micro or retrognathia (Bird-face, Pigeon jaw)
   (d) Macroglossia
4. Sleeping posture
5. Physical fatigue
6. Idiopathic (unknown cause)

There is a significant individual variability as to the onset, duration, intensity and acoustic features of snoring. The snoring can vary or modify by sleeping postures, amount of physical activities during the day (physical fatigue), alcohol, CNS suppressant drugs, bedding condition, general physical condition, environmental factors, etc. Snoring may occur at any stage of sleep (not related to the depth of sleep).

EVALUATION AND TREATMENT OF SNORING

1,979 patients were evaluated for snoring at the author's clinic from 1970 through 1983. 694 were males (35%) and 1,285 were females (65%). They were referred by nationwide sources; physicians, former patients treated for snoring or news media.

Underlying reasons for snoring evaluation are listed in Table 3. The most common reason is their concern over a disrupted marital life (24%) or family life (20%), frequently causing sleepless nights of their spouses or family members. Anxiety over participating in group trips (camping, golfing, etc.) is the next common reason (17%), followed by their concern over health (13%). Evaluation requests for snoring are far more frequent in women than in men (65% vs 35%). The patients of age group 21 - 30 are the most frequent visitors at a snoring clinic. (Table 2, 3)

The evaluation of snoring patients begins with a careful history of snoring, its onset, duration, search for contributing factors, system review and family history.

The physical examination includes measurements of height and weight, observation of facial appearance - profile (retro or micro-gnathia) and ENT examination. Above all, the inspection of the orpharynx is vitally important. It is performed first without a tongue depressor to see the soft palate in relation to the tongue. The tongue is then gently depressed with a blade to inspect the uvula and soft palatal arch with respect to size, shape, and position in the oropharyngeal space. The free margin of the soft palate is then observed while at rest and at phonating a letter "A". Gag-reflex can be minimized by a gentle touch or a spray of local anesthetic.

DIMENSIONS OF OROPHARYNX (SOFT PALATE & UVULA)

The dimensions of oropharyngeal anatomy, soft palate, uvula and oropharyngeal space are illustrated in figures (2, 3). These measurements represent the mean value of oropharyngeal dimension based on the study of 50 Japanese adults.

    The antero-posterior dimension of hard palate .... 50 mm
    The antero-posterior dimension of soft palate .... 40 mm
    (Distance from the posterior margin of the hard palate to the root of the uvula)
    The uvula length .... 10 mm
    The uvula width .... 7 mm
    The width of posterior pillar .... 4 mm

The oropharyngeal dimension during phonating "Ah" (Fig. 3)
    The distance between the root of uvula and the dorsum of tongue .... 30 mm
    The distance between the right and left anterior pillar (arch) .... 30 mm
    The distance between the right and left posterior pillar (arch) .... 20 mm
    The distance between the posterior sufrace of uvula and the posterior pharyngeal wall .... 10 mm

ANATOMICAL VARIATIONS OF SOFT PALATE AND UVULA IN SNORING PATIENTS

The following observations were made in snoring patients with regard to the dimension of oropharyngeal structures. These were classified basically to 6 types (A, B, C, D, E, F) based on the shape and size of the soft palate or the uvula. The combination of more than two types are frequently seen.

(1) Type A. (Long soft palate): The antero-posterior dimension of soft palate is greater than 50 mm.
(2) Type B. (Elongated uvula): The length of uvula greater than 11 mm.
(3) Type C. (Enlarged uvula): The width of uvula is greater than 10 mm.
(4) Type D. (Redundant posterior pillar mucosa or posterior palatal arch): The width of pillar mucosa is greater than 5 mm.

Type D is subdivided into 4 groups: (Fig. 4)
    (a) Type DI (parallel type): The anterior palatal arch curves parallel with the posterior palatal arch.
    (b) Type DII (Webbing type): The posterior palatal arch forms a web-like appearance.
    (c) Type DIII (Imbedded type): Uvula imbedded in the posterior palatal arch.
    (d) Type DIV (Emerging type): Uvula emerges from the posterior platal arch.

(5) Type E. (Narrowing of the oropharynx) (Fig. 5)
    (a) Type EI (Anterior arch narrowing): The distance between the anterior palatal arches is less than 20 mm.
    (b) Type EII (Posterior arch narrowing): The distance between the posterior arches is less than 15 mm.
    (c) Type EIII (Shallow oropharynx): The distance between the posterior surface of the uvula and the posterior pharyngeal wall is less than 5 mm.

(6) Type F. (Large dorsum tongue): The oropharyngeal space cannot be visualized at phonating "Ah" sound.

TREATMENT PLAN FOR SNORING

The treatment of snoring is generally directed to three major categories. (1) Counseling of snoring control. (2) Treatment of underlying physical conditions. (3) Partial uvulectomy and palatopharyngoplasty.

The change of sleeping position from the supine to the side or the prevention of mouth breathing (taping the mouth) may prove to be helpful. The abuse of alcohol or certain drugs predisposing to snoring should be avoided. Underlying physical condition either systemic or local should be treated accordingly (obesity, endocrine or metabolic disease, upper airway obstruction).

PLASTIC SURGERY OF SOFT PALATE AND UVULA FOR SNORING
(palatopharyngoplasty and partial uvulectomy)

1) The criteria for selection of surgical candidate
If the patients snoring should persist after adequate treatment of upper airway disease, the following criteria is used to select the patient for the operation.
    (a) The tape recorded snoring is suggestive of uvular origin. (The length of the uvula is greater than 10 mm (Type B).
    (b) The A-P dimension of the soft palate is greater than that of the hard palate.
    (c) The width of posterior pillar mucosa is greater than 5 mm.
    (d) The distance between the posterior palatal arches is less than 25 mm.
    (e) Webbing of the posterior pillar mucosa (Type DII).
    (f) Enlarged Uvula (Type C).

2)   Surgical Technique
The technique of this surgery was previously reported. (Ikematsu, T. Study of Snoring, 4th Report. Therapy (in Japanese) J. Jap Oto-Rhino-Laryngol 64: 434-435.) The basic technique is illustrated in Figure 6. A wedge section is made in the posterior pillar mucosa adjacent to the root of the uvula. The mucosa of the pillar between the palatal arches is removed. The mucosal edges of the anterior and posterior palatal arches are approximated by interrupted sutures. A small partial resection of mucosa and submucosal tissues from the root of the uvula would cause anterior displacement of the uvula. (Fig. 6)

3)   Result
Total 152 patients underwent this surgery in 1963 through 1967. 81.6% reported improvement of snoring after the surgery. (46.1% - marked, 35.5% - moderate) No significant complications were noted.

Between 1970 and 1983, 1,979 patients were seen for snoring evaluation and treatment at Ikematsu ENT Clinic. 1,690 cases were considered as surgical candidates, however, 1,646 underwent the surgery, 1,007 cases were lost for followup (61%) since the majority of these patients came from various parts of Japan far from Noda City. 584 reported an improvement (30%) while 55 indicated no positive effect (3.6%).

CONCLUSION

Based on my observations and studies of snoring on more than 4,000 snorers since 1952, I have become convinced that habitual heavy snoring is neither a symbol of good health nor a physiological respiratory sound. The heavy snoring is a pathological respiratory noise caused by an increased resistance to air flow in the upper airway tract during sleep.

The following conclusions are reached from this study:
(1)   Snoring is caused by a multitude of factors.
(2)   Specific anatomy of soft palate and uvula plays a significant role in geneses of snoring.
(3)   Snoring may cause social disaster and potential hazard to health.

Out of 4,000 patients, the data of snorers examined in the year of 1961 is as follows.

①   Total Number of Snorers: 292
      Number of Snorers of Soft Palate Disorders: 206 (male: 110, female: 96)

②   Age Distribution of Snorers:
      10 yrs to 20 yrs   2 persons
      21 yrs to 30 yrs   34 persons
      31 yrs to 40 yrs   38 persons
      41 yrs to 50 yrs   47 persons
      51 yrs to 60 yrs   62 persons
      61 yrs to 70 yrs   19 persons
      71 yrs and older   4 persons

As an additional factor, there were more female patients in the age group of under 30 years old, and more male patients in the older age group. This means that men become more conscious about their snoring as they become older. Until 10 years before, the percentage of female patients among the older age group was higher.

The structures of soft palates of the heavy habitual snorers are classified into 15 groups as shown in the illustration. It can be said that forms of soft palates have some relevancy to snoring, however, there are no relations found between snoring and snorer's sex, age, facial structure, etc.

③ Result of V.P.P.P.

Extremely effective 43 persons = 21%
Very effective   62 persons = 30%   87%
Effective   75 persons = 36%
Not effective   26 persons = 13%

Another conclusive factor is that 70.5% of habitual snorers had disorders in their soft palates.

④ 87% of patients were recognized of their improvement through V.P.P.P. This treatment was also found very effective for non-respiration-syndrome-asleep.

<u>Classified Soft Palates</u>

I   Normal   II   Enlarged uvula   III   Elongated uvula

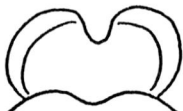 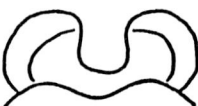 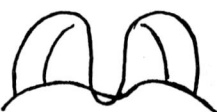

IV   Twin-shaped uvula   V   Parallel palatal archs   VI   Horizontal posterior palatal arch

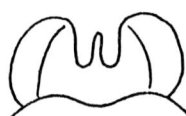 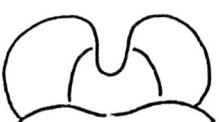 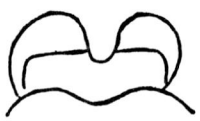

VII   Embedded uvula   VIII   Emerging uvula   IX   Anterior arch narrowing

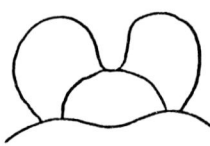 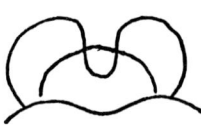 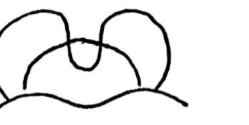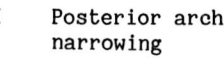

X   Posterior arch narrowing   XI   Shallow oropharynx   XII   Large dorsum tongue

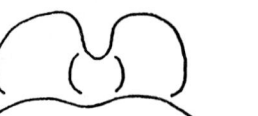 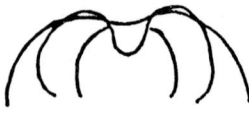

XIII Wide soft palate   XIV Enlarged side pharyngeal walls   XV Enlarged tonsils

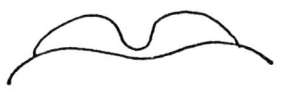  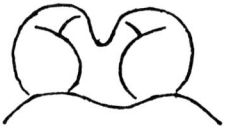

XVI Deformed soft palates

TABLE 1
INCIDENCE OF SNORING

Light habitual snorer	52%
Heavy habitual snorer	10%
Non-habitual snorer	30%
Non-snorer (hardly any snore)	8%

TABLE 2
UNDERLYING REASONS FOR SNORING EVALUATION

1. Disrupting marital relationship (24%)
2. Disrupting family life (20%)
3. Anxiety over joining group trips (17%)
4. Anxiety over health (13%)
5. Concern for living at nursing home or admission to the hospital (10%)
6. Anxiety over disturbing others on the job (8%)
7. Restless sleeper (7%)
8. Concern of living in apartment (.2%)
9. Others (.8%)

TABLE 3
AGE DISTRIBUTION OF SNORERS EVALUATED

AGE GROUP	CASES
0-10	14
11-20	31
21-30	484
31-40	263
41-50	289
51-60	310
61-70	92
71-80	2
	1485

Male   -   694 (35%)
Female - 1,285 (65%)
Total   - 1,979
        (494 - not included)

TABLE 4
RESULT OF UPPP (1963-1967)

Total 152 cases (49 males, 103 females)
Subjective response

Snoring markedly improved	70 cases	46.1%
Snoring moderately improved	54 cases	35.5%
Snoring unimproved	8 cases	5.3%
Snoring unknown	20 cases	13.1%

81.6% reported improvement

TABLE 5
TREATMENT OF SNORING AT IKEMATSU ENT CLINIC
NODA CITY CHIBA PREF. (1970-1983)

Total cases	1,979
Male:	694
Female:	1,285

Counseling of snoring control alone	204 cases
Palatopharyngoplasty and partial uvulectomy	1,646 cases
Surgery canceled	44 cases
Those reported improvement by surgery	584 (30%)
Those reported no improvement by surgery	55 (3.6%)
Those lost for followup	1,007 (61%)

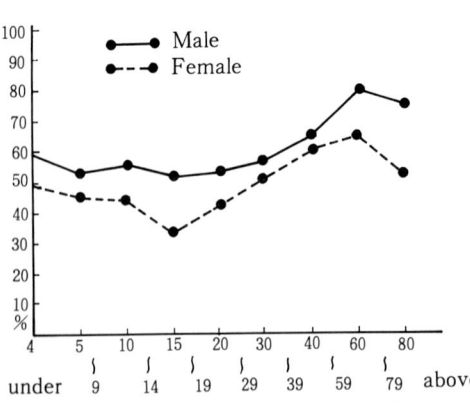

Fig. 1 (A)
INCIDENCE OF SNORING AND AGE

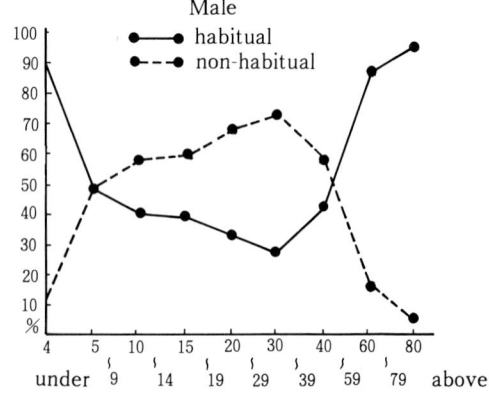

Fig. 1 (B)
HABITUAL & NON-HABITUAL SNORING

Fig. 1 (A) : INCIDENCE OF SNORING
            AGE & SEX DISTRIBUTION

Fig. 1 (B) : INCIDENCE OF SNORING HABITUAL
            & NON-HABITUAL (MALE & FEMALE)

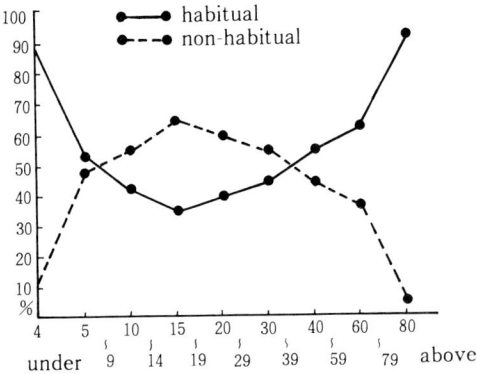

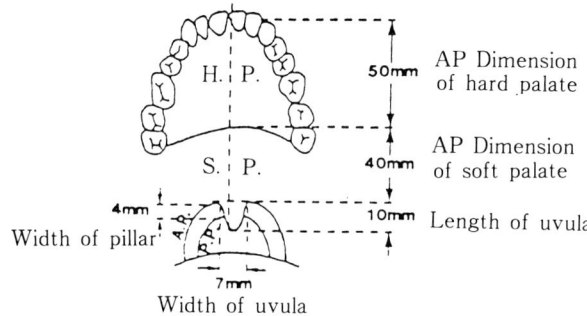

Figure 2. Dimension of soft palate (adult)
H. P. (hard palate) S. P. (soft palate) U (Uvula)
A. P. (anterior pillar) p. p. (posterior pillar)

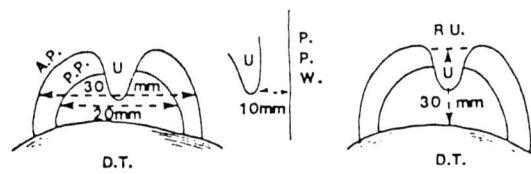

Figure 3. Dimension of oropharynx
U. (uvula) R. U. (root of uvula) A. P. (anterior pillar)
P. P. (posterior pillar) P. P. W. (posterior pharyngeal wall)
D. T. (dorsum of tongue)

PALATO - PLASTY & Partial Uvulectomy
IKEMATSU

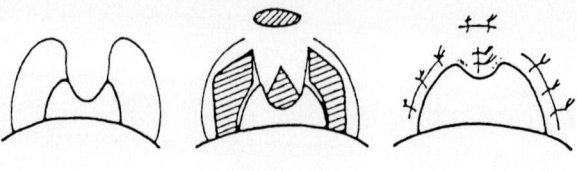

Fig. 6

SOFT PALATE (TYPE D)

TYPE D-(1) : (Parallel Type)

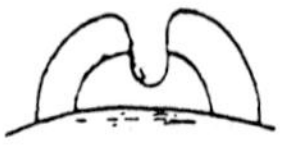

TYPE D (2) : (Webbing Type)

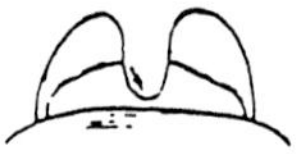

TYPE D (3) : (Imbedded Uvula)

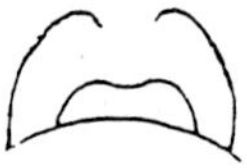

TYPE D (4) : (Emerging Uvula)

Fig. 4

TYPE E (1) (Ant-PA-Nar) <20mm

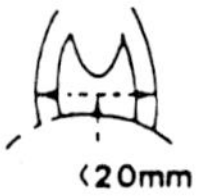

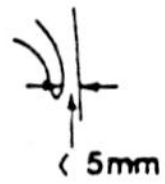

TYPE E (2) (Post-PA-Nar) <15mm

TYPE E (3) (Shallow O-P) <5mm

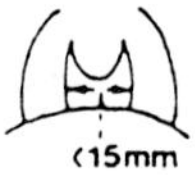

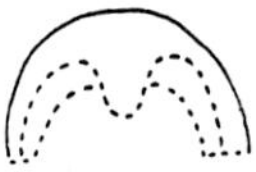

TYPE F (S. P. behind T)

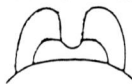

Fig. 5

Anatomic mechanism of snoring

F. Chabolle

Service O.R.L., Hôpital Saint-Antoine, 184 rue du faubourg Saint-Antoine, 75012 Paris, France

ABSTRACT

Snoring is due to soft palate vibration secondary to the opposed and conjugated action of gravity and Bernouilli's effect induced by upper aerial tracts narrowing. Assay methods of the anatomic site relie on clinical examination and numerous complementary investigations, more or less complex and invasive. In certain cases, it is possible to find local or general congenital causes of obstruction. But very often, determination of exact obstructive site is difficult in spite of the numerous complementary investigations described in litterature. In total, two privileged sites seem to exist, located at soft palate lower part or at tongue base.

KEYWORDS

Anatomy ; Oral cavity ; Oro-pharynx ; Sleep Apnea Syndrome ; Snoring.

INTRODUCTION

Since 1952, when Ikematsu opened new therapeutic perspectives in the field of snoring or rhonchopathy, very numerous authors have studied its mechanism and especially its anatomic bases. It is now asknowledged that an obstacle sits at the level of the upper aerial tracts, responsible of this sonorous manifestation due to the vibration of soft palate. Since the early eighties, the necessity of discovering exactly the obstructive anatomic sight became more eager when the S.A.S was identified like being a serious evolutionary complication of snoring, with severe physio-pathological consequences.

MECHANISM

Rhonchopathy is due to vibration of soft palate when it bumps against the oropharyngeal wall and involves a sonorous effect (Chouard, 1986).

Snoring demands a narrowing of the upper aerial tracts, often associated to soft palate abnormality.

During sleep, a loss of tonicity in the muscles of oro-pharynx appears, beginning by soft palate tensor muscle, as evidenced by different electro-myographic tests. On the opposite, phrenic muscle conserves the same activity as when awake. Oro-pharyngeal muscular hypotonicity increases progressively during the four stages of R.E.M sleep and persists during non R.E.M sleep. It is maximum in the last stage of R.E.M sleep.

A back drop of tongue and of soft palate occurs when normal subject is in supine position, soft palate spreads itself on posterior pharyngeal wall under the effect of gravity, explaining then efficience of posture therapy of snoring.

Snoring requires the presence of another obstacle in the upper aerial tracts. This obstacle can have numerous causes, variously associated (tonsils, base of tongue, pharyngeal wall ...). It is then created a narrowing of the upper aerial tracts, changing gazeous fluids displacement mode, and creating turbulence. Soft palate vibrates during the inspiration period under conjugated action of two opposite effects : on the one hand, gravity pushes soft palate against posterior wall, on the other, Bernouilli's effect has the opposite effect by taking soft palate off posterior wall and putting it back in the middle of the upper aerial tracts. At the oro-pharyngeal level, Bernouilli's effect is due to combined action of upper aerial tracts narrowing and persistance of phrenic inspiration activity during sleep. Air presents an increase of flow speed at that level and a reduction of pressure tending to create a negative pressure zone in the narrowing area and then taking soft palate off posterior wall and putting it back at the narrowing center.

Soft palate is thus submised to two forces of opposite activity making it vibrate during inspiration and causing a noise with an intensity possibly reaching 70 Db and of various frequencies.

Snoring intensity depends on soft palate surface, length, elasticity and thickness, but also on the other oro-pharyngeal structures dimension and tonicity.

INVESTIGATION METHODS OF OBSTACLE MECHANISM

Anatomic causes must be looked for first, in order to eliminate obvious snoring factors. Organic functional nose obstruction, abnormality of head and neck morphology as retrognathia, tongue, soft palate and tonsil hypertrophy, or any soft palate morphologic abnormality must be searched.

Complementary investigations are useful especially in snoring complicated with S.A.S in order to determinate the exact obstructive sight. Some are considered to be invasive, even in the opinion of their authors, because they introduce a foreign body in the upper aerial tracts and then modify sleep and anatomic configuration, despite miniaturisation possibilities. It consists most often in an assay with a fibroscope introduced in the nasal tract and placed at the various levels of the upper aerial tracts and coupled with video recording. It can also consist in a method using acoustic reflexion requiring the presence of a buccal nozzle or a nasal probe with staged pressure sensors, allowing to situate maximum pressure level (Bradley, 1986 ; Hudgel, 1986).

On the opposite, non invasive methods are closer to pathologic reality and essentially call upon medical imagery. Profile teleradiography appreciates a possible abnormality of the head. Radiocinema and sleep fluoroscopy can allow a dynamic approach of rhonchopathy anatomic mechanisms. CT scan examination shows aerial tracts dimensions in axial sections at various levels and appreciates hypertrophy of various structures of the area, as well as any possible repartition of fat infiltration. CT scan with 3 dimensions study was proposed in order to carry out tongue volumetric reconstructions and quantify a possible hypertrophy. More recently, M.R.I allowed to obtain, with appropriated surface aerials, a sagittal section very useful to study the respiratory tract and connections of oro-pharyngeal structures (Haponik, 1983 ; Katsantonis, 1986 ; Kryger, 1983 ; Suratt, 1983).

ANATOMIC CAUSES OF SNORING

Anatomic causes of snoring involve on the one hand soft palate abnormalities and on the other, an obstacle of the upper aerial tracts.

Soft palate abnormalities

We must quote in anatomic causes of snoring, various anatomic variations of soft palate vibrator by differentiating, very schematically, two types :
- Soft palate of a young subject having been snoring since adolescence, due to soft palate muscle system hypertrophy often associated with an inferior mucosa palmation with two tonsils joining at the uvula level with disappearance of the muscles of the soft palate lower part, giving a mucous membran. In this case, soft palate length is sub-normal with, frequently, a very large and non narrowed pharynx.
- On the opposite, soft palate of the aged plethoral subject with a lengthening and a congestive hypertrophy of soft palate and uvula palatina. This lengthening of soft palate goes often with an hypertrophy of the various structures of hypopharynx as macroglossia, posterior wall congestive mucosa with false posterior pillars apt to meet on the posterior medium line during nauseous reflex (Chouard, 1986).

Obstruction of upper aerial tracts

According to recent publications, it appears that this obstacle is especially located at the level of oro-pharynx. Nasal fossae or intra-laryngeous narrowings are unusually involved (Cole, 1984).

In the normal subject, there is a variation of pharyngeal resistances depending on sex, age, weight and sleep depth. In the female, pharyngeal resistances are lower, especially before menopause; in the same way, they increase in the aged, explaining more frequent rhonchopathy in that soil.

The obstacle of upper aerial tracts can appear in the context of a general systemic disease or of an isolated pathology of upper aerial tracts.

It may also involve congenital anomaly such as Pierre ROBIN's syndrome, with micrognathia and glossoptosis, where the obstacle is located at the base of the tongue. In the same way, isolated micrognathia can be involved where backing of genioapophyses and thus of tongue insertion is the reason of low oro-pharynx narrowing (Spier, 1986 ; Davies, 1983).

But, most often this anomaly is acquired. Some local causes appear to be obvious but unusual in the narrowing genesis : lymphoma of lingual tonsils (Lugarest, 1975), basi lingual ectopic thyroïd, upper aero-digestive tracts cancer, especially of tongue base in its proliferating form, acquired micrognathia with glossoptosis due to temporo-mandibular rheumatoïd arthritis. It is also true for laryngeal pathologies such as paralyses of nervus recurrens or tumors. Tonsils hypertrophies are much less frequent in the adult than in the child where they contribute to change aerial flux with a turbulence appearance due to preponderant noctural buccal respiration responsible of the vibration of soft palate (Orr, 1981).

Beside these local causes, there are many general favouring factors. Alcohol and narcotics worsen rhonchopathy by increasing sleep depth and the intensity of release of oro-pharyngeal muscles (Issa, 1982).

Age increases risks of snoring that can however occur in young subject as soon as adolescence. In this case, one must look for a soft palate congenital anomaly consisting in a muscular disappearance in the soft palate lower part.

Obesity plays a particularly important role. Weight increase by fatty infiltration of all tissues contributes in increasing widely oro-pharyngeal resistances. Fat repartition is still discussed but CT scan examinations demonstrated that this infiltration is diffuse and not only located in a single fat coat at the level of sub-mucosa region of upper aerial tracts. Obesity role is demonstrated by frequent disappearance of reduction of rhonchopathy when back to a satisfactory weight balance. More unusual are endocrin causes as acromegalia, gonadotrophine insufficiency in the female or even hypothyreosis, treatement allowing a disappearance of rhonchopathy, thus contra-indicating surgical therapy (Mezon, 1980).

All previously described causes are easy to find and to treat when obvious.

But very often determinating the obstructive site is much more difficult. In these cases, complementary investigations allow to find roughly two privileged obstructive sites of upper aerials tracts, isolated or associated. The first one is located at the higher part of oro-pharynx, between soft palate and tongue, second lies under the other, between tongue base and posterior part of oro-pharynx. Knowing this obstructive site allows to predict success or failure of UPPP in case of rhonchopathy associated to S.A.S. Dynamic assays recently achieved try to find, in case of an obstruction, which of these two sites is in first involved.

However numerous questions still haven't found a good answer in the field of anatomy of upper aerial tracts in the snorer :
- Does pharynx narrowing involve the lengthening of soft palate by creating a negative pressure zone and then a suction phenomenon or is it first the excessive length of soft palate that is responsible of this narrowing ?
- Is glossoptosis secondary to the fall of mouth floor and hyoid bone or is it due to a primary macroglossia secondarely responsible of a fall of the floor ? (Guilleminault, 1984).

Answering these questions governs success of the therapic gests to propose in case of snoring with S.A.S (Billiard, 1984 ; Lugarest, 1975 ; Rivlin, 1984).

CONCLUSION

Knowing anatomic causes of snoring still stays perfectible. Respective roles of soft palate and tongue base must still be determined precisely because they govern the success of different therapies proposed for simple snoring and especially when complicated with S.A.S. Knowledge of rhonchopathy anatomy can't however be dissociated from dynamic physiologic assays and must be integrated in a wider study aiming to separate the primary mechanism from the numerous and ill known consequences of this pathology.

REFERENCES

BILLIARD M., BESSET A., BRISSAUD L. (1984) : Le syndrome d'apnées récurrentes au cours du sommeil. Rev. Med. Intern. 142 - 151

BRADLEY T.D., BROWN I.G., GROSSMAN R.F., ZAMEL N., MARTINEZ D. (1986) : Pharyngeal size in snorers, non-snorers, and patients with obstructive sleep apnea. N. Engl. J. Med. 315, 1327 - 1331

CHOUARD C.H. (1986) : La ronchopathie chronique ou ronflement, "Aspects cliniques et indications thérapeutiques". Ann. Oto-Laryng. 103, 319 - 327

COLE P., HAIGHT J.S.J. (1984) : Mechanisms of nasal obstruction in sleep. Laryngoscope 94, 1557 - 1559

DAVIES S.E., IBER C. (1983) : Obstructive sleep apnea associated with adult-acquired micrognathia from rheumatoid arthritis. Am. Rev. Respir. Dis. 127, 245 - 247

GUILLEMINAULT C., RILEY R., POWELL N. (1984) : "Implications for treatement", Abnormal cephalometric measurements. Chest 86 (5), 793 - 794

HAPONIK E.F., SMITH P.L., BOHLMAN M.E., ALLEN R.P., GOLDMAN S.M., BLEECKER E.R. (1983) : "Correlation of airway size with physiology during sleep and wakefulness", Computerized tomography in oustructive sleep apnea. Am. Rev. Respir. Dis. 127, 221 - 226

HUDGEL D.W. (1986) : Variable site of airway narrowing among obstructive sleep apnea patients. J. Appl. Physiol. 61 (4), 1403 - 1409

ISSA F.G., SULLIVAN C.E. (1982) : Alcohol, snoring and sleep apnea. J. of Neurology, Neurosurgery and Psychiatry 45, 353 - 359

KATSANTONIS G.P., WALSH J.K. (1986) : Somnofluoroscopy : its role in the selection of candidates for uvulopalatopharyngoplasty. Otolaryngol. Head Neck Surg. 94, 56 - 60

KRYGER M.H. (1983) : "From the Needles of Dionysius to continuous positive airway pressure", Sleep Apnea. Arch. Intern. Med. 143, 2301 - 2303

LOWE A.A., GIONHAKU N., TAKEUCHI K., FLEETHA J.A. (1986) : Three dimensional CT reconstructions of tongue and airway in adult subjects with obstructive sleep apnea. Am. J. Orthod. Dentofac. Orthop. 90, 364 - 374

LUGAREST E., COCCAGNA G., FARNETI P., MANTOVANI M., CIRIGNOTTA (1975) : Snoring. Electroencephalography and Clinical Neurophysiology 39, 59 - 64

MEZON B.J., WEST P., MACLEAN J.P., KRYGER M.H. (1980) : Sleep apnea in acromegaly. Am. J. Med. 69, 615 - 618

ORR W.C., MARTIN R.J. (1981) : Obstructive sleep apnea associated with tonsillar hypertrophy in adults. Arch. Intern. Med. 141, 990 - 992

RIVLIN J., HOFFSTEIN V., KALBFLEISCH J;, McNICHOLAS W., ZAMEL N., BRYAN A.C. (1984) : Upper airway morphology in patients with idiopathic obstructive sleep apnea. Am. Rev. Respir. Dis. 129, 355 - 360

SPIER S., RIVLIN J., ROWE R.D., EGAN T. (1986) : Sleep in Pierre ROBIN Syndrome. Chest 90 (5), 711 - 715

SURATT P.M., DEE P., ATKINSON R.L., ARMSTRONG P., WILHOIT S.C. (1983) : Fluoroscopic and computed tomographic features of the pharyngeal airway in obstructive sleep apnea. Am. Rev. Respir. Dis. 127, 487 - 492

ZORICK F., ROTH T., KRAMER M., FLESSA H. 1980) : Exacerbation of upper airway sleep apnea by lymphocytic lymphoma. Chest 77 (5), 689 - 690

Chronic rhonchopathy. Ed. C.H. Chouard. © 1988, John Libbey Eurotext Ltd. pp.20-29.

Elements de physiologie du sommeil

M. Minz

Service du Professeur HP Cathala, Explorations Fonctionnelles – Neurologie, Hôpital de la Salpétrière, 75651 Paris Cedex 13, France

RESUME

Cet exposé résume quelques données récentes concernant la physiologie du sommeil, rappelle les structures nerveuses impliquées et certaines de leurs relations anatomiques et fonctionnelles. Il est également rappelé que la régulation de fonctions physiologiques essentielles peut être différente selon l'état de vigilance considéré, en soulignant le caractère souvent aggravant ou révélateur du sommeil paradoxal sur les syndromes d'apnées. Enfin, la question est posée des relations entre le ronflement et les syndromes d'apnées (les réponses ne sont pas fournies).

MOTS CLEFS

Sommeil, physiologie, apnée, ronflement.
Sleep, physiology, apnea, snoring.

INTRODUCTION

C'est avec une grande satisfaction que l'on constate l'intérêt croissant que portent les médecins à une partie importante et longtemps négligée de la vie de leurs patients : le temps pendant lequel ils dorment. Est-ce parcequ'on a longtemps considéré le sommeil comme un phénomène passif de déconnection ? est-ce parceque le médecin ne voit pas son malade dormir puisque le sommeil s'observe le plus souvent en dehors des heures de consultation et de visite ? peu importe ! On sait maintenant que de très nombreux évènements se produisent au cours du sommeil et surtout qu'ils peuvent avoir une incidence déterminante sur l'état de santé de très nombreux malades. Toutes les spécialités médicales sont évidemment concernées et comme le ronflement est le type même de phénomène directement lié au sommeil , il a semblé utile de rappeler de manière très schématique quelques données concernant la physiologie du sommeil.

On distingue donc trois différents états de vigilance (veille sommeil lent et sommeil paradoxal) depuis la mise en évidence de ce dernier état par Aserinsky et Kleitman (1953). La polygraphie permet l'identification de ces états selon des critères précis admis de tous. Le sommeil paradoxal en particulier est constitué de phénomènes "toniques" comme l'activation du tracé E.E.G., la suppression de l'activité tonique au niveau de la musculature axiale, une érection etc... et de phénomènes "phasiques" parmi lesquels : des mouvements oculaires rapides, des irrégularités respiratoires , des variations de la pression artérielle, du débit sanguin cérébral, de la pression intra-crânienne, etc... En même temps que ces "évènements, on peut enregistrer chez l'animal des pointes ponto-géniculo-occipitales (P.G.O). Veille-Sommeil Lent - SommeiL Paradoxal réalisent un continuum avec une organisation temporelle et rythmique, comme d'ailleurs toutes les autres grandes et moins grandes fonctions physiologiques. Le sommeil, phénomène actif nécessite pour se produire un niveau d'éveil suffisamment bas (nous y reviendrons) et est soumis à l'influence de rythmes circadiens et de rythmes ultradiens avec des interactions multiples , des phénomènes d'inhibition et de facilitation souvent complexes.

Les variations avec l'âge sont importantes de même que les différences interindividuelles ; l'influence du milieu et de l'environnement est également essentielle mais ne sera pas abordée ici.

Le modèle monoaminergique du sommeil élaboré dans les années 60 par M.Jouvet repose sur :
1°) Les résultats à court terme de lésions de certaines structures : la destruction du raphé médian qui est le point de départ de 80 % des neurones sérotonénergiques (5HT) provoque une insomnie totale pendant trois jours ; les huit jours suivants on ne recueille que de la somnolence (stade I du sommeil) puis le sommeil paradoxal (SP) réapparait. Le sommeil à ondes lentes n'est restauré qu'après trois semaines, sans phénomène de rebond . Cette insomnie est donc réversible!

2°) Les résultats d'expérimentations pharmacologiques : l'administration de Parachlorophénylalanine (PCPA), inhibiteur de la synthèse de la 5HT qui empêche la transformation du tryptophane en 5-Hydroxytryptophane(5HTP) provoque après un délai de 24 heures une insomnie avec chez l'animal, enregistrement de pointes PGO. L'administration de 5 HTP a pour conséquence une disparition immédiate des pointes PGO (ce qui est tout à fait compatible avec une neurotransmission) mais il faut trente minutes pour que réapparaisse le sommeil lent et soixante minutes pour que réapparaisse le sommeil paradoxal, ce qui est incompatible avec une neurotransmission ou même une neuromodulation.

Ce modèle qui admet la 5HT comme neurotransmetteur direct du sommeil et qui privilègie certaines structures tout en en negligeant d'autres comme l'hypothalamus qui pourtant n'avait pas démérité n'est plus retenu tel quel.Cela d'autant que l'enregistrement de l'activité unitaire de neurones 5HT du raphé et l'étude de la libération de 5HT au niveau des vesicules synaptiques ont montré que : les décharges des cellules 5HT sont maximum pendant la veille, diminuent au cours du sommeil lent et sont au niveau le plus bas pendant le sommeil paradoxal. La quantité de 5HT libérée diminue également au cours du sommeil lent.

iL faut toutefois rappeler que ce modèle marque la naissance de l'hypnologie moderne et que la sérotonine conserve un rôle essentiel dans la physiologie du sommeil.

Les expériences montrant la possible existence et intervention de neuromodulateurs de nature peptidique arrivent à point pour remettre au goût du jour l'idée très ancienne d'une ou de plusieurs substances "hypniques". Depuis quelques années des substances plus souvent peptidiques se portent candidats au titre et on peut déjà en compter plus que de candidats potentiels à l'election présidentielle.Chacun défend son champion avec acharnement et souvent d'ailleurs des arguments très convaincants.

On peut citer entre autres le Facteur S qui est un muramyl peptide et le SPS (Sleep Promoting Substance) qui ont été isolés à partir du cerveau puis de l'urine d'animaux privés de sommeil.

Le DSIP (Delta-Sleep Inducing Peptide) extrait du sang après stimulation thalamique (stimulaton thalamique qui induit le sommeil comme cela avait été signalé par Hess dès 1943).
Le VIP (Vasoactive Intestinal Peptide) ou encore l'AVT (Arginine Vasotocine). Le calcium mérite également une mention puisqu'il est possible de modifier l'organisation du sommeil en modifiant le contenu en calcium du liquide céphalo-rachidien.
Mais pour être accepté comme facteur induisant physiologiquement le sommeil il ne suffit pas qu'une substance soit endogène, c'est à dire retrouvée dans le cerveau, le sang ou le L.C.R., qu'elle s'accumule et soit augmentée par la privation de sommeil, qu'elle agisse directement sur les mécanismes exécutifs du sommeil; il faut aussi et surtout que son inactivation soit suivie d'une insomnie durable sans phénomène de rebond !
Or aucun peptide à ce jour ne répond à ce dernier critère !
Il n'en reste pas moins que l'intervention de substances de nature peptidique est plus que vraisemblable et de toute manière leur intérêt pharmacologique est évident, même si la plupart d'entre elle ne sont que des facteurs facilitants.
Le problème se complique un peu si on tient compte des très nombreux travaux qui depuis longtemps (Nauta 1946) montrent que des lésions ou stimulations de diverses régions de l'hypothalamus altèrent profondément le rythme veille-sommeil.
En particulier il a été mis en évidence récemment au niveau de l'hypothalamus postérieur ventro-latéral des neurones contenant surtout de l'histamine mais aussi du GABA et une substance peptidique, réalisant un système à connections multiples en particulier avec la région préoptique (hypothalamus antérieur), le cortex et le raphé. Ce système est actif pendant l'éveil et cesse de fonctionner pendant le sommeil. Sa destruction est suivie d'une remarquable hypersomnie (l'éveil restant possible).
Donc et pour résumer et intégrer ce qui précède (Fig.1): on a de bonnes raisons de penser que la 5HT puisse agir sur la région préoptique qui elle-même exerce une action inhibitrice sur le système d'éveil hypothalamique postérieur (peut-être histaminergique) ; ce dernier devant être bloqué pour que le sommeil puisse s'installer.

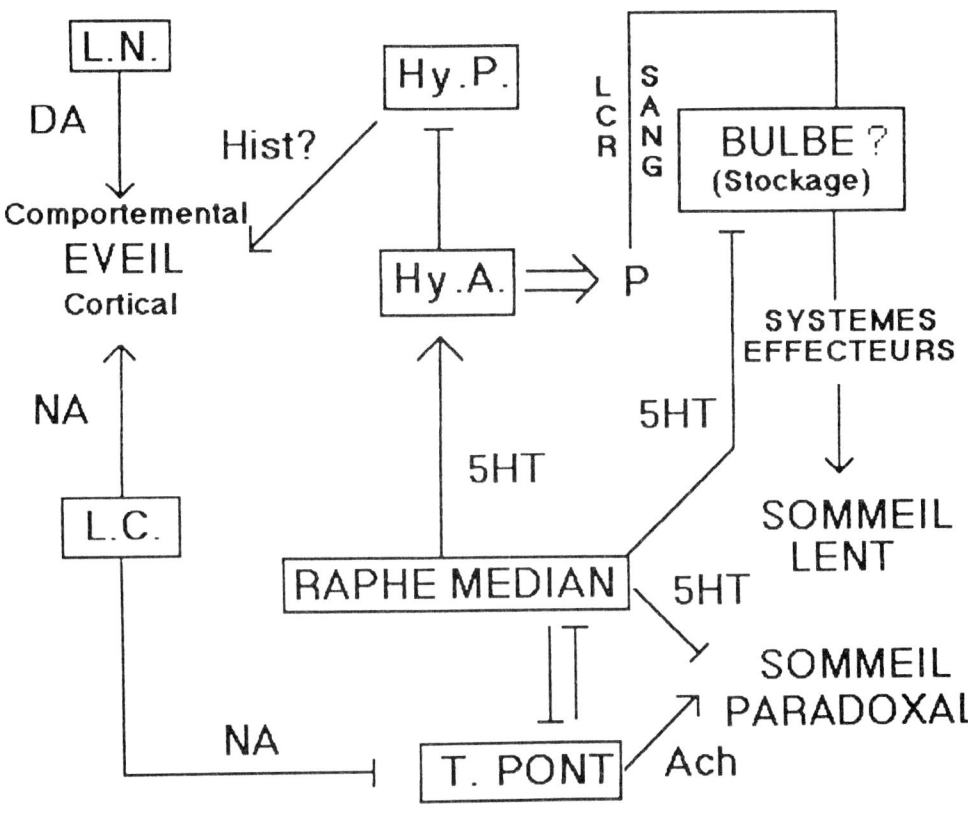

D'après M. JOUVET

LN : Locus niger ; LC : complexe coeruleus ; HyA : région préoptique ;
HyP : hypothalamus postérieur ventro-latéral ; P : substance peptidique
→ : activation   NA : neurone noradrénergique ; DA : neurone dopaminergique
⊣ : inhibition   5HT : neurone serotoninergique ; Ach : neurone cholinergique
                  Hist : neurone histaminergique

Fig. 1

D'autre part la 5HT pourrait agir sur l'hypothalamus antérieur (peut-être aussi sur l'hypophyse) et favoriser pendant la veille la synthèse, la libération, l'accumulation de substances de nature peptidique qui véhiculées par le L.C.R. et / ou le sang seraient stockées dans la région bulbaire où l'activité 5HT de vieille empêcherait sa libération. La diminution de l'activité 5HT aurait pour conséquence de lever l'inhibition s'exerçant sur la région où est stockée le peptide qui pourrait alors agir sur les systèmes effecteurs du sommeil.

En ce qui concerne le sommeil paradoxal, il n'y a pas actuellement de modèle qui intègre toutes les données des expérimentations neurophysiologiques, les résultats de lésions à différents niveaux, les enregistrements d'activités cellulaires et les résultats d'expérimentations pharmacologiques qui semblent parfois difficilement conciliables. Plusieurs systèmes sont vraisemblablement impliqués avec des phénomènes d'inhibition réciproque.

Certains groupes de neurones 5HT (P.S."off") pourraient avoir un rôle permissif sur la commande du SP (par levée d'une inhibition?). Le ou les systèmes exécutifs seraient sous la dépendance de groupes de neurones de nature cholinergique (PS"on") que l'on trouve au niveau du champ latéral du tegmentum pontique. Il existe des connections noradrenergiques entre le complexe coeruleus et ces neurones mais leur mise en jeu ne semble pas nécessaire à l'expression du sommeil paradoxal.

On peut observer sur le schéma que la région hypothalamique apparaît comme stratégique pour l'ensemble du système et s'il existe une "horloge" réglant l'alternance veille-sommeil, c'est bien dans cette région qu'il faut la chercher. Comme cette même région intervient aussi dans la régulation de la température centrale, cela nous amène à la question qui reste controversée d'une "horloge unique réglant l'alternance veille-sommeil et les variations circadiennes de la température ou de deux systèmes oscillants independants, tous les autres paramètres mesurables étant soumis à l'un ou l'autre de ces oscillateurs?

Pour arriver à des problèmes plus pratiques et plus proches des préoccupations du jour, nous présentons quelques documents :

N1) Enregistrement nocturne continu de la SAO2 chez un patient présentant un syndrome d'apnées du sommeil (SAS) où on peut remarquer les différences importantes des variations de ce paramètre entre le sommeil lent et le sommeil paradoxal.
N2) Patient de 54 ans venant consulter pour des endormissements diurnes invincibles depuis 6 mois chez qui on constate une baisse importante de la SAO2 uniquement pendant les phases paradoxales.
Ceci pour illustrer le fait que comme cela a été montré chez l'animal, le contrôle de la ventilation s'exerce vraisemblablement aussi chez l'homme de manière différente selon l'état de vigilance considéré :
Au cours du sommeil lent la ventilation est étroitement dépendante du système de contrôle métabolique, avec une tendance spontanée à la périodicité respiratoire pour le sommeil léger (stades I et II) et une respiration plus régulière dans le sommeil lent plus profond (stades III et IV). En revanche, au cours du sommeil paradoxal et particulièrement du SP phasique, la sensibilité des centres respiratoires à l'hypercapnie seraient nettement moindre et peut-être même absente ; seule persisterait une certaine sensibilité à l'hypoxie. Or le facteur éveillant semble être avant tout l'hypercapnie, l'éveil permettant la mise en jeu d'une régulation ventilatoire plus efficace.
Ces deux observations concernent des sujets considérés comme de "gros ronfleurs" mais le document suivant montre un ronflement important et particulièrement sonore en sommeil lent profond, sans aucune incidence notable sur la ventilation, le rythme cardiaque ou la SAO2 ! ce qui amène à se poser la question non pas de l'existence d'un lien entre ronflement et apnées, qui semble communément admis mais sur la nature de ce lien : tous les sujets présentant un syndrome d'apnées du sommeil de type obstructif ont une reprise respiratoire (inspiratoire) bruyante en fin d'apnée, ce qui explique que l'on trouve plus de SAS chez les ronfleurs que dans la population générale. Cela montre que le ronflement est un signe d'appel important devant faire chercher un SAS mais cela ne démontre pas que les ronfleurs sont plus aptes à developper un SAS, même si chez certains d'entre eux on trouve des baisses significatives de la SAO2 pendant le sommeil, parfois même sans apnées.
Seule une étude prospective sur une grande échelle, qui à ma connaissance n'a pas été réalisée permetrait d'éclaircir ce point essentiel.

REFERENCES

Aserinsky, Kleitman : Regularly occuring periods of eye motility and concomitant phenomena during sleep. Science 1953 118, 273,274.

Jouvet M. : The role of monoamines and acetylcholine-containing neurons in the regulation of the sleep-waking cycle. Ergebnisse der Physiologie 1972 64, 166-307.

Nauta W.J.H. : Hypothalamic regulation of sleep in rats. J. Neurophysiol. 1946 9, 285-316.

Pappenheimer J.R., Miller T.B., Goodrich C.A. : Sleep-promoving effects of cerebrospinal fluid from sleep-deprived goats. Proc. Nat. Acad. Sci. USA 58, 513-517.

Phillipson C.A. : Control of breathing during sleep. Am. Rev. Resp. Dis. 1978 118, 909-939.

Rechtschaffen A., Kales A. : A manual of standardized Terminology, Techniques and scoring system for sleep states of human subjects. US Government Printing Office Washington D.C. 1968.

SLEEP PHYSIOLOGY AND SNORING.

M. MINZ
Service Pr H.P. CATHALA-Explorations Fonctionnelles-Neurologie
Hôpital de la Salpêtrière-Paris 75651 Cedex 13.

SUMMARY

This lecture summarizes some recent data on sleep physiology, recalls the neurological structures involved and some of their anatomical and functional relationships. Recall is also made of the fact that control of essential physiological functions like breathing can be sleep stage dependant, specially underlining the aggravating and sometimes revealing character of REM sleep on sleep apnea syndromes. It then brings up the subject (without giving the answers) of the relationship between snoring and sleep apnea.

Correlation of structure and mechanics in pharyngeal obstruction during sleep

J.E. Remmers, T. Feroah, J.R. Perez-Padilla and W.A. Whitelaw

University of Calgary, Health Sciences Centre, Calgary, Alberta, Canada

ABSTRACT

Pharyngeal narrowing or complete closure occurs during sleep in patients with obstructive sleep hypopnea or obstructive sleep apnea, respectively. While the broad outlines of the pathogenesis of airway obstruction and airway occlusion in the pharynx are understood, the specific details in individual patients are not available. In order to identify exactly why and precisely where the pharyngeal lumen narrows in patients with obstructive sleep apnea and hypopnea, fiberoptic examination of the pharynx was performed in patients while asleep. Intrapharyngeal pressure and airflow were recorded while positive pressure was applied to the nose. Variations in pressure allowed the pharynx to narrow. The site of narrowing was observed to occur at the nasopharynx, oropharynx, or hypopharynx. Nasopharyngeal narrowing was characterized by a concentric reduction in aperture. Oropharyngeal narrowing was produced by a backward movement of the tongue and soft palate. Hypopharyngeal narrowing was produced by a dorsal rotation of the epiglottis.

KEY WORDS

Sleep disordered breathing, snoring, pharyngeal mechanics, nasal airway positive pressure, obstructive sleep apnea, obstructive sleep hypopnea

INTRODUCTION

Sleep is normally associated with a rise in upper airway (UA) resistance due to a decrease in neural outflow to UA muscles that act to enlarge the lumen of the nares, pharynx and larynx. Sleep is associated with much larger increases in UA resistance in heavy snorers (1) and, when associated with a reduction in alveolar ventilation, is referred to as obstructive sleep hypopnea (OSH). Sleep can also be associated with complete closure of the upper airway, referred to as obstructive sleep apnea (OSA). While the narrowing and closure of the airway in these disorders is known to occur in the pharynx (2,3), the precise locus of airway collapse has not been identified. Similarly, while the mechanics of pharyngeal compression is understood in a general sense, the factors responsible for stable narrowing of the pharynx in OSH and for complete closure in OSA remain to be elucidated. In order to elucidate these structural and mechanical factors, we have measured pharyngeal pressure, flow and lumen size in patients with OSH and OSA while asleep.

METHODS

All patients reported daytime hypersomnolence and all displayed episodes of hypoxemia during sleep with decreases in arterial O_2 saturation exceeding 5%. Patients slept with a custom fitted nose mask connected to a pneumotachograph and a controllable positive pressure source. Naris and intrapharyngeal pressures were recorded, together with arterial O_2 saturation (ear oximeter), breath sounds (chest microphone) and standard bioelectric signals for sleep staging. Intrapharyngeal images were obtained using a small fiberscope (O.D.2.7mm Olympus PF-27L). These images were recorded on videotape, together with a time code, which allowed identification of analogue signals recorded coincident with the image. The patient slept while receiving relatively high nasal airway positive pressure (7-12 cm H_2O). Naris pressure was then reduced for several breaths while images and analogue signals were recorded. Narrowing or occlusion of the lumen was classified anatomically with reference to three subdivisions of the pharynx; namely, the nasopharynx, the oropharynx, and the hypopharynx.

RESULTS

Obstructive Sleep Hypopnea
Stable narrowing of the pharyngeal lumen was observed in all three subdivisions of the pharynx in patients with OSH. This narrowing appeared during the 1-3 inspirations after naris pressure was reduced to near atmospheric levels and was associated with an abrupt increase in UAR to values exceeding 75 cm $H_2O \cdot \ell^{-1} \cdot min^{-1}$. This narrowing was also associated with flow limitation; i.e., inspiratory airflow remained constant at a low level (0.15-0.3 $\ell \cdot sec^{-1}$) despite a progressive decrease in pressure caudal to the site of narrowing. This behavior is displayed in Fig. 1 and was associated with circumferential constriction at the level of the soft palate during inspiration, as shown in center image of this figure. The occurrence of inspiratory flow limitation by constriction of the nasopharynx was uniformly associated with three other findings: heavy snoring, high frequency oscillation in supraglottic pressure and airflow, and vibration of the margin of the constricted lumen as shown in the rightmost photo of Fig. 1. The frequency of the last was usually 40-60 Hz, and this corresponded to the fundamental frequency observed on the simultaneously recorded power spectra of breathing sounds.

Although less common, stable narrowing was also observed in the other two pharyngeal subdivisions. In the case of oropharyngeal narrowing, the tongue was often observed to move dorsally and contact the posterior pharyngeal wall, leaving only a small lumen. In other cases, inward movement of the lateral walls was most apparent. Finally, stable hypopharyngeal narrowing during inspiration was observed, caused by dorsal rotation of the epiglottis (Fig. 3A).

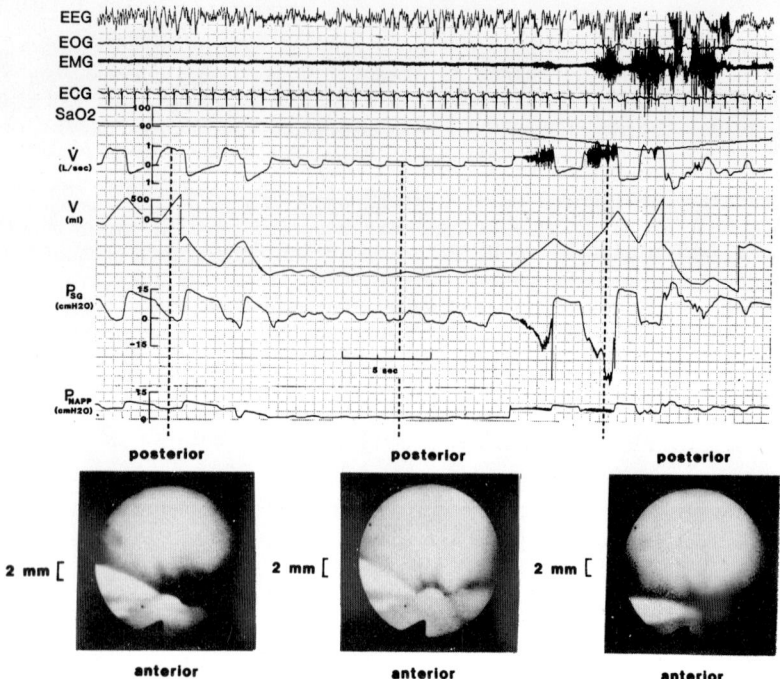

Fig. 1. Polygraphic tracing (above) and simultaneously observed nasopharyngeal images (below) during a period of obstructive hypopnea caused by reducing nasal airway positive pressure (NAPP). Supraglottic pressure (P_{sa}) displays rhythmic fluctuations during the hypopnea and airflow ($\dot{V}$) reveals flow limitation at this time. The left photo shows a patent nasopharynx for P_{NAPP} equal to 8-10 cm H_2O. The center photo shows collapse of this segment when P_{NAPP} is reduced. The right photo shows the nasopharynx during loud snoring. The blurred margin in the last photo results from high frequency oscillation of the lumen margins.

Obstructive Sleep Apnea

Complete occlusion of the pharynx was also observed in the nasopharynx, the oropharynx and the hypopharynx. The nasopharynx displayed a concentric closure, as shown in Fig. 2. A 2 mm orifice was present at the beginning of inspiration and this was obliterated shortly after inspiratory flow began, leaving the airway occluded at the level of the soft palate. The hypopharyngeal occlusion was related to posterior displacement of the tongue.

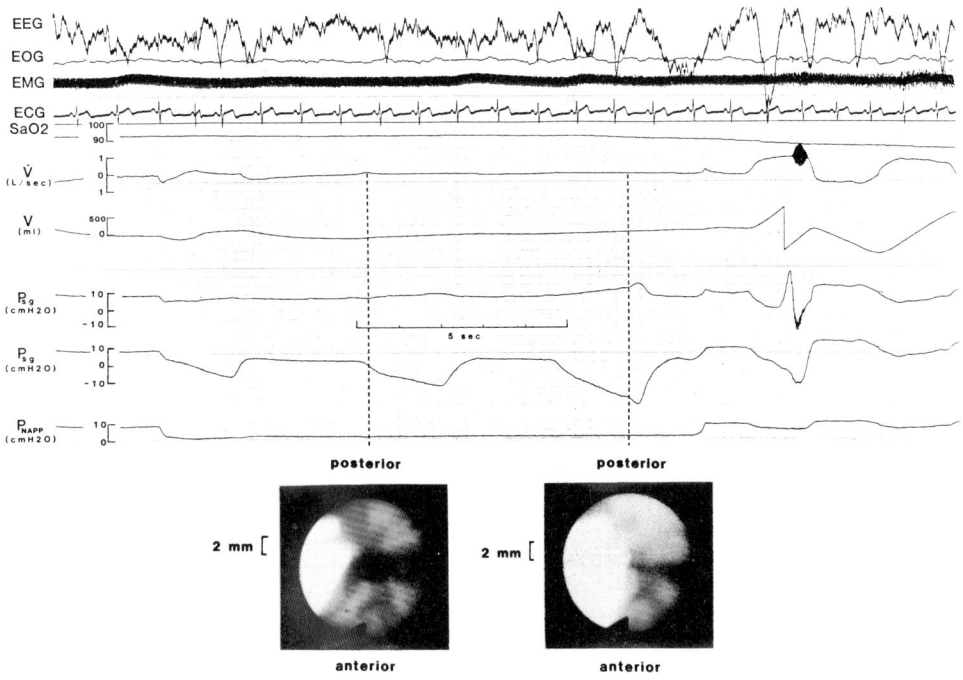

Fig. 2. Complete occlusion of the nasopharynx caused by reduction of P_{NAPP} from 8 to 2 cm H_2O.

The uvula and free margin of the soft palate also appeared to participate; i.e., these structures became wedged between the tongue and the posterior pharyngeal wall. Occlusion of the hypopharynx was related to posterior rotation of the epiglottis, which displayed a flap-valve type of behavior, apparently being sucked down over the larynx, as shown in Fig. 3A. As in the case of stable narrowing caused by narrowing of the hypopharyngeal lumen, a period of airflow preceded occlusion of the hypopharynx. Recordings of pressure below the epiglottis but above the vocal cords reveal a negative deflection in pressure during inspiration, indicating that the laryngeal lumen was patent (Fig. 3B).

DISCUSSION

Patients with sleep disordered breathing display either OSH or OSA. The former is associated with incomplete closure of the pharynx and the latter is caused by pharyngeal occlusion. The present results reveal that pharyngeal narrowing with incomplete or complete closure can occur during sleep in all three subdivisions of the pharynx. To the extent that pharyngeal muscles were only minimally active while nasal airway positive pressure was applied, the observed narrowing or closure of the pharynx reflect movements of passive structures. After several breaths at lower pressure, chemical stimuli to breathing probably increased, and the UA muscles were probably activated. Several muscles of the pharynx and mouth promote mouth closure (medial pterygoid), ventral motion of the hyoid (geniohyoid and sternohyoid), protrusion of the tongue (genioglossus) and stiffening of the soft palate (tensor palatini). All of these muscles display rhythmic inspiratory activity, and the resulting contraction tends to

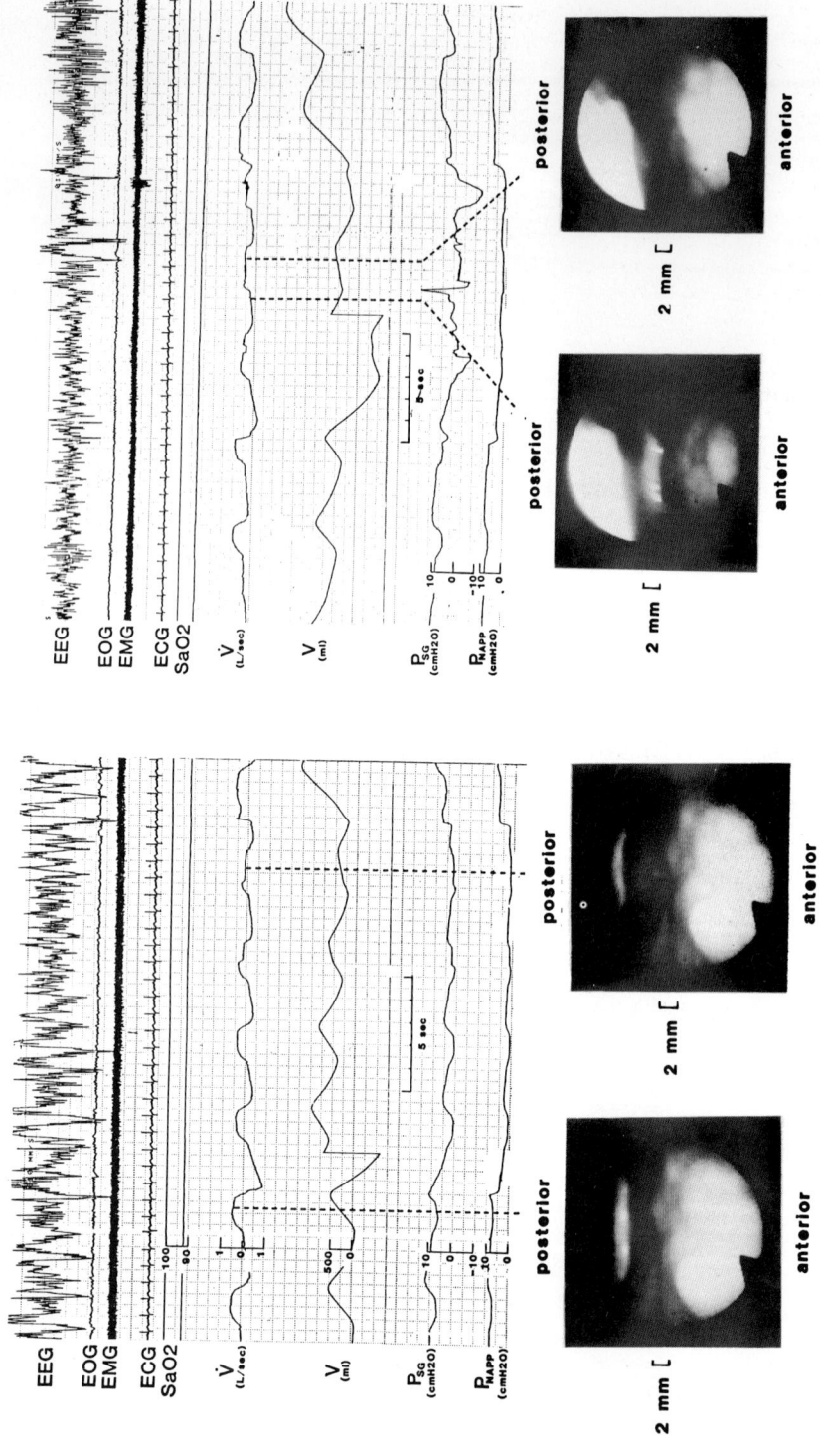

Fig. 3A and 3B. Closure of the epiglottis caused by reduction of P$_{NAPP}$. P$_{sg}$ was recorded above the epiglottis. The epiglottis rotates dorsally during inspiration, causing a reduction of airflow ($\dot{V}$) midway through this phase (right photo). Fig. 3B shows similar events when P$_{sg}$ was recorded below the epiglottis.

reduce the compliance of the pharynx, allowing it to resist pharyngeal suction pressure developed during inspiration. The size of the pharyngeal lumen, therefore, depends upon the interaction of the "effective" compliance of the pharynx and the pharyngeal suction pressure. Pharyngeal suction pressure; i.e., subatmospheric pharyngeal luminal pressure, has two components; one related to flow resistance of the nose and pharynx and one related to the velocity of the airstream in the pharynx. The former depends upon flow rate in relation to upstream resistance; the latter varies with velocity and, hence, lumen size in relation to flow rate.

In OSH, the behavior of the pharynx resembles that of a Starling resistor. Intraluminal pressure decreases during inspiration, causing airflow through the nose and nasopharynx. This appears to reduce the size of the lumen in one or more pharyngeal sequents, thereby increasing velocity of airflow through the segment. This engenders further narrowing since it reduces lateral wall pressure, in turn causing further narrowing. This segment of the airway appears to be highly compliant under the conditions of our study, since a pinhole lumen finally results. The high frequency vibration presumably reflects the instability of this airway in which the airway virtually collapses, flow ceases, the intraluminal pressure increases, a tiny lumen is reestablished, flow resumes, the intraluminal pressure decreases, and the airway collapses.

REFERENCES

Skatrud, J.B. (1985): Airway resistance and respiratory muscle function in snorers during NREM sleep. J. Appl. Physiol. 59, 328-335.
Remmers, J.E., deGroot, W.J., Sauerland, E.K. and Anch A.M. (1978: Pathogenesis of upper airway occlusion during sleep. J. Appl. Physiol. 44, 931-938.
Katsantonis, G.P. and Walsh, J.K. (1986): Somnofluoroscopy: its role in the selection of candidates for uvulopalatopharyngoplasty. Otolaryngol. Head Neck Surg. 94, 56.

RESUME

Durant le sommeil, un étranglement du pharynx peut induire, chez des patients, des hypopneés ou des apneés obstructives. Le but de la présente étude est de localiser précisement cet étranglement chez ces patients. Un étranglement fut observé aux trois differents niveaux du pharynx, soit au niveau du nasopharynx, de l'oropharynx ou de l'hypopharynx. Chez certains patients, nous avons observé un seul site étranglement, alors que chez d'autres patients, deux au trois sites d'étranglement furent observés. Dans tous les cas, la dimension du segment étranglé depend de la pression transpharyngienne. Dans certains cas, un étranglement du pharynx sans obstruction complète était associé au ronflement et à une limitation des debits respiratoires. Le ronflement est associé à une oscillation à haute frequence des segments collapsibles du pharynx.

Epidemiology of snoring and obstructive sleep apnea syndrome

E. Lugaresi, F. Cirignotta and P. Montagna

Institute of Neurology, University of Bologna, Bologna, Italy

ABSTRACT

The clinical and polysomnographic evidence for a relationship between trivial snoring and OSAS has been confirmed by several epidemiological surveys. These have also confirmed that snoring and OSAS exert harmful effects, on the heart and the circulation. The exact pathogenic mechanisms responsible for the self-aggravating process of OSAS remain however poorly defined, and require future studies.

KEY-WORDS

Snoring, sleep apnea, epidemiology, arterial hypertension, heart disease.

INTRODUCTION

In our studies on obstructive sleep apnea syndrome (OSAS) we have always been impressed by the fact that patients had been heavy snorers for years or decades prior to the full development of the syndrome (Lugaresi et al. 1978). In a sample of 118 patients, affected with OSAS, snoring was reported by all patients and, as a mean, it preceded the onset of symptoms and signs typical of OSAS (e.g. intermittent snoring and daytime somnolence) by 20 years (Fig. 1).

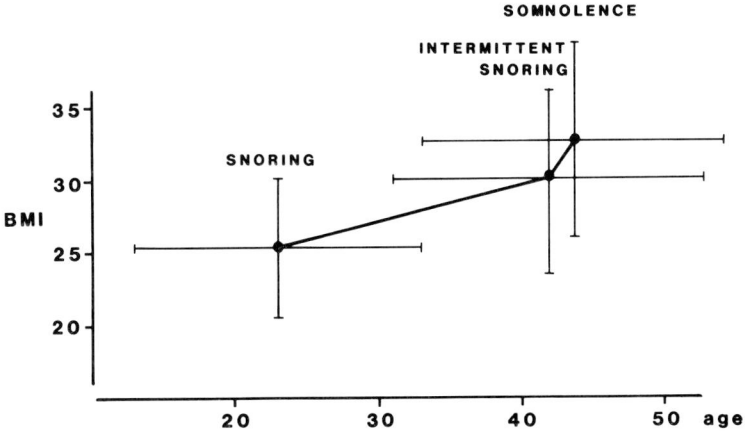

FIG.1 - Snoring antedates the onset of intermittent snoring (i.e. snoring interrupted by obstructive apneas) and daytime somnolence by about 15-20 years. Bars represent SD; BMI represents body mass index.

This close clinical relationship between snoring and OSAS could be confirmed by polysomnographic findings (Lugaresi et al, 1975).

Polysomnography shows that snoring is an inspiratory noise, due to narrowing of the upper airways. It is associated with increased activity of inspiratory muscles and with a marked increase in endothoracic negative pressure. Heavy snorers however may display obstructive apneas, sporadically or in clusters during light and REM sleep. These obstructive apneas are favoured by transient weakening of central breathing. This is shown by a decrease in EMG activity of inspiratory muscles during the apneas.

Heavy snoring is also associated with a decrease in alveolar ventilation, which may exceed the normal limits, and with a slight rise in pulmonary arterial pressure over the physiological values.

Systemic arterial pressure, contrary to what is normally seen in healthy non-snoring people, also progressively increases and reaches the highest values during REM sleep (Lugaresi et al, 1975).

These ventilatory and haemodynamic changes seen on polysomnography in heavy snorers are quite comparable to those which are observed, in a worse degree, in patients with full-blown OSAS. The polysomnographic studies thus confirm the clinical evidence for a link between snoring and OSAS. They furthermore suggest that persistent snoring may have deleterious effects for the heart and the circulation.

EPIDEMIOLOGICAL STUDIES

Spurred by the clinical and polysomnographic evidence, we tried to verify our hypothesis of a link between snoring and OSAS by conducting two epidemiological surveys in San Marino, an ancient independent republic of 22.000 people in Northeastern Italy (Mondini et al, 1983). In the general population we found snoring to be a widespread phenomenon, with 24% of men and 14% of women always or nearly always snoring. The number of habitual snorers rose with age, but a decrement was seen after 65 years age, especially among males. At age 60 years, about 60% of men and 40% of women were habitual snorers. Snoring was favoured by obesity. In the age range 30-59 years, 16% of thin, 32% of moderately obese and 45% of frankly obese people were habitual snorers. Apart from the high prevalence figures however, one most relevant finding came out of our survey. We found systemic arterial hypertension more frequently among habitual snorers than among non-snorers. This association between snoring and hypertension was independent of obesity. In fact in the age range 30-59 years hypertension was found in markedly overweight, moderately overweight as well as in thin snorers. In our first survey, a link between snoring and heart disease was also found. This however could not be substantiated in a second epidemiological study.

Following our first reports, several other epidemiological studies confirmed our findings and also established snoring as a risk factor for the heart and circulation.

Snoring was reported by 42% of an unselected population of 6.000 people in a Canadian study (Norton and Dunn, 1985). According to responses given by their spouses it was reported that 70% of the men and 50% of the women were habitual snorers. Both hypertension and heart disease were more common among snorers. These both rose with heavier snoring. The association between snoring and hypertension or heart disease was independent of smoking and obesity.

A relationship between snoring and hypertension was again found in a Finnish study. This relationship was proportional to the severity of snoring. It was also noticed that among males aged 40-69 years, snoring was found to correlate with angina pectoris (Koskenvuo et al, 1985). More recently, in a 3-year prospective study on 388 men aged 40-69 years, Koskenvuo et al (1987) found that both heart disease and stroke were more frequent among snorers and especially habitual snorers as compared to occasional snorers.

The risk for ischemic heart disease associated with snoring was also independent of body mass index (BMI), hypertension and smoking

Conversely, research groups in the USA reported increased incidence of apneas during sleep in hypertensive patients. Thirty percent of 50 hypertensive patients had high apnea index (22.4) during sleep, while apneas were absent or occasional in the normotensive control group (Kales et al, 1984). These findings were reproduced by Fletcher et al (1985) who suggested a causal relationship between OSAS and hypertension. Williams et al (1985) also concluded that more than half of patients with essential hypertension had OSAS and that sleep apnea could play a role in the development of essential hypertension.

In our opinion the sum of these data, firmly establish that snoring represents a risk factor for the heart and the circulation. The question now arises whether the cause of greater cardiocirculatory risk is snoring per se or rather the increased apneas which are displayed by heavy snorers.. Apneas during sleep are found with increased incidence in male subjects of advancing age and the exact prevalence of sleep apneas among heavy snorers is unknown. It is customary to accept 5 or more apneas per hour of sleep as the upper limit of normal, characterizing the beginning of OSAS, but this figure is arbitrary and some authors, more conservatively, put the upper limit of normal at 10 apneas per hour.

Gislason (1987) has recently addressed the problem of the prevalence of OSAS in an at-risk population of males aged 30-69 years. By selecting those patients with clinical evidence for OSAS and studying a sample with polysomnography, he found that 1.3% of 3100 interviewed people had OSAS when an apnea index 5 was accepted as criterion of disease. Most patients fell within 50 and 59 years of age. We are currently conducting a similar survey on a sample of 3479 randomly chosen males aged 30 to 69 years. In our 32 habitual snorers aged 40-69 years who have already undergone full polysomnographic studies the apnea index remained below 5 in a third, reached values between 5 and 12 in another third and was over 25 in the remaining third (Fig. 2).

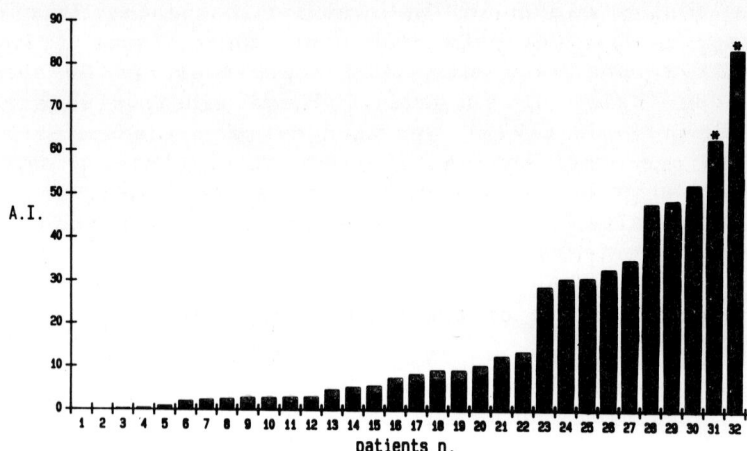

FIG. 2 - Apnea Index (AI) in 32 unselected habitual snorers.

The index was progressively distributed in the first 22 patients, but rose sharply and disproportionately in the last 10 patients.
We found a similar pattern for the desaturation events index indicating the number of pathological desaturationn events during sleep (Fig. 3).

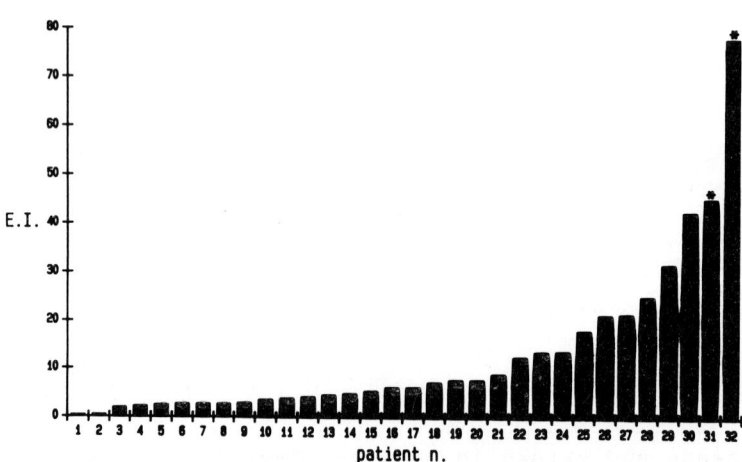

FIG. 3 - O_2 desaturation events index (EI) in 32 unselected habitual snorers.

The highest values of Apnea Index were found in the age range 50-59 years. No correlation was found between severity of OSAS and BMI. Our preliminary data suggest that, accepting as pathological an apnea index of 10, the prevalence of OSAS in males aged 40-69 years was about 3%. Apneas were more frequent between 50 and 59 years, while persistent snoring was more common between 40 and 49 years. Heavy snoring and sleep apneas both decreased after 60 years of age. Moreover, the disproportionate increase in apneas in our group of habitual snorers (Figg. 2, 3) could, in our opinion, suggest that, beyond a certain critical value, there begins a self-aggravating process, leading to a faster progression of the disease. The mechanisms responsible for this vicious circle, could be the fragmentation of sleep and/or the hypoxic events induced by the apneas. Both phenomena in fact reduce the excitability of the respiratory centers.

CONCLUSION

In the last 20 years we have slowly realized, that OSAS and snoring represent just the end of a spectrum of continuous clinical conditions. OSAS represents just the tip of an iceberg, which has more complex and far-reaching hidden parts. It is these "hidden" questions we have to address if we are going to tackle in an effective way the prevention and treatment of respiratory and cardiocirculatory disorders in the future.

REFERENCES

Fletcher E.C., De Behuke R.D., Lovoi M.S., Gorin A. (1985): Undiagnosed Sleep Apnea in Patients with Essential Hypertension. Am. Int. Med. 103, 190-195.
Gislason, T. (1987): Sleep apnea. Clinical symptoms, epidemiology and ventilatory aspects. Thesis, Upsala University, pp.1-48.
Kales A., Bixler E.O., Cadieux R.J., Schneck D.W., Shaw L.C., Loke T.W., Vela-Bueno A., Soldatos C.R. (1984): Sleep apnoea in a hypertension population. The Lancet, ii, 1005-1008.
Koskenvuo M., Kaprio J., Partinen M., Langinvainio H., Sarna S., Heikkilä K. (1985): Snoring as a risk factor for hypertension and angina pectoris. The Lancet, i, 893-895.
Koskenvuo M., Kaprio J., Telakivi T., Partinen M., Heikkilä K., Sarna S. (1987): Snoring as a risk factor for ischaemic heart disease and stroke in men. Br. Med. J. 294, 16-19.
Lugaresi E, Coccagna G., Farneti P., Mantovani M., Cirignotta F. F. (1975): Snoring. Electroencephal. Clin. Neurophysiol. 39, 59-64.

Lugaresi E., Coccagna G., Mantovani M. (1978): Hypersomnia with Periodic Apneas. Spectrum, New York.
Mondini S., Zucconi M., Cirignotta F., Aguglia U., Lenzi P.L., Zauli C., Lugaresi E. (1983): Snoring as a risk factor for cardiac and circulatory problems: an epidemiological study. Sleep/Wake Disorders: Nocturnal Hystory, Epidemiology and Long-term Evolution. ed Guilleminault C., Lugaresi E., Raven Press, New York, pp. 99-105.
Norton P.G., Dunn E.V. (1985): Snoring as a risk factor for disease: an epidemiological survey. Br. Med. J. 291, 630-632.
Williams A.J., Houston D., Finberg S., Lam C., Kinney J.L., Santiago S. (1985): Sleep Apnea Syndrome and Essential Hypertension. Am. J. Cardiol. 55, 1019-1022.

II CHRONIC RHONCHOPATHY GENERAL FEATURES

Chairman: B. Fleury

Chronic rhonchopathy. Ed. C.H. Chouard. © 1988, John Libbey Eurotext Ltd. pp.45-49.

Detection of the partial upper airway obstruction by the SCSB-method

O. Polo, M. Tafti and P. Vaara

The Department of Physiology, University of Turku, Finland, and The Sleep Disorders Center, University of Montpellier, France

RESUME

Le rétrécissement partiel des voies aériennes supérieures au cours du sommeil entraîne dans certains cas une hypoxie, qui à son tour, stimule l'effort respiratoire. Ce dernier peut provoquer par une dépression au niveau du pharynx une aggravation du rétrécissement et de l'hypoxie. Une obstruction, même partielle, des voies aériennes au cours du sommeil peut être détectée par la méthode non invasive du Matelas Electrostatique, dont le principe est décrit. Les patterns de l'obstruction partielle et les données d'enregistrements de 44 ronfleurs par cette méthode sont présentés.

KEYWORDS

snoring, partial obstruction, Static Charge Sensitive Bed (SCSB)

INTRODUCTION

Sleep related partial obstruction of the upper airways may result in hypoxia that stimulates respiration until normoxia is restored. The reserves of the respiratory muscles permit to increase the inspiratory effort so that up to 5 times the normal intrathoracic pressures may be registered (Krieger, pers. com.). A severe partial obstruction may cause snoring, daytime somnolence or cardiovascular complications and in the long run develop into obstructive sleep apnea syndrome. Since the airflow is not necessarily modified, special methods are needed to detect this partial obstruction.

The Static Charge Sensitive Bed (SCSB) is a movement sensor that permits longterm monitoring of ballistocardiogram, respiration and body movements without attaching any electrodes or cables on the subject (Alihanka et al. 1981). The ballistocardiogram (BCG) displays even the slight variations of the heart contractility, that are due to small changes of the intrathoracic pressure during the respiratory cycle. An increase of the intrathoracic pressure variation due to respiratory efforts against airway obstruction is immediately mirrored by increased variations of heart contractions and thus registered by the BCG. The respiratory channel of the SCSB displays the changes of the respiratory movement amplitude.

SUBJECTS AND METHODS

44 subjects (37 males, 7 females, mean age 52,4 years) referred from the ORL consultation to the Montpellier Sleep Disorders Center because of snoring, underwent all-night Static Charge Sensitive Bed (SCSB) and ECG recording with a video/sound monitoring.

The SCSB tracing was scored in 2 min epochs according to Alihanka's (1987) principles. Of special interest is the Increased Respiratory Resistance (IRR) -pattern (Alihanka 1987) that refers to an increasing respiratory movement amplitude as during the rising phase of periodic breathing, but which, instead of waning, retains high for a longer period (up to 5 - 30 minutes). The pattern is accompanied by increasing respiratory variation of the SCSB-ballistocardiogram and often by a slow progressive arterial oxygen desaturation (fig. 1 - 2). Finally an arousal body movement or a spontaneously waning respiratory amplitude can be observed.

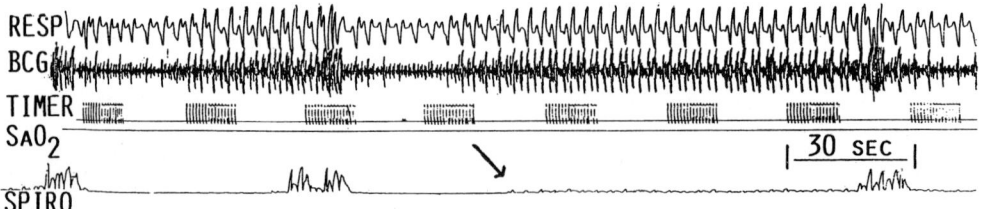

FIGURE 1: The Increased Respiratory Resistance Pattern (IRR) following obstructive sleep apneas. Airflow starts at the arrow.

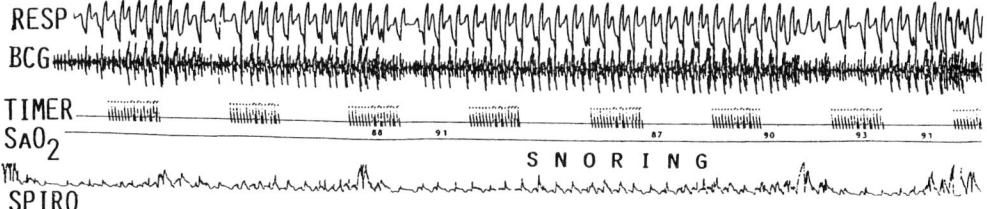

FIGURE 2: IRR without concomitant sleep apneas.

In the figures short IRR-patterns are presented with spirometer recordings. Fig. 1 shows an IRR-pattern that follows obstructive sleep apneas: during the increased respiratory efforts there is some air exchange (the arrow) but a resumption of proper airflow is needed. The longer the IRR periods are, the less the tidal volume is diminished and more the resumption delayed. The IRR without concomitant sleep apneas is illustrated in fig. 2.

RESULTS

In our series of 44 snorers 18 complained of excessive daytime somnolence (EDS, Table I). The IRR-pattern was observed without important number of obstructive sleep apneas in 6 patients, out of which 4 complained of daytime somnolence. Among the somnolents 50 % had obstructive sleep apneas (OIII type) during more than 25 min a night (about 5 % of time in bed) while in the nonsomnolent group the percentage was only 4. In 6 subjects no respiratory anomalies were revealed.

Table I: The occurrence of different SCSB patterns in the somnolent and nonsomnolent groups.

The SCSB-patterns		EDS	N-EDS	TOTAL
number of subjects		18	26	44
no resp. anomalies	< 25 min	1 (6%)	5 (19%)	6 (14%)
OI with BCG +	> 25 min	9 (50%)	13 (50%)	22 (50%)
OII	> 25 min	7 (39%)	9 (35%)	16 (36%)
OIII	> 25 min	9 (50%)	1 (4%)	10 (23%)
IRR > 25 min and OIII > 25 min		1 (6%)	0 (0%)	1 (2%)
IRR > 25 min and OIII < 25 min		4 (22%)	2 (8%)	6 (14%)

DISCUSSION

Obstructive sleep apneas (OIII) were present in important quantity in half of the patients complaining of daytime somnolence. The IRR-pattern was a common finding during heavy snoring. In four somnolent and in two nonsomnolent patients few obstructive apneas were recorded, the IRR being the predominant breathing anomaly.

The IRR-phenomenon could be explained as follows: hypoxia during sleep stimulates the respiratory effort until normoxia is restored. In the case of IRR hypoxia develops because of partial upper airway obstruction. The increasing respiratory efforts manage to prevent aggravation of hypoxia, but cannot reestablish normoxia because forced inspiration worsens the partial obstruction. Hence, breathing is constantly stimulated and therefore continues for longer periods at high amplitude proportional to hypoxia.

Theoretically, a constant hypoxia induced respiratory stimulation could be harmful to the upper airway anatomy. In the long run the soft tissues may get flaccid and stretched until they cause a complete occlusion. According to this hypothesis a therapeutic intervention could be more effective if done before appearance of important anatomical changes of the upper airways. Therefore, the early detection of a relative upper airway obstruction during sleep would be of primordial importance.

REFERENCES

ALIHANKA, J, VAAHTORANTA K. and SAARIKIVI, I. (1981): A new method of longterm monitoring of the ballistocardiogram, heart rate and respiration. **Am. J. Physiol. 240: 384-392**

ALIHANKA, J, (1987): Basic Principles for Analyzing and Scoring Bio-Matt (SCSB) Recordings. **Annales Universitatis Turkuensis (in press)**

POLO, O, BRISSAUD, L, SALES, B, SENEGAS, E, BESSET, A, ALIHANKA, J, PARTINEN, M. and BILLIARD, M. (1986): The validity of The Static Charge Sensitive Bed (SCSB) in detecting obstructive sleep apneas. **Abstr, 8th European congress on sleep, Szeged**

AKNOWLEDGEMENTS: The authors wish to express their gratitude to Professor Billiard and the personal of the Montpellier Sleep laboratory.

SUMMARY

DETECTION OF THE PARTIAL UPPER AIRWAY OBSTRUCTION BY THE SCSB-METHOD

O. Polo, M. Tafti and P. Vaara

The Department of Physiology, University of Turku, Finland, and
The Sleep Disorders Center, University of Montpellier, France

Sleep induced narrowing of the upper airways may result in hypoxia that is compensated by increasing the inspiratory effort, until enough oxygen is obtained. A severe partial obstruction may cause snoring, daytime somnolence or cardiovascular complications and in the long run develop into obstructive sleep apnea syndrome. It cannot be detected by the conventional polysomnography and special methods are therefore needed.

A partial upper airway obstruction can be registered in a noninvasive manner by the Static Charge Sensitive Bed (SCSB) as a rising respiratory movement amplitude and increasing respiratory variation of the SCSB-ballistocardiogram (IRR-pattern described by Alihanka). In our series of 44 snorers 18 complained of daytime somnolence. Among those 18 four showed IRR-patterns, sometimes associated with a progressive oxygen desaturation but without important quantity of obstructive sleep apneas.

Because continuous IRR-breathing may cause daytime somnolence and could be harmful for the upper airway anatomy, it should be detected and eventually treated before an obstructive sleep apnea syndrome develops.

Cinematographic X-ray study on snoring

C. Hannig, A. Wuttge-Hannig and H.W. Mahlo

Institut für Röntgendiagnostik der Technischen Universität München, HNO-Klinik und Poliklinik der Technischen Universität München, München, FRG

RESUME

Onze malades avec une respiration obstructive pendant le sommeil ont été examinés par une radiographie cinématographique de l'oropharynx et du nasopharynx. Cette procédé permet une localisation exacte de l'obstruction au niveau des voies respiratoires superieures; elle constitue un examen essentiel pour indiquer la nécessité d'une intervention chirurgicale (palatopharyngeoplastie).

MOTS CLEFS/ KEY WORDS

Rhonchopathie chronique, cinématographie radiographique, oropharynx, nasopharynx phonation, palatopharyngeoplastie

Chronhic rhonchopathie, cinematographiy, x-ray, oropharynx, nasopharynx palatopharyngeoplastic

INTRODUCTION

The oro-nasopharynx-cinematography is a method taken from the esophagus diagnostic which can be used to study the reacxtion of muscular structures in mouth and throat during physiological activity. The oro-nasopharynx is essential to the production of sounds, to swallowing and also, as a part of the upper respiration tract, to breathing.
The oro-nasopharynx-cinematographie is an important method for the study of muscular and mucosal tissue in mouth and pharynx of habitual snorers especially when compared with the classical method which consists solely of inspection of this regions.

SUBJECTS, MATERIALS, METHODS

The oro-nasopharynx-cinematographie was performed on 11 patients with habitual snoring or with obstructive sleep-apnea-syndrome. We examined the mouvements of the oro- and nasopharynx during the production of sounds by using test words (which generated throat sounds) and the movements of the soft palate by forced nasal and oral inspiration and the act of swallowing.

At the beginnging of the examination we impregnated the nasopharynx and the nasopharyngeal part of the soft palate with an barium suspension via nasal aspiration. Following this we contrasted the oropharynx and the oropharyngeal part of the soft palate and the base of the tongue by application of the barium suspension.

The x-ray picture was taken after centering the apparatus on the oropharynx and nasopharynx so that the x-rays followed a strictly lateral path.
We used a target apparatus generally taken for gastro-intestinal diagnostic containing a picture-amplifier and a television-receiver and also an pulse transformator. The picture that emerged on the pulse transformator was separated by a mirror-optic and a part was sent to the television monitor and the other to the attached cinema camera.

PRESENTATION OF THIS METHOD IN A VIDEO FILM

RESULTS

By the oro- nasopharynx-cinematographie an accurate localisation and description of the obstruction in the upper respiration tract can be obtained; for example a narrow oropharynx or nasopharynx , a macroglossie, a neurogenic or myogenic insufficiency of the soft palate or an excessively long velum can be diagnosed. By the production of throat sounds the proportion of hard to soft palate can be registered, also an excess of mucose parts of the soft palate can be seen which are not involved in the production of sounds.

CONCLUSION

This method thus facilitates the decision for or against a surgical intervention (palatopharyngeoplastic). By given indication the exact size of the tissue resection can be accurately dtermined and a reduction of postoperative complications can be achieved.

REFERENCES

Fairbanks DN (1985): effect of nasal surgery on snoring. South medical journal.
          March 1985   78 (3): 268-270
Hannig C   (1986): cineradiographic examination of the pharyngeoesophageal
          motility. Reported at the " International Esophageal Week" in
          München, 1986, 15-19 september.

ABSTRACT

CINEMATOGRAPHIC X-RAY-STUDY ON SNORING

11 patients with chronic rhonchopathy were examined by the cineradiography of
the nasopharynx and oropharynx. This method provide an accurate localisation
and description of the obstruction in the upper respiration tract . It is
performed during the production of sounds by using test words (which produce
throat sounds) and during the movements of the soft palate by forced nasal
and oral inspiration and during the act of swallowing. This procedure is helpful
at the indication of the surgical therapy of habitual snoring (palatopharyngeoplastic).

Videoradiography of obstructive sleep apnea, OSAS: technical description with a case report

Birgitta Hillarp

Department of Diagnostic Radiology, Malmö General Hospital, S-214 01 Malmö, Sweden

ABSTRACT

In patients with snoring disease videoradiography of pharynx during speech, deglutition, simulated snoring and natural or induced sleep can profitably be performed preoperatively. This permits evaluation of the morphological and functional state of the naso-, oro- and hypopharynx.

A 66-year-old man with snoring, excessive daytime sleepiness and anamnestically apnea periods during sleep was subjected to videoradiography. Besides a somewhat long and thick soft palate there were no significant abnormalities present when awake. During sleep, however, repeated apnea periods due to obstruction at the epiglottic level were recorded.

As videoradiography can reveal morphological as well as functional abnormalities in the pharynx and even visualize the site of obstruction, it is an appropriate method in the evaluation of snoring disease.

KEY WORDS

Snoring, sleep apnea, operation, videoradiography, pharynx, obstruction

INTRODUCTION

Social snorers, i.e. patients with a socially disturbing snoring but no hypersomnia, are common especially in the elderly of whom it has been suggested that as much as 60 to 85 per cent of the men and 40 to 60 per cent of the women snore habitually (Norton 1983; Lugaresi et al 1980). The incidence of snoring and apnea periods during sleep augments normally with age as the incidence of obstructive sleep apnea syndrome (Krieger 1986). The true incidence is a matter of question and has been estimated to 1-10% in the general population (Krieger 1986) resulting in a significantly higher percentage in snorers (Fairbanks 1984).

Obstructive sleep apnea syndrome is due to intermittent collapse of the upper airway due to muscular hypotonia and/or anatomic abnormalities of the

airway. Reports, however, disagree regarding the site of obstruction with
the naso-, oro- and hypopharynx, all being implicated. A simple answer is
probably that the site differs interindividually and that there also might
exist multiple sites of obstruction in the same individual.

Since the precise site of obstruction could help in choosing appropriate
therapy, operative or non-operative, its true visualization, and not mere
indication, might be valuable. By videoradiography this is possible as shown
in the case report below.

Radiologic technique
For the examination an ordinary manually controlled fluoroscopic tiltable
table with image intensifier and video-television system is used. Lateral
and frontal views of the pharynx with simultaneous sound reproduction on a
video-taperecorder are obtained. The patient is examined in the recumbent
position and, if necessary, in the erect position. The examination starts
with the patient supine swallowing a sip of contrast medium (barium 60 w/v %)
and the motor activity of the pharynx and esophagus is registered in AP
projection. The same procedure is repeated in lateral projection with a
magnified, coned-down view over the pharynx. The soft palate and pharyngeal
walls are hereafter coated with contrast administered by a pipette in both
nostril. The morphological and functional state is then recorded in breathing,
speech, Mullerian maneouvre and simulated snoring in both frontal and lateral
views.

Henceforth, the patient is studied supine with horizontal beam direction as
above, and, in natural or induced sleep. For sleep induction Dormicum^R is
given intravenously.

Finally, films in the lateral view of the oropharynx in quiet breathing and
fonation are taken with the patient standing.

This examination reveals central dysfunction as well as morphological abnormalities. An overall esteem of motor activity, size and configuration of the
soft palate and tongue and the pharyngeal depth and width is obtained. In
quiet breething, Mullerian maneouvre, simulated and, if possible, natural
snoring the pliability of the soft tissues is seen as well as the site of
possible or true obstruction. When central dysfunction is present a cineradiography is performed for its evaluation.

The dose equivalent for a videoexamination as scheduled above is about 3 mSv,
which is less than an upper gastrointestinal study.

CASE REPORT

A 66-year-old man suffering from snoring and constant feeling of sleep
deprivation since many years consulted his doctor after a television program
on snoring disease. He is socially handicapped as he cannot travel by train
in the sleeping compartment or stay overnight at a hotel because of complaints
about his loud snoring. During conversation he occasionally falls asleep if
the subject is of little interest to him and he has even fallen asleep at
red light when driving. Subjectively, however, he has no sleep apnea periods.
He is of average bodybuild, 1.70 m and 75 kg, takes no medicines, denies
drugs and alcohol disuse. He is a heavy smoker and has, since some time, an
irritating non-productive cough, especially when supine but is else in good

physical shape and still at work running his own business. In the early 1930s he was in hospital for two months because of epidemic encephalitis of which he has no known sequelae.

He is planned to have uvulo-palato-pharyngo-plasty (UPPP) done and preoperatively he was subjected to rhinomanometria, sleep latency test, polygraphic sleep registration and videoradiography. The rhinomanometria was normal. The sleep latency test showed typical findings of hypersomnia and the polygraphic three-hour sleep registration verified obstructive sleep apnea syndrome (OSAS). He had an apnea index of 46.6 (apneas/hour) and an apnea duration of 10-56 seconds (average 25 sec) indicating that he spent 32.5 % of his sleep in apnea. The apnea periods were mainly of the obstructive type.

An ordinary chest X-ray examination revealed infiltrates in the left upper lobe, which mainly resolved on conventional antibiotic therapy.

The videoradiography and the films in the lateral view showed a somewhat long and thick soft palate and a normal pharyngeal depth (Fig 1 and 2). The space between the posterior pharyngeal wall and the thick soft palate was somewhat reduced at rest with the mouth closed and the tongue against the palate (Fig 2).

At deglutition and speech (Fig 3) the functional state of the pharynx appeared normal. At inspiration there was, due to a pushback of the tongue, a slight reduction of the pharyngeal anterior-posterior diameter. This reduction was more pronounced at forced inspiration. When supine, the anterior-posterior diameter diminished still more, even at quiet breathing, when the tongue, due to gravity, approached the posterior pharyngeal wall (Fig 4).

In simulated snoring the velar activity could not be properly assessed because of deficient relaxation. The pharyngeal diameter, however, diminished moderately due to adduction of the lateral pharyngeal walls and retroposition of the tongue, but when awake no obstruction was seen.

The patient was left alone supine with the light out during 15 minutes and fell asleep. His sleep behaviour was then registered in the lateral view. During the time of observation (about 10 minutes), no loud snoring was heard but mixed apnea periods were recorded as follows: after a brief central apnea of 5-10 seconds duration the tongue progressively approached the posterior pharyngeal wall. Finally complete obstruction of the hypopharynx followed. The site of obstruction was observed to be at the epiglottic level. This induced an obstructive apnea of 20-40 seconds duration. During the apnea 6-10 inefficient breathing efforts were seen. This was terminated by arousal, when the pharynx regained normal depth. Normal breathing of short duration, i.e. 20-30 seconds, then followed.

The above observed pattern was seen repetitively. However, the obstructive apnea was not always preceded by a central apnea, neither was the central apnea always followed by the obstructive type.

DISCUSSION

The patient presented in this report has, anamnestically and according to physiological tests, a mainly obstructive sleep apnea syndrome. Videoradiography, when awake, revealed findings suggesting obstruction between the posterior pharyngeal wall, soft palate and the tongue. During sleep, however, an obstruction is seen at the epiglottic level well below the soft palate.

The patient is planned to undergo a UPPP which probably will reduce or abolish his social handicap. In several reports (deBerry-Borowiecki et al 1985; Harmon et al 1986; Editorial 1986; Afzelius et al 1986) on UPPP in OSAS the results on snoring seems to be very good. However, the results on the apneas are reported to be less successful. This suggests an obstructive level below the site of operation.

How the UPPP will affect the obstructive apneas in our patient is still to be seen.

CONCLUSION

In the preoperative evaluation of patients with snoring disease, polygraphic sleep registration will reveal if obstructive sleep apnea syndrome is present. The morphological and functional state of the pharynx and the site of the obstruction, however, are not available with these methods but can profitably be demonstrated by videoradiography.

REFERENCES

Afzelius, L.-E. et al (1986): Treatment of obstructive sleep apnea syndrome with palatopharyngoplasty. Läkartidningen 83, 4099-4101.
deBerry-Borowiecki, B. et al (1985): Indications for palatopharyngoplasty. Arch Otolaryngol 111, 659-663.
Editorial (1986): Snoring in perspective. Clin Otolaryngol 11, 53-54.
Fairbanks, D.N.F. (1984): Snoring: Surgical vs non-surgical management. Laryngoscope 94, 1188-1192.
Harmon, J.D. et al (1986): Uvulopalatoplasty and obstructive sleep apnea. South Med J 79, 197-200.
Krieger, J. (1986): Les syndromes d'apnées du sommeil de l'adulte. Bull Eur Physiopathol Respir 22, 147-189.
Lugaresi, E. et al (1980): Some epidemiologic data on snoring and cardiocirculatory disturbances. Sleep 3, 221.
Norton, P.G. et al (1983): Snoring in adults: Some epidemiologic aspects. Can Med Assoc J 128, 674-675.

RESUME

Les patients atteints de rhoncopathie chronique seront choisis pour l'enregistrement polygraphique au cours du sommeil. Cet examen révèle ou exclut le syndrome d'apnée du sommeil, SAS, mais il ne peut apprecier ni le lieu d'obstruction ni l'etat morphologique ou fonctionel du pharynx. Dans ce but la videoradiographie se trouve appropriée et est une méthode simple et rapide. Un enregistrement polygraphique du sommeil a été realisé chez un homme, qui a 66 ans, avec un tableau clinique évocateur de SAS. Ceci a montré un index d'apnées superieur à 40. A l'etat de veille la videoradiographie présente un palais moux allongé et épais et aucune autre anomalie de la morphologie ou de la fonction. Lors de l'endormissement et pendant une brêve apnée centrale on voit une obstruction au niveau de l'epiglotte, celle-ci provoque une apnée obstructive de 20 à 40 secondes suivi d'un eveil. Cet enchainement se répète de façon stéreotypée tout au long du sommeil avec quelques variations.

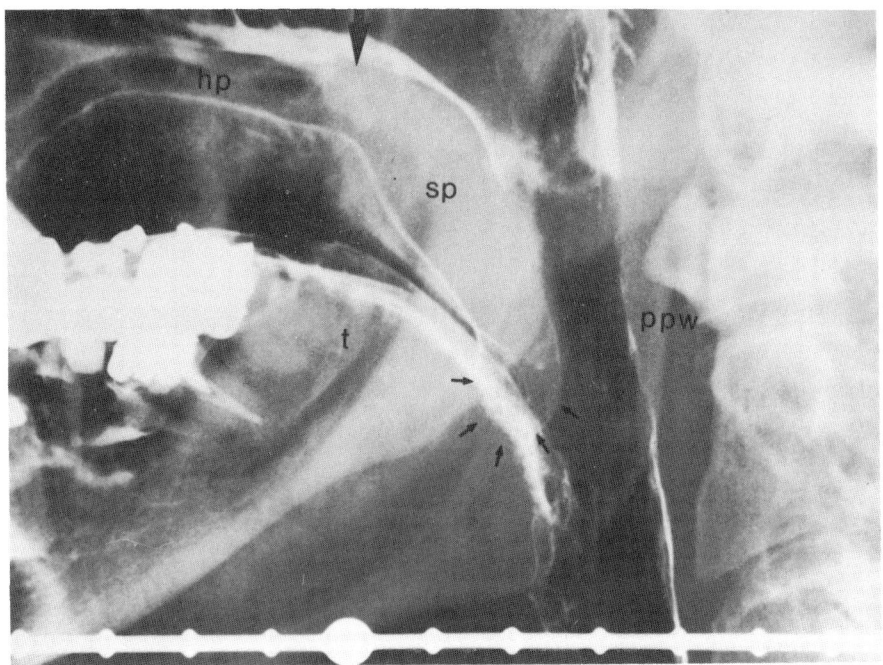

Fig 1. Lateral view with contrast medium in the nasal and oral cavity. At rest with lowered tongue (t). The soft palate (sp) is long and fairly thick. The uvula (small black arrows) is partially conceiled resting at the tongue. The distance between the soft palate and the posterior pharyngeal wall (ppv) is normal. The pharyngeal depth as measured from the posterior limitation of the hard palate (thick arrow) to the posterior pharyngeal wall is normal. The prevertebral tissue is of ordinary thickness (hp - hard palate).

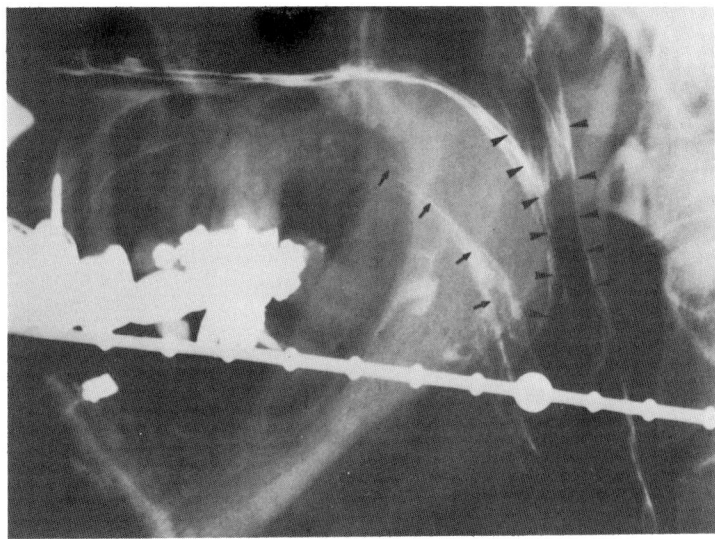

Fig 2. Lateral view at rest with the surface of the tongue (small arrows) against the hard and the soft palate. In this position the distance between the soft palate and posterior pharyngeal wall (arrow heads) is diminished.

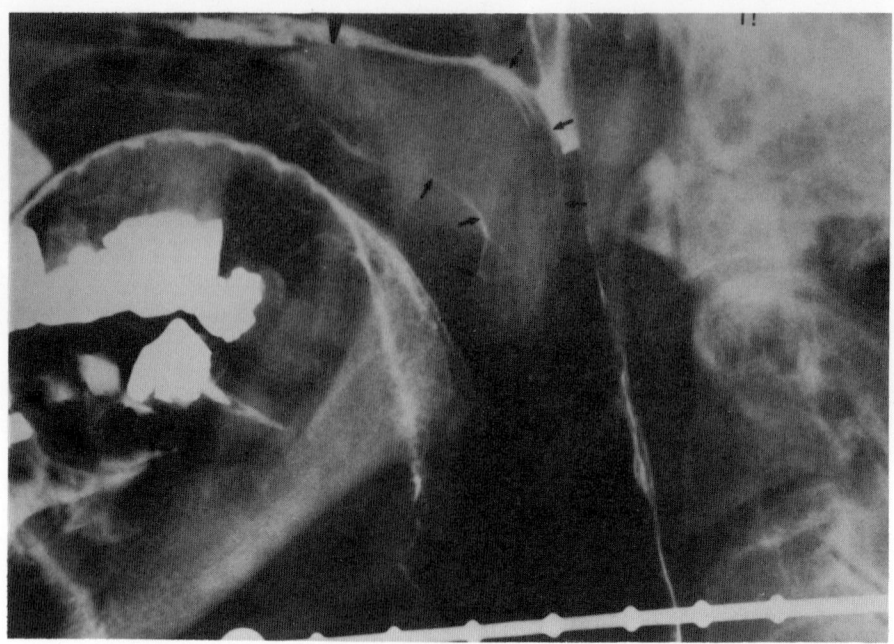

Fig 3. Lateral view during fonation of "e". The soft palate (small arrow) is seen at full length when slightly elevated and approaching the posterior pharyngeal wall in a normal way.

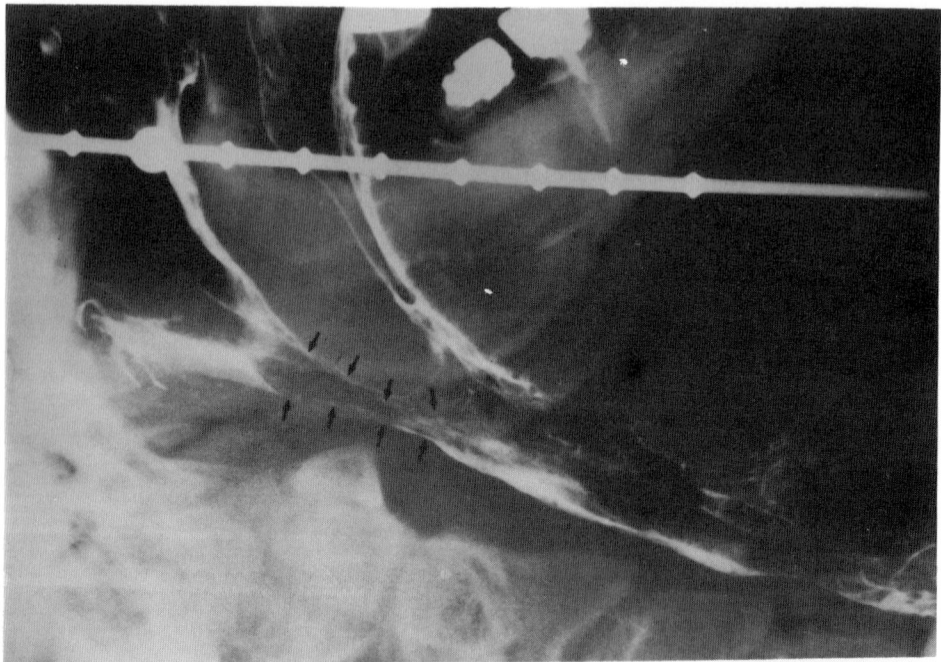

Fig 4. Lateral view in the supine position during rest. The anterior-posterior pharyngeal diameter is diminished, especially at the uvular level due to retroposition of the tongue.

Respiratory muscles activity in children with sleep obstructive apnea syndrome

J.P. Praud, J.P. Monrigal, M.F. Delaperche, A.M. d'Allest, H. Nedelco and C.H. Gaultier

Laboratoire de Physiologie, CNRS UA 1159, Hôpital Antoine Béclère, 92141 Clamart, France

ABSTRACT

We studied electrical activity (EMG) of respiratory muscles in 13 children (6 mo- 15yr) with sleep obstructive apnea syndrom (SOAS), apart from apneic events. During natural sleep, we monitored sleep stages (neurophysiological criteria), nasal and oral airflow (thermistors), rib cage and abdominal anteroposterior diameter variation (magnetometers), transcutaneous blood gases (PO_2 and PCO_2), EMG of inspiratory muscles (diaphragm (Di), 2th and 3th parasternal muscles (PS), sternocleidomastoïd (SCM), expiratory muscles (lateral abdominal wall muscles (AB)) and pharyngeal dilators (genioglossus (GG)) (cutaneous electrodes). Analysis of EMG traces apart from apneic events showed permanent phasic activity of all the studied muscles during inspiration (Di, PS, SCM, GG) or expiration (AB). Analysis of muscles recruitment according to sleep stages allows for a better analysis of thoracic and abdominal motions. We conclude that apart from apneic events, respiratory muscles are recruited to support Di inspiratory contraction in children with SOAS. This muscle recruitment increases the work of breathing.

KEY WORDS

Sleep obstructive apnea syndrome, children, respiratory muscles work of breathing, thoraco-abdominal movements.

INTRODUCTION

The sleep obstructive apnea syndrome (SAOS) is characterized in children, as in obese adults, by intermittent upper airways (UA) occlusions. Nevertheless, between obstructive apneas (OA), periods of incomplete obstruction occur, with clinical evidence of increased recruitment of respiratory muscles. This study was designed in children to investigate the recruitment of the respiratory muscles, i.e. the diaphragm (Di), the second and third parasternal muscles (PS), the sternocleidomastoïd (SCM), the genioglossus (GG) and the lateral abdominal muscle group (AB). The only study published on this subject gave no information about differences on recruitment of respiratory muscles with sleep stages (JEFFRIES, 1984).

MATERIAL AND METHODS

Thirteen children (6mo - 15yr) were tested. Etiology of their SOAS is listed in table I. Parental informed consent was obtained in each case. Sleep study was conducted under the surveillance of a physician during an afternoon (seven children)

or a night (six children). Results of sleep study concerning repartition of sleep
stages and characteristics of apneas are listed in the table I. No premedication
nor sleep deprivation were used, because of their depressive effect on UA muscle
activity (HERSHENSON, 1984 ; LEITER, 1985). Sleep stages were scored according to
neurophysiological criteria (electroencephalogram, electrooculogram and submental
electromyogram). The following respiratory parameters were recorded : 1) nasal and
oral airflow (thermistors) 2) rib cage and abdominal anteroposterior diameters
(magnetometers) 3) transcutaneous partial pressures of O_2 and CO_2 (Radiometer).Moreover, from surface electrodes we recorded electrical activity (EMG) of respiratory muscles : inspiratory muscles i.e. Di, PS and SCM ; expiratory muscles, i.e.
AB ; pharyngeal dilator muscle, i.e. GG. EMG_{Di} was recorded from two electrodes
placed in the eight right intercostal space, one on the anterior axillary line,
the other on the midaxillary line. EMG_{PS} was recorded from two electrodes positionned near the sternum in the second and third intercostal space. EMG_{SCM} was recorded by two electrodes one centimeter apart on the middle third of the muscle.
EMG_{AB} was recorded with two electrodes placed one centimeter apart midway between
umbilicus and iliac crest. EMG_{GG} was recorded from two electrodes positionned in
the middle line, one just under the lower lip, the other midway between the chin
and the hyoïd bone (SAUERLAND, 1981). Raw EMG signals were filtered (30-1000Hz)and
amplified (Universal GOULD Amplifier). All variables were simultaneously displayed
on a 16 channel recorder (ALVAR). Analysis of respiratory muscles EMG was made
qualitatively during the non-occlusive periods.

TABLE I : CHARACTERISTICS OF THE SLEEP OBSTRUCTIVE APNEA SYNDROME

Cases	Age (mo)	Sex	Etiology	Night (N) Nap (n)	TST (mn)	% REM	Index of apnea	% of OA
1	45	M	Micrognathism	N	423	9	11	85
2	51	F	Franchescetti	N	390	12	12	45
3	65	F	E.T.	N	295	15	5	79
4	60	F	Crouzon	N	384	19	36	46
5	180	F	Osteopetrosis	N	320	7	11	97
6	90	M	E.T.	N	409	15	13	64
7	41	M	E.T.	n	81	18	5	84
8	12	F	Pierre Robin	n	127	8	17	100
9	6	M	E.T.	n	90	14	17	100
10	30	M	E.T.	n	116	15	15	96
11	30	M	E.T.	n	76	8	10	50
12	24	M	E.T.	n	145	30	108	98
13	42	M	E.T.	n	194	10	27	32

M : male ; F : female ; E.T. : enlarged tonsils ; TST : total sleep time ; OA :
obstructive apnea ; Index of apnea : number of apneas and hypopneas ≥ 5s per hour
of sleep.

RESULTS

Respiratory muscle activity changes with sleep stage
NREM sleep in all the children was associated with regular phasic respiratory muscle activity : inspiratory activity was recorded from Di and PS muscles, from SCM
and also from GG ; expiratory phasic activity was recorded from AB muscles. In all
these muscles, tonic activity persisted between two bursts of phasic activity. An
exemple of recording obtained in NREM sleep is given in figure 1.During REM sleep,
respiratory muscles activity was different from NREM sleep : inspiratory activity
persisted during the whole REM sleep period in Di, PS and GG muscles, with decreased or absent tonic activity; phasic inspiratory EMG_{SCM} was decreased or absent.
EMG_{AB} was studied in ten children during REM sleep : phasic expiratory EMG_{AB} was
absent in eight children, and persisted only in two others (cases 7 and 8).

Thoraco-abdominal motions

During REM sleep, paradoxical inward movement of rib cage (PIRC) during inspiration was seen in all the children with absent EMG_{AB}, i.e. all but children 7 and 8. On the contrary, during NREM sleep, abdominal motions seemed to be modified by presence of expiratory EMG_{AB} : indeed, asynchronous abdominal movements with airflow were present in all children but two (cases 3 and 9) ; in addition, PIRC during inspiration was associated in six of them.

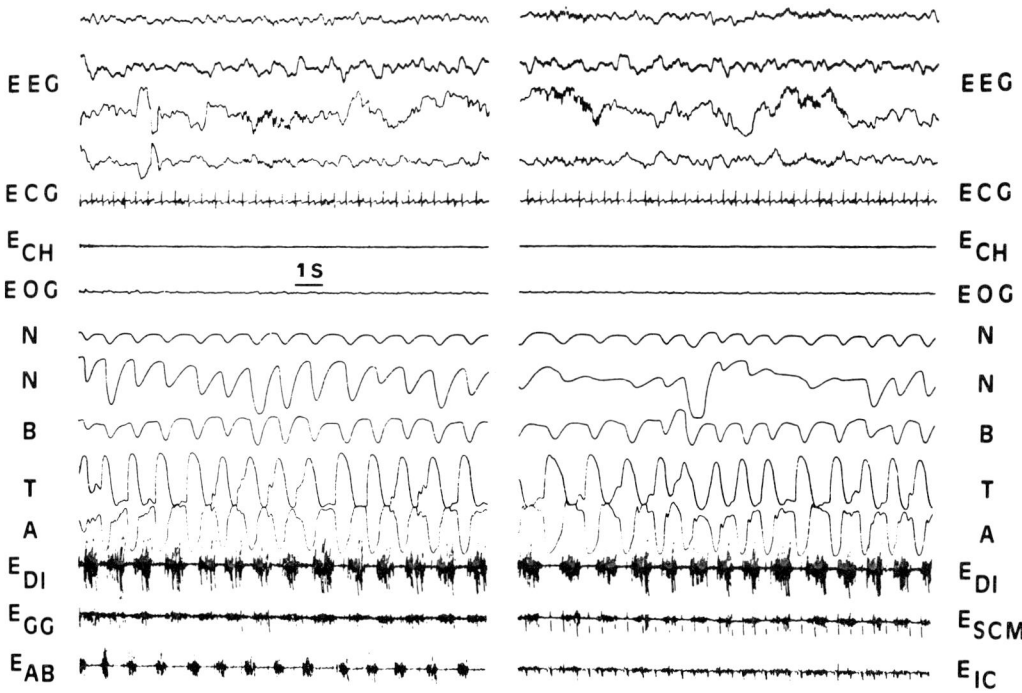

Figure 1 : Representative traces in patient 9 during NREM sleep. From top to bottom : 1st to 7th traces, electroencephalogram (EEG), electrocardiogram (ECG), chin electromyogram (E_{CH}), electrooculogram (EOG) ; 8th to 10th traces : nasal (N) and buccal (B) airflow ; 11th and 12th traces : rib cage (T) and abdominal (A) anteroposterior diameters ; 13th to 15th traces : electrical activity of respiratory muscles, on the left : diaphragm (E_{DI}), genioglossus (E_{GG}), lateral abdominal wall muscles (E_{AB}) ; on the right : E_{DI}, sternocleidomastoïd (E_{SCM}), interchondral part of 2th and 3th intercostal muscles (E_{IC}). Phasic inspiratory (DI, IC, SCM, GG) or expiratory (AB) contraction is present in all studied respiratory muscles. Paradoxical inward rib cage movement during inspiration was recorded during the whole sleep period in this patient.

DISCUSSION

This study in children with SOAS showed recruitment of respiratory muscles apart from OA, i.e. during inspiration rib cage (Di, PS ans SCM) and UA dilator muscles (GG) and during expiration AB. The recruitment of respiratory muscles varied with sleep stages and was associated with different abdomino-thoracic motions.

Recruitment of respiratory muscles and sleep stages

During NREM sleep, inspiratory muscles (PS and SCM) were recruited to support Di contraction against the increased UA resistance. Moreover, AB expiratory activity had the same effect, by placing the Di on a better part of its force-lenght curve (MARTIN, 1982). Nevertheless, respiratory muscles recruitment leads to increase in the work of breathing. At the UA level, GG must contract to counteract the highly negative intraluminal pressure created by Di, PS and SCM contraction (REMMERS, 1979). *During REM sleep,* Di contraction was not supported by SCM and AB any more ; REM sleep inhibition of postural muscles as SCM and AB has been previously reported in adults (JOHNSON, 1984 ; ISSA, 1985). At the UA level, GG inspiratory contraction is now of crucial importance to maintain pharyngeal patency in absence of expiratory tone. Finally, Di must contract alone against a still higher UA resistance than during NREM sleep. This may partially explain the aggravation of the SOAS reported in children during REM sleep (GUILLEMINAULT, 1980).

Thoraco-abdominal motions

Previous data on SOAS showed that children exhibited inspiratory PIRC during REM and NREM sleep, what is different from controls (GAULTIER, in press). Asynchronous abdominal movement with respiration has also been observed (PRAUD, 1984). In the present study we recorded the latter in most of the children during NREM sleep ; the expiratory contraction of AB seems to be responsible for the outward abdominal movement during expiration, both of them disappearing simultaneously during REM sleep.

CONCLUSION

In children with SOAS, our data showed respiratory muscles recruitment during NREM sleep to support Di contraction against UA obstacle, apart from apneic events. This recruitment leads to increase in the work of breathing. On the contrary, during REM sleep, Di often appeared to be the only respiratory muscle to contract ; in this situation, Di should be close to its fatigue threshold, especially in infants.

REFERENCES

GAULTIER Cl, PRAUD JP, CANET E, D'ALLEST AM. Paradoxical inward rib cage motion during rapid eye movement in infants and young children. J. Dev. Physiol. In press

GUILLEMINAULT C. (1980): Sleep apnea syndromes : impact of sleep and sleep states. Sleep 3, 227 - 234.

HERSHENSON M, BROUILLETTE RT, OLSEN E, HUNT CE (1984): The effect of chloral hydrate on genioglossus and diaphragmatic activity. Pediatr. Res. 18, 516-519.

ISSA FG and SULLIVAN CE (1985) : Respiratory muscle activity and thoracoabdominal motion during acute episodes of asthma during sleep. Am. Rev. Respir. Dis. 132, 999-1004.

JEFFRIES B, BROUILLETTE RT, HUNT CE (1984) : Electromyographic study of some accessory muscles of respiration in children with obstructive sleep apnea. Am. Rev. Respir. Dis. 129, 696-702.

JOHNSON MW and REMMERS JE (1984) : Accessory muscle activity during sleep in chronic obstructive pulmonary disease. J. Appl. Physiol. Respirat. Environ. Exercise Physiol. 57, 1011-1017.

LEITER JC, KNUTH SL, BARTLETT JR (1985) : The effect of sleep deprivation on activity of the genioglossus muscle. Am. Rev. Respir. Dis. 132, 1242-1245.

MARTIN JG and DE TROYER A. (1982) : The behaviour of the abdominal muscles during inspiratory mechanical loading. Respiration Physiol. 50, 63-73.

PRAUD JP, GAULTIER Cl, BUVRY A, BOULE M, GIRARD F. (1984) : Lung mechanics and breathing pattern during wakefulness and sleep in children with enlarged tonsils. Sleep 7, 304-312.

REMMERS JE, DE GROOT WJ, SAUERLAND EK, ANCH AM (1978) : Pathogenesis of upper airway occlusion during sleep. J. Appl. Physiol. Respirat. Environ. Exercise Physiol. 44, 931-938.

SAUERLAND EK, SAUERLAND BAT, ORR WC, HAIRSTON LE (1981) : Noninvasive electromyography of human genioglossal (tongue) activity. Electromyogr. Clin. Neurophysiol. 21, 279-286.

ACTIVITE DES MUSCLES RESPIRATOIRES DANS LE SYNDROME D'APNEES OBSTRUCTIVES DU SOMMEIL.

JP. Praud, JP Monrigal, MF Delaperche, AM D'Allest, H Nedelco, Cl. Gaultier.

L'obstruction des voies aériennes supérieures durant le sommeil se caractérise par la survenue intermittente d'apnées obstructives (AO). Cependant les signes cliniques de lutte respiratoire en dehors des AO chez l'enfant évoquent le recrutement d'autres muscles respiratoires que le diaphragme (Di). Le but du travail est d'étudier en dehors des AO l'activité électromyographique (EMG) des muscles respiratoires chez 13 enfants de 6 mois à 15 ans ayant un syndrome d'AO. Au cours du sommeil naturel les stades de sommeil (critères neurophysiologiques), le flux nasal et buccal (thermistances), les variations des diamètres antéro-postérieurs du thorax et de l'abdomen (magnétomètres), les gaz du sang transcutanés ($SatO_2$, PO_2, PCO_2), l'EMG des muscles inspiratoires (Di, sternocléidomastoïdien (Scm), 2è et 3è parasternaux (Ps)), expiratoires (larges de l'abdomen (Ab)) et dilatateurs du pharynx (génioglosse (Gg)) par électrodes cutanées ont été monitorés. L'analyse des signaux EMG bruts 1) montre en dehors des AO une activité phasique permanente de tous les muscles étudiés à l'inspiration (Di, Scm, Ps, Gg) ou à l'expiration (Ab) 2) permet d'analyser les différents types de respiration paradoxale, thoracique ou thoraco-abdominale. En conclusion, cette étude montre au cours du sommeil chez l'enfant ayant un syndrome d'AO que d'autres muscles respiratoires que le Di sont recrutés ce qui est en faveur d'une augmentation permanente du travail ventilatoire en dehors des AO.

ACKNOWLEDGMENTS

This work was supported by CNRS UA 1159 and le Comité national des Maladies respiratoires.

The authors wish to thank, N. BAALA, S. HAQUEBERGE, C. LEBRETONNIC, A. VIRASSAMY for their technical assistance and S. ROUCHAVILLE for typing the manuscript.

Prognostic value of magnetic resonnance imaging cephalometric study in snorers with or without sleep apnea syndrome

F. Chabolle*, B. Fleury**, M.T. Ibazizen*** and A.E. Cabanis***

*Service O.R.L. Hôpital Saint-Antoine, 184 rue du faubourg Saint-Antoine, 75012 Paris, France
**Service de Pneumologie, Hôpital Saint-Antoine, 75012 Paris, France
***Service de Radiologie, Hôpital des Quinze Vingt, 75012 Paris, France

ABSTRACT

The authors achieved a cephalometric study using I.R.M imagery in 30 patients : 10 snorers without S.A.S ; 10 snorers with S.A.S and 10 controls. They quoted a more important verticalization of mouth floor when snoring was associated with severe sleep disorders. Comparative measure of tongue and oro-pharynx areas allows to find a more important macroglossy when there exists S.A.S. At last, the measure of various oro-pharynx diameters allows to define a tongue base morphology guiding therapeutic strategy in S.A.S.

KEYWORDS

Cephalometric ; Magnetic Resonnance Imaging ; Oro-pharynx ; Sleep Apnea Syndrome ; Snoring.

INTRODUCTION

Exact determination of the obstructive site in case of isolated or associated to Sleep Apnea Syndrome (SAS) snoring, still remains imperfectively resolved in spite of numerous modern investigation methods. If some causes are obvious, respective roles of soft palate and tongue are difficult to evidence, the incomplete and unpredictable success of Uvulopalatopharyngoplasty (UPPP) in S.A.S surgical therapy made us incriminate tongue basis. Magnetic Resonnance Imaging nowadays constitutes the only method of non invasive medical imagery allowing a sagittal section showing both bone and soft structures of the head and neck region.

MATERIAL

An I.R.M study has been achieved in 30 patients from 34 to 69 years old with an average age of 51. It concerns 27 men and 3 women homogeneously divided in 3 groups : first two are constituted by 10 non apneic snorers, and 10 apneic snorers all having been submitted to a polygraphic sleep recording. Patients of the apneic group have an apneic index between 36 and 81 for non REM sleep and between 8 and 45 for REM sleep, with mean indexes respectively of 66 for non REM sleep and 36 for REM sleep.

These two first groups have been compared to a third group of 10 non snoring patients.

These 3 populations are comparable for height, but there exists an overweight v.s. theoretical weight more important when the snorer is apneic. The mean overweight is of 7 % in the control group, 28 % in the non apneic snorers, and 40 % in the apneic snorers. This confirms the wellknown role of obesity in sleep apnea syndrome.

At last 8 of the patients in the apneic group have gone through U.P.P.P and 2 were treated by C.P.A.P.

METHOD

M.R.I examination was carried out with a CGR 1 500 MAGNISCAN device by realising joining sagittal, axial and frontal sections with adapted zone aerial. First part of the examination was achieved in 350/30 echo spin taken in T2 in order to make sure of brainstem integrity. Head extremity was immobilised in the same position for all patients.

However, certain limits of this examination have shown : i.e. 7 patients previously planned for this procedure had to be rejected : 3 of them showed such an obesity that they could not enter the machine, another had heart insufficiency and didn't bear to be closed in the machine, and finally 3 suffered from claustrophobia and refused the examination.

The other limit of the investigation is constituted by the presence of artefects due to ferromagnetic elements, especially in teeth, changing M.R.I results. This artefect has been quoted in 11 cases, and made us reject 2 patients from the procedure.

For each examination, 3 sorts of measurings have been planned with a mediane sagittal section.

First of all, distance between the posterior part of tongue and oro-pharynx posterior wall has been measured at 3 levels : soft palate inferior edge, epiglottis superior edge, and the level of maximum narrowing of upper airway tract respectively. Second measure achieved was the angle between first the line joining mandibula inferior edge and C2 C3 vertebral disk and secondely the line joining mandibula inferior adge and the middle of hyoid bone. Measure of this angle has been completed with vertical distance between hyoid bone and bone palate. Third and last measure was surface determination. Tongue area recorded as well as oro-pharynx and oral cavity areas, the limits of which passing by palate, oropharynx, posterior wall, then at the level of hyoid bone superior edge, mouth floor superior edge (genio-hyoidis muscle) and at last at the back of dental region.

RESULTS

Control population
Angle measure showed values between 0 and 17° with a mean angle of 8°, +/- 5 S.M. Vertical distance between hyoid bone and palate was between 53 and 69 mm with a mean value of 61 mm, +/- 5 S.M.

Tongue areas went from 25.6 to 34.1 cm2 with an average area of 29.8 cm2, +/- 2.9 S.M, and those of oro-pharynx from 35 to 51.8 with a mean value of 43.6, +/- 5.9 S.M, the average rate of the two areas was of 68 %.

Average width of the upper airway respiratory tract was of 9.2 mm, +/- 2.0 S.M, at the level of soft palate lower edge and of 11.4 mm, +/- 3.2 S.M, at the epiglottis superior edge. Average width of maximum narrowing was of 9.2 mm, +/- 2.2 S.M.

Non apneic snorers

All patients had an angle value between 9° and 33° with an average angle of 19°, +/- 8 S.M, i.e. 11° more than the control group. Average vertical distance value is 70 mm, +/- 9 S.M, with extremes from 53 to 82 mm, i.e. 9 mm more than control group.

Tongue area went from 24.2 to 34.5 cm2 with an average value of 31.5 cm2, +/- 4.2 S.M, i.e. 1.60 cm2 more than control group.

Oro-pharynx average surface was of 46.1 cm2, +/- 7.8 S.M, i.e. 2.4 cm2 more than control group. The rate of those two areas is of 68 %, the same as control group.

Average width of upper airway respiratory tract was of 12.3 mm, +/- 5.3 S.M, at the level of soft palate lower edge, and of 11.6 mm, +/- 4.6 S.M, at epiglottis superior edge.

Apneic snorers

Angle measure shows an important increase, each patient having an angle going from 25° to 46° with an average angle of 31°, +/- 8 S.M, i.e. 23° more than control group and 12° more than non apneic snorers.

In the same way, height increases parallely with an average of 79mm, +/- 8 S.M, i.e. 18 mm more than control and 9 mm more than non apneic snorers. Tongue area has a mean value of 33.7 cm2, +/- 3.6, +/- 4.5, i.e. 4 cm2 more than control group. Oro-pharynx area is of 50.3 cm2, +/- 7.2, i.e. 7 cm2 more than control group.

But the rate of these two areas is still 67 % and the same as the two previous groups.

Average width of upper airway respiratory tract was of 12.5 mm, +/- 5.4 S.M, at the level of soft palate lower edge, and of 9.2 mm, +/- 5.1 S.M, at epiglottis superior edge. Average width of maximum narrowing was of 11.4 mm, +/- 3.2 S.M.

	CONTROLS	SNORERS	S.A.S
MEAN ANGLE	8 +/- 5	19 +/- 8	31 +/- 8
OROPHARYNX MEAN HEIGHT	61 +/- 5	70 +/- 9	79 +/- 8

RESULTS : ANGLES MEASURING

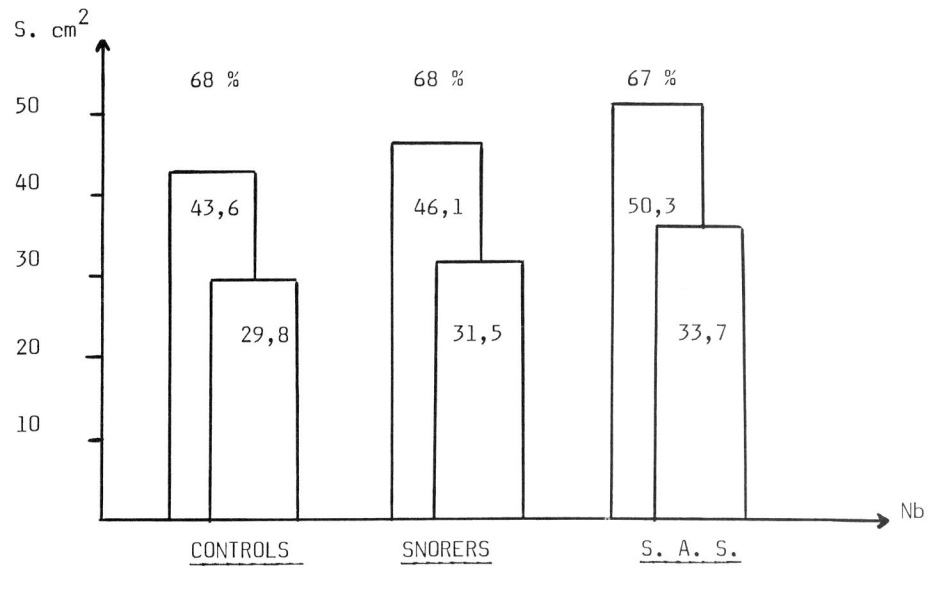

COMPARISONS
of TONGUE and OROPHARYNX SURFACES

	CONTROLS	SNORERS	S.A.S.
SOFT PALATE LOWER EDGE (mm)	9,2 ± 2,0	12,3 ± 5,3	12,5 ± 5,4
MAXIMUM REDUCTION (mm)	9,2 ± 2,2	10,4 ± 5,0	9,2 ± 5,1
EPIGLOTTIS HIGHER EDGE (mm)	11,4 ± 3,2	11,6 ± 4,6	11,4 ± 3,2

RESULTS :

OROPHARYNGEAL AIRWAY MEASURING

DISCUSSION

The results lead to a first remark : the measure of the angle determined by mandibula lower edge, C2 C3 vertebral disk and hyoid bone body shows a greater lowering of hyoid bone when snoring is complicated with S.A.S. This result is corroborated by parallele increase of oro-pharynx height. This observation must be compared to the one of GUILLEMINAUT who also found a lowering of hyoid bone by cephalometric study with sagittal teleradiography. This author concludes to the necessity of mandibular advancement or hyoid bone suspension surgery in this case due to a floor of the mouth release, especially of genio-hyoid muscle, (Guilleminault, 1984).

However if the mouth floor fell, thus constituting the initial mechanism, the rate of tongue and oro-pharynx areas should reduce, content becoming to small for container.

But this rate stays remarquably constant at 68 % in the 3 groups. There exists then a measurable parallele increase of tongue area, that representes 30 % more than control group.

This tongue hypertrophia is certainly the base of incomplete result of U.P.P.P in sleep apnea syndrome. As a matter of fact, tongue muscle is contained in an oropharynged cavity with solid bone structure on the anterior, posterior, superior and lateral walls. Only muscle ligamentery floor of the mouth is apt to move by lowering under the effect of tongue muscle pushing, which is one of the most powerfull of the organism (Haponik, 1983 ; Lowe, 1986).

This phenomenon could explain low electromyographic activity of this muscle found by some authors in obeses.

A second point must be underlined : measure of various posterior respiratory tracts should allow to define a more efficient therapeutic strategy. Analysis of posterior respiratory tracts diameter values doesn't evidence any significant difference between the 3 groups, in absolute values. On the opposite, studying each level reveals several points :
- diameter at epiglottis higher edge is roughly the same in the 3 groups and never represents maximum narrowing.
- On the other hand, comparative assay of airway section at soft palate lower edge level and at maximum narrowing level shows that this narrowing is located at soft palate lower edge in control group, i.e. there is a verticalization of tongue base (Haponik, 1983 ; Suratt, 1983). On the opposite, the more snoring is complicated with S.A.S, the more maximum narrowing goes down and gets further from soft palate lower edge. Tongue base then looses its verticality by getting round in the back with an anterior concavity. This degree of postero-inferior tongue projection has been appreciated in function of therapeutic results of U.P.P.P. 7 out of the 10 patients of S.A.S group have gone through surgery and had post-operative sleep recording. In the 3 other patients, 2 were treated by C.P.A.P and one refused his post-U.P.P.P recording.

The objective efficience of U.P.P.P measured by the rate of reduction of the apnea/hour index has been compared to the rate of maximum narrowing of upper aerial tracts V.S. soft palate lower edge section. We then evidenced that the more tongue base was vertical, with a soft palate lower edge diameter equivalent to maximum narrowing diameter, the more U.P.P.P was efficient. On the opposite, the more maximum narrowing is located down and further from soft palate lower edge, the less U.P.P.P is efficient.

Then, sagittal M.R.I sections allow to assay tongue base anatomic morphology and to define a more efficient therapy of S.A.S.

If tongue base :
- is vertical and maximum narrowing diameter is the same as soft palate lower edge diameter, U.P.P.P must treat snoring and S.A.S.
- on the opposite, if tongue base is round and presents an anterior concavity and if maximum narrowing diameter is very lower than soft palate lower edge diameter, U.P.P.P is apt to lead to incomplete or complete failure. In this case, absence of retrognathia must be evidenced by cephalometric assay. If there is an associated retrognathia, surgical mandibular advancement must be proposed. On the opposite, if articulate is normal and there is no retrognathia as often, it seems useful to us to prefer basi lingual glossectomy to hyoid bone suspension, this one not solving the problem of tongue pushing due to muscular hypertrophy (Powell, 1983 ; Rivlin, 1984 ; Spire, 1983).

CONCLUSION

According to a study including 30 patients in 3 groups : control, non apneic and apneic snorers, all having gone through R.M.I examination, it is then possible to evidence that the floor of the mouth lowering is due to tongue hypertrophia. This examination should contribute to predict success or failure of U.P.P.P in apneic patients by the exact determination of maximum narrowing of the airway. Therapeutic indication depends on its situation   at tongue base level, or a soft palate inferior edge level.

REFERENCES

GUILLEMINAULT C., RILEY R., POWELL N. (1984) : "Implications for Treatement", Abnormal Cephalometric Measurements. Chest 86 (5), 793 - 794
HAPONIK E.F., SMITH P.L., BOHLMAN M.E., ALLEN R.P., GOLMAN S.M., BLEECKER E.R. (1983) : "Correlation of Airway Size with Physiology during Sleep and Wakefulness", Computerized Tomography in Obstructive Sleep Apnea. Am. Rev. Respir. Dis. 127, 221 - 226
LOWE A.A., GIONHAKU N., TAKEUCHI K., FLEETHAM J.A. (1986) : Three dimensional CT reconstructions of tongue and airway in adult subjects with obstructive sleep apnea. Am. J. Orthod. Dentofac. Orthop. 90, 364 - 374
POWELL N., GUILLEMINAULT C., RILEY R., SMITH L. (1983) :Mandibular advancement and obstructive sleep apnea syndrome. Bull. europ. Physiopath. resp. 19, 607 - 610
RIVLIN J., HOFFSTEIN V., KALBFLEISCH J., McNICHOLAS W., ZAMEL N., BRYAN A.C. (1984) : Upper airway Morphology in Patients with Idiopathic Obstructive Sleep Apnea. Am. Rev. Respir. Dis. 129, 355 - 360
SPIRE J.P., KUO P.C., CAMPBELL N. (1983) : Maxillo-Facial surgical approach : an introduction and review of mandibular advancement. Bull. europ. Physiopath. resp. 19, 604 - 606
SURATT P.M., DEE P., ATKINSON R.L., ARMSTRONG P., WILHOIT S.C. (1983) : Fluoroscopic and Computed Tomographic Features of the Pharyngeal Airway in Obstructive Sleep Apnea. Am. Rev. Respir. Dis. 127, 487 - 492

III CHRONIC RHONCHOPATHY GENERAL FEATURES
Chairman: J.F. Derenne

Computerized analysis of snoring

Alberto Leiberman and Arnon Cohen

Department of Otolaryngology, Soroka University Hospital and Faculty of Health Sciences; and Department of Electrical and Computer Engineering Biomedical Program, Ben-Gurion University of the Negev, Beer-Sheva, Israel

ABSTRACT

The nature and characteristics of the snoring sounds may depend on the level and the degree of the obstruction. Sophisticated sound analysis may be of value to estimate these characteristics. Computerized analysis of snoring sounds was performed by two main methods: 1) The Power Spectral Density function, where the power distribution of the signal is plotted against frequency yielding the relative percentage of the signal power in each frequency band, and 2) The Estimated Cross-section area. Using a model of the airway with varying cross-sectional area, starting in the trachea and ending in the nose and lips, the cross-sectional area was estimated from the snoring signal. Different patterns appeared depending upon the site of the pathology. The computerized algorithm may automatically distinguish and classify the various types of snoring signals. The results of these analyses in patients suffering from chronic rhonchopathy are presented.

Key words: Snoring; computerized analysis of sound; location of airway obstruction

INTRODUCTION

Snoring is a non-stationary random process. The acoustic signal is generated by an excessive air turbulence as a result of nocturnal upper airway obstruction (Simmonds, 1983). Many factors have been attributed to be the cause of snoring (Fairbanks, 1981; Heiner, 1983; Moran, 1985). Effective surgical procedures depend on the understanding of the mechanism involved in the airway obstruction in each individual and the ability to identify and locate the type of obstruction (Simmonds, 1983; Fujita, 1981). This goal may be achieved by a sophisticated analysis of the snoring sounds, which may provide important information concerning the source of the sound. The snoring signal is characterized by changes of the amplitude (energy) and the frequency during inspiration and expiration. This signal, as other stochastic signals, are better characterized by their Power Spectral Density (PSD) function rather than by their time records. The power distribution of the signal is plotted against frequency yielding the relative percentage of the signal power in each frequency band (Cohen, 1986). The purpose of this preliminary report is to describe a new technique for digital processing of snoring in order to estimate the source and location of the snoring sounds.

MATERIAL AND METHODS

The snoring signal was picked by a microphone hand held in front of the patient at a distance of about 20 cm. The acquisition and processing of the signal are schematically described in Fig. 1. No attempt was made to record absolute sound pressures. An effort was made to get a low background noise. The time domain energy envelope of the signal was found to be one of the characteristics of the snoring signal. An algorithm for inspiratory/expiratory boundaries detection was developed based on the energy envelope signal (Cohen and Leiberman, 1986). Analysis was then performed separately for inspiratory and expiratory periods. For further analysis of the signal we assumed an extremely simple model of the airway. The upper airway tract was assumed to be an acoustic tube with varying cross sectional aea, starting from the trachea, vocal cords and ending at the lips and nose. The tube was arbitrarily divided into sections each with equal length, but different cross sectional area. We further assume that the sections length was small enough and the tube was rigid with negligible losses (Fig. 2).

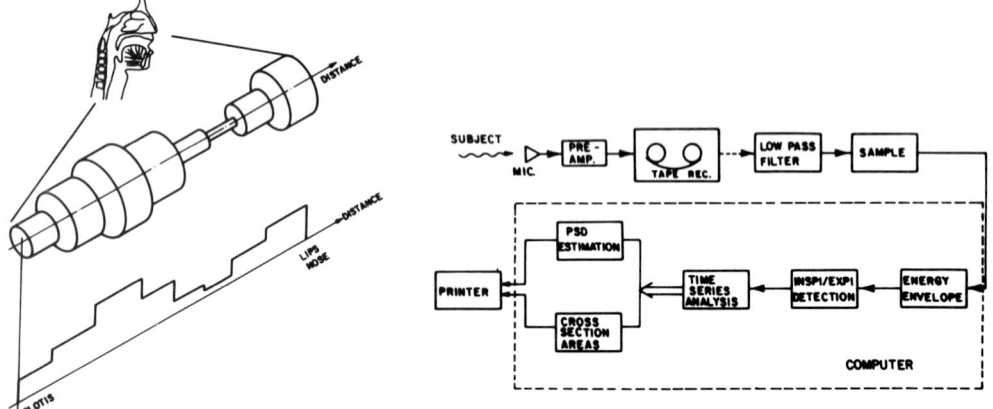

Fig. 1. Squematic diagram of the analysis system

Fig. 2. Upper airway tube model

With these assumptions, the cross sectional area can be estimated from the snoring signal. Using time series analysis methods, linear prediction parameters were estimated from the signal. With the help of these parameters the PSD function was estimated, as well as the cross sectional area (ECSA). Because the non stationarity of the signals, these were calculated every 20 milliseconds and presented in three dimensional plots. Several case studies will be presented to illustrate the different patterns according to the level of the obstruction. In all patients the snoring sound disappeared after surgery, thus we assume that the pathology removed had a cardinal role in the pathogenesis of the snoring sounds. In all cases the snoring signal was recorded and analyzed before surgery.

Case 1. A 35-year-old woman presented with a history of snoring which disturbed her husband's sleep. She also suffered from recurrent tonsillitis. During an overnight screening no signs of sleep apnea were found. A tonsillectomy was performed. The PSD function and estimated cross sectional area are shown in Fig. 3a and 3b.

Case 2. A 19-year-old soldier presented with a history of loud snoring. He had been asked by other soldiers sleeping in the same room to leave the dormitory because of his snoring. On physical examination, hypertrophy of both inferior turbinates with marked impairment of nasal breathing was found. Edema and redness of the pharyngeal mucosa associated with an elongated uvula were seen. A bilateral turbinectomy and uvulopalatopharyngoplasty (UPP) was advised, but since the patient was reluctant to submit to the UPP, only a bilateral turbinectomy was performed. One month following surgery during an overnight screening no snoring sound was heard. The PSD function and ECSA are seen in Fig. 4a and b.

Case 3. A 55-year-old male was admitted because of loud snoring. His physical examination demonstrated a long uvula and a redundant pharyngopalatine mucosa. In addition, a septal deviation with impairment of nasal breathing was seen. An overnight polysomnography showed 200 obstructive apnea episodes with an average duration of 25 sec. Under general anesthesia an UPP and a submucous nasal septoplasty were performed. Subsequently the snoring sound disappeared. The PSD function showed the sound energy concentrated in the low frequency. The ECSA showed obstruction of the airway from the nose up to the laryngeal area.

Case 4. A 56-year-old female was admitted because of loud snoring, daytime somnolence and nocturnal apneic episodes. On physical examination a redundant pharyngopalatine mucosa and an elongated uvula were found. A polysomnographic study showed 420 obstructive apnea episodes of 15-25 seconds duration. Following surgery (UPP) the snoring sounds and the daytime somnolence disappeared.
The PSD function showed the energy concentrated at the low frequency and some energy at the middle and high frequency range. The ECSA showed the airway obstructed at the level of the oropharynx at the beginning of the inspiration. Later on the airway collapsed at the supralaryngeal and laryngeal level.

Case 5. A 5-year-old boy was seen because of difficulty in breathing through the nose and loud snoring during sleep. Physical examination revealed hypertrophic adenoids. Following an adenoidectomy he was able to breathe through the nose and the snoring sounds disappeared. The PSD function showed the sound energy concentrated at the low frequency band. The ECSA showed the airway tube collapsed from the nose until approximately the supraglottic area.

DISCUSSION

The characteristics of the produced sound may be related to the level and degree of the obstruction. We have presented the preliminary study of the snoring signal and its sound analysis using computerized digital signal processing. Two main analysis methods were applied: 1) The PSD function, and 2) ESCA. The PSD figures showed a different pattern dependant on the site of the pathology, as shown in the presented cases. The level of the obstruction may be estimated from the acoustic signal. For this purpose, a model of the airway was used. Several problems arise when this model is applied to the problem at hand. The

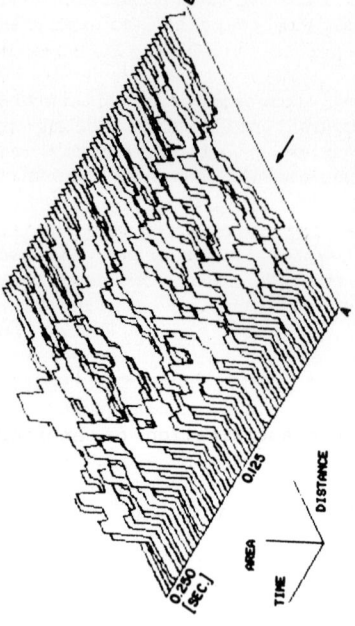

FIG. 3$_a$: PSD FUNCTION DURING INSPIRATION IN CASE 1.
THE ENERGY IS CONCENTRATED IN TWO FREQUENCY BANDS.

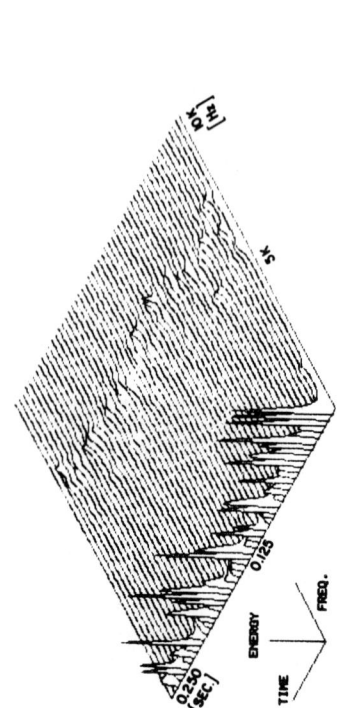

FIG. 4$_a$: PSD FUNCTION IN CASE 2 SHOWING THE SOUND
ENERGY AT A LOW MIDDLE RANGE FREQUENCY.

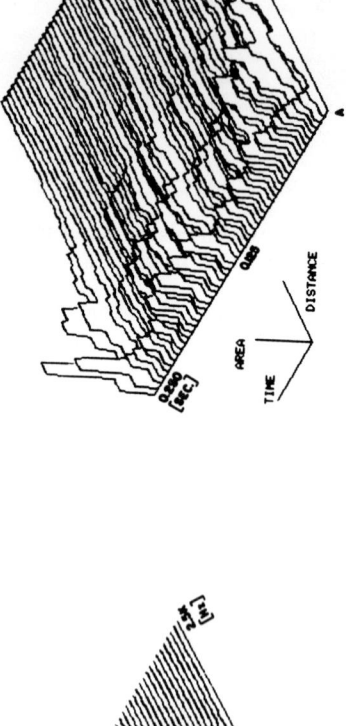

FIG. 3$_b$: ECSA IN CASE 1 IS SHOWN BY THE HEIGHT OF
THE CURVE. THE LOW CURVE SHOWS THE OBSTRUCTION AT
THE PHARYNGEAL AND SUPRALARYNGEAL AREA (ARROW).
A – SUBGLOTTIS; B – NOSE AND LIPS.

FIG. 4$_b$: THE ECSA IN CASE 2 SHOWING THE OBSTRUCTION
IN ITS UPPER PORTION (ARROW).
A – SUBGLOTTIS; B – NOSE AND LIPS.

assumptions that the airway is rigid, with no losses, are not entirely true and is one of the reasons we cannot locate the site of the obstruction very accurately. However, this simplification is successfully applied to estimate vocal tract shape in speech application (Wakita, 1973; Kuc, 1985). Further improvement of this model is needed to get better estimations of the level of obstruction. In all examples, the ECSA successfully estimates approximately the area of obstruction. Digital acoustic analysis has many advantages. The signal is easily recorded, the sound may be recorded at bedside, in the hospital or at home. It is non invasive and does not require skilled personnel. The data obtained may be stored as an objective document. As has been stressed by Moran and Orr (1985), "one of the main failures at the present time has been the inability to develop site of lesion testing as we have in the field of audiology". The data obtained from these preliminary studies showed a consistent pattern according to the site of the produced sound.

REFERENCES

Cohen, A. and Leiberman, A. (1986): Analysis and classification of snoring signals. Proc. Int. Conf. Acous. Speech and Sin. Proc. ICASSP -86, Japan.
Cohen, A. (1986): Biomedical signal processing. CRC Press Boca-Raton, Fl.
Fairbanks, D.N. (1981): Snoring: surgical vs. nonsurgical management. LARYNGOSCOPE 94, 923-924.
Fujita, S., Conwan, W., Zorick, F. et al. (1981): Surgical correction of anatomical abnormalities in obstructive sleep apnea syndrome: uvulopalatopharyngoplasty. Otolaryngol. Head Neck Surg. 89, 923-924.
Heimer, D., Scharf, S., Leiberman, A. et al. (1983): Sleep apnea syndrome treated by repair of deviated nasal septum. Chest 84, 184-185.
Moran, W.B. and Orr, W.C. (1985): Diagnosis and management of obstructive sleep apnea. Arch. Otolaryngol. 111, 650-658.
Kuc, R., Tuteur, F. and Vaisnys, R. (1985): Determining vocal tract shape by applying dynamic constraints. Proc. ICASSP-85, pp 1101-1103.
Simmonds, F.B., Gilleminault, C. and Silvestri, R. (1983): Snoring and some obstructive sleep apnea, can be cured by oropharyngeal surgery. Arch. Otolaryngol. 109: 503-507.
Wakita, H. (1973): Direct estimation of the vocal tract shape by inverse filtering of the acoustic speech waveforms. IEEE Trans ASSP-21, pp 417-427.

Résumé

La nature et les caractères du son dans le ronflement dépendent du niveau et du degré de l'obstruction. Une analyse sophistiquée des sons pourrait apprecier ces caractères. L'analyse des sons faite sur ordinateur a été effectuée par 2 principales methodes: 1) la fonction du spectre de densite qui donne la distribution de l'intensite du signal en rapport a la frequence, et le pourcentage relatif de l'intensité du signal pour chaque bande de frequences, et 2) l'estimation de la surface de coupe. La surface de coupe du signal-ronflement est définie en utilisant un model de voies respiratoires depuis la trachea jusqu'aux lèvres et nez. Il existe des modèles differents en fonction du niveau de la pathologie. l'algorithme donne de facon automatique une classification des differents types de signaux sonores. Les resultats de ces analyses chez les patients souffrant de chronic rhonchopathy y sont présentés.

Upper respiratory tract resistance and snoring in dogs

J.G. Widdicombe and A. Davies

Department of Physiology, St George's Hospital Medical School, Cranmer Terrace, London SW17 0RE, UK

ABSTRACT

We have developed a model to study snoring in supine, anaesthetised dogs (greyhounds). The trachea was cannulated both low in the neck and also 1-2 cm below the larynx, and the two cannulae were connected via a Fleisch pneumotachograph. Thus the dog breathed through the upper respiratory tract (URT). We recorded airflow, pharyngeal pressure via an oesophageal catheter, and tracheal pressure below the larynx, so that URT and oronasal resistances could be assessed from pressure/flow relationships. We also recorded the e.m.g. from genioglossus (airway dilator) muscle and the sound of snoring. In some dogs snoring was spontaneous, in others it was induced by gentle manual closing of the nares, and in others it could not be induced at all. Recording the same variables in the same dogs we measured URT resistances by passing air through the upper tracheal cannula and the URT from a gas cylinder via a rotameter while the dogs breathed through the lower tracheal cannula; flow/pressure curves were constructed. Insertion of 0.5-1 ml of Sonarex (0.2 g benzalkonium chloride, 2 g polysorbate 80, 2 g glycerol, 9 g NaCl, per litre) into the oropharynx promptly lowered URT and oropharyngeal resistances, increased genioglossus e.m.g. and decreased snoring when present. All results are statistically significant. 0.5 to 1 ml of 0.9 per cent saline had similar but smaller actions. Flow/pressure in the isolated URT measured 5-20 min before and after introduction of liquid into the oropharynx showed decreases in resistance due to Sonarex and increases in resistance due to saline. We conclude that Sonarex decreases snoring and URT resistance partly by a direct mechanical action and partly by reflex constriction of airway dilator muscles; saline has a smaller and more transient effect.

KEY WORDS

Snoring, genioglossus, dogs, oropharyngeal resistance, Sonarex.

INTRODUCTION

We have developed a model to study snoring, upper airway resistance and upper airway dilator muscle activity in anaesthetised dogs. We have used this model to test the effect of Sonarex (0.2 g benzalkonium chloride, 2 g polysorbate 80, 2 g glycerol and 9 g NaCl, per litre) introduced into the pharynx.

METHODS

Ten adult greyhounds of either sex were used, anaesthetised with intravenous pentobarbitone sodium (30 mg.kg^{-1} initially) and placed supine. The caudal cervical trachea was cannulated low in the neck, and a similar cannula was inserted cranially pointing towards the larynx (Fig. 1). The cannulae were connected to a Fleisch pneumotachograph so that the animal breathed through the pneumotachograph and the URT. A plastic catheter was inserted through the oesophagus into the oropharynx, where its tip could be observed via the mouth. Sometimes a small balloon was tied over the tip of the catheter. This catheter was used for measuring pharyngeal pressure. Tracheal pressure was measured from the upper tracheal cannula. The records of airflow and the two pressures allowed measurement of upper airways resistance either including the larynx (from the tracheal cannula) or excluding the larynx (from the pharyngeal catheter). At intervals during recording the two nares were gently closed by hand so that the dog breathed through the mouth. This method allowed assessment of upper airways resistances during spontaneous breathing through the upper airways, from the pressure/flow relationships. The results could be divided into resistances in the various components of the URT.

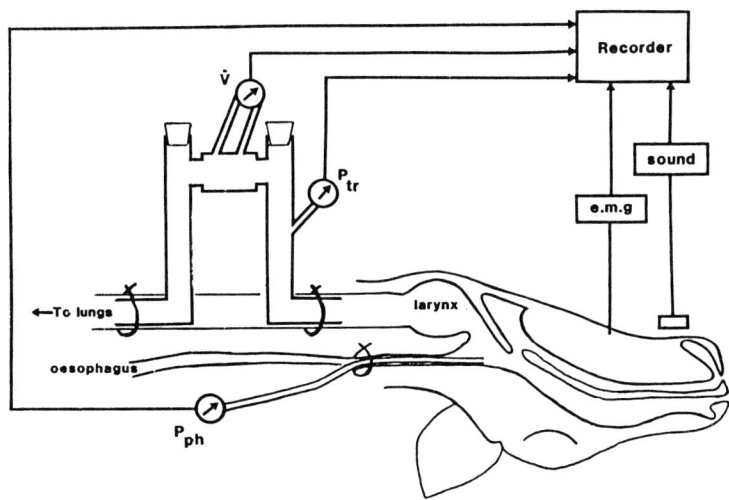

Fig. 1. Diagram of experimental arrangement

A modification of the method was to allow the dog to breathe through the lower tracheal cannula, and to have continuous airflow through the upper tracheal cannula and URT. Flow was measured with a rotameter and, by varying flow, flow/pressure curves could be constructed for the upper airways.

Additional measurements included an e.m.g. from wire-hook electrodes in the genioglossus muscle, the sound of snoring or upper respiratory airflow from a microphone taped to the neck of the dog, and systemic arterial blood pressure.

To test the effects of Sonarex the solution was injected through the catheter in the oropharynx in 0.5-1 ml volumes, during recording of respiratory variables. Controls with 0.9 per cent NaCl solution were also performed and randomised with tests of Sonarex. At least 2 h were allowed between injections of liquids.

All variables were recorded on magnetic tape and on a chart recorder. The records of genioglossus e.m.g. and snoring were later integrated using half-way rectification and a moving average integrator with a time constant usually 200 ms. Peak changes in e.m.g., sound and upper airway conductances are reported. Conductance is used rather than resistance (its reciprocal) because complete closure of the upper airways would lead to infinite resistance and this would invalidate averaging of results.

RESULTS

Administration of Sonarex into the pharynx while the dog was breathing through the URT caused a prompt increase in upper airway conductance. This varied with the respiratory phase since the upper airway dilates during inspiration because of contraction of the dilator muscles. When the nose was open resistance measured from the trachea increased conductance by $+48 \pm 18.2$ per cent in expiration, and by $+18 \pm 7.2$ per cent in inspiration ($p < 0.05$, $n = 15$). When the nose was closed corresponding increases in conductance were $+37 \pm 22.1$ and $+24 \pm 8.6$ per cent ($n = 13$). Administration of saline into the pharynx caused variable effects, although there was often an increase in upper airway conductance usually smaller than that seen with Sonarex.

Analysis of the pressure/flow curves of the upper airways show that before Sonarex the curves were remarkably alinear, presumably due to sudden changes in upper airway geometry. After Sonarex the curves were not only more smooth in appearance but also the upper airway resistance estimated from the curves was consistently reduced except at very high and very low flow rates. By contrast, when saline was administered into the oropharynx the pressure/flow curves were usually displaced upwards, i.e. indicating a higher resistance to airflow.

Analysis of the integrated e.m.g. from genioglossus muscle showed that administration of Sonarex increased the activity during inspiratory phases by $+55.2 \pm 15.4$ per cent ($p < 0.01$, $n = 14$). By contrast, saline had a far smaller effect ($+17.0 \pm 6.0$ per cent, $p < 0.05$, $n = 5$). Analysis of the integrated records of the sound of snoring showed that this was significantly reduced by Sonarex (-19.4 ± 8.0 per cent, $p < 0.05$, $n = 10$). In three experiments saline had inconsistent effects on the sound of snoring.

DISCUSSION

Our results show that both saline and Sonarex administered into the oropharynx decrease the sound of snoring and the resistances of the URT, and increase genioglossus muscle activity. However the results with saline are smaller and usually far less consistent that those with Sonarex.

By contrast, when pressure/flow curves were obtained for the URT, Sonarex consistently produced far smoother pressure/flow relationships and a decrease in upper airway resistance whereas saline, if anything, increased resistance. The difference between the results described in the previous paragraph and those here may be that the former give the immediate response to agents in the pharynx whereas the pressure/flow curves were obtained at a considerable interval (5-20 min) before and after the administration of Sonarex or saline. In other words Sonarex seems to have a maintained action in increasing upper airways conductance whereas the effect of saline is very brief.

The mode of action of Sonarex has not been established, but the fact that genioglossus usually contracted more forcibly suggests that there may be reflex activation of this muscle and stimulation by the injection of fluids into the pharynx. Another possibility is that the adhesiveness of the oropharyngeal walls may be lessened by agents such as Sonarex or saline, although this in itself should not increase genioglossus activity. Sonarex contains four constituents as well as water, and our results suggest that sodium chloride and water are not the most active of these. Which of the other three is or are the most important in this respect requires further experiments.

RESUME

Nous avons developpé une methode pour étudier le ronflement sur des chiens (levriers) anesthésiés et couchés sur les dos. La trachée a été canulée bas dans le cou et aussi 1-2 cm au-dessous du larynx, et les deux canules ont été jointes par un pneumotachographe (Fleisch). Le chien donc respirait par les aériennes supérieures. Nous avons enregistré le débit aérien, la pression pharyngienne par un cathéter oesophagien, et la pression trachéale au-dessous du larynx pour dériver les résistances des aériennes supérieures et nasobuccales des relations débit/pression. Nous avons aussi enregistré l'e.m.g. du muscle genioglossus (dilatateur des aériennes) et le son du ronflement. Quelques chiens ont présenté un ronflement spontané, des autres ont ronflé quand leurs naseaux ont été fermées gentiment avec le main, et les autres n'ont pas ronflé n importe quelle leur condition. Nous avons aussi enregistré les mêmes variables dans les mêmes chiens, et nous avons measuré les résistances des aériennes superieures et nasobuccales; nous avons introduit de l'air dans la canule trachéale craniale et l'aérienne supérieure à l'aide d'un cylindre de gaz et un rotametre, lorsque les chiens respiraient par la canule trachéale inférieure. Nous avons donc derivé les curbes débit/pression. L'injection de 0.5-1 ml de Sonarex (0.2 g benzalkonium chloride, 2 g polysorbate 80, 2 g glycerol et 9 g NaCl, per litre) dans l'oropharynx a réduit rapidement les résistances des aériennes supérieures, a augmenté l'e.m.g. du genioglossus et a réduit le ronflement quand il se presentait. Tous les résultants étaient significatifs du point de vue de la statistique. 0.5-1 ml de saline 0.9 per cent ont montré des réponses similaires mais plus petites. Les curbes débit/pression des aériennes supérieures isolées, measurées 5-20 min avant et après l'injection du liquide dans l'oropharynx, ont montré une baisse de la résistance pour l'action du Sonarex et une augmentation de la résistance pour l'action de saline. Notre conclusion est que le Sonarex baisse le ronflement et la résistance des aériennes supérieures en partie par une action méchanique et directe, et en partie par la contraction reflexe des muscles dilatateurs des aériennes supérieures. La saline a un effet moins marqué et plus transitoire.

Upper airway anatomic abnormality of chronic snorers with obstructive sleep apnea (methods of evaluation and classification)

Shiro Fujita, Eugene Potesta and Jack L Clark

Henry Ford Hospital, Detroit, Michigan, USA

Upper airway anatomic abnormality of chronic snorers with or without clinically significant obstructive sleep apnea was investigated. The methods of investigation include 1) routine otorhinolaryngological examination, 2) fiberoptic scope findings of upper airway with Mueller's maneuver and 3) dynamic cephalometric analysis. Three types are classified based on the major site of airway narrowing and the position of palatal arch relative to the tongue base. Type I represents a group whose airway narrowing involves predominantly oropharynx with a normal palatal arch position. Type II represents a group with low palatal arch position. It is divided into two subgroups, IIa and IIb, depending on the extent of airway narrowing - IIa oropharyngeal, IIb oro-hypopharyngeal. Type III includes a group in which airway narrowing involves only the hypopharynx with normal oropharynx. The presence or absence of nasal obstruction is added to this classification.

The anatomical abnormalities or variations to look for during routine ENT examination include 1) redundant oropharyngeal tissue (large edematous uvula, wide pillar mucosa or redundant lateral or posterior pharyngeal wall), 2) low palatal arch with a low-hanging soft palate, 3) relatively large tongue at the base, 4) floppy epiglottis with redundant ary-epiglottic folds, and 5) hypertrophic lingual tonsils. Since upper airway patency changes during respiratory cycles, the dynamic range of the airway must be observed during the different phases of the respiratory cycles.

This paper presents a new system for the classification of the upper airway anatomy of chronic snorers. This is based on Mueller's maneuver with fiberoptic scope as well as dynamic cephalometrics (upper airway x-rays taken in both upright and supine positions during inspiration and exhalation).

REFERENCES

1. Wilm D, Conway WA, Fujita S et al. "Anatomic abnormalities in obstructive sleep apnea". Ann Otol Rhinol Laryngol 91 (1982), 595-96.

2. Fairbanks D, Fujita S, Simmons B, and Ikematsu T. Snoring and Sleep Apnea. New York: Raven Press, 1987 (in press).

Classification of Upper Airway Anatomy (OSA)
(based on major site of airway compromise)

UPPP			MUELLER'S MANEUVER	
			(Oropharynx)	(Hypopharynx)
Type I		Oropharyngeal type	3+, 4+	0 , 1+
Type II	(a)	Low palatal arch (Predominantly orophar.)	3+, 4+	1+, 2+
	(b)	Low palatal arch (Both oro- & hypophar.)	3+, 4+	3+, 4+
Type III		Normal oropharynx Posteriorly positioned tongue base (Retrognathia, Micrognathia)	0 , 1+	3+, 4+

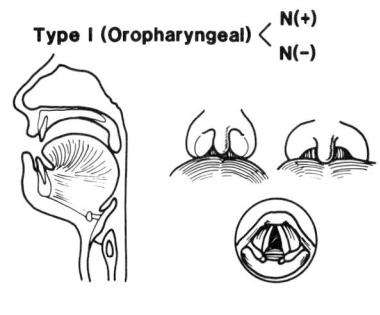

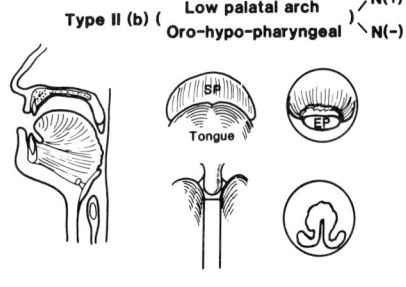

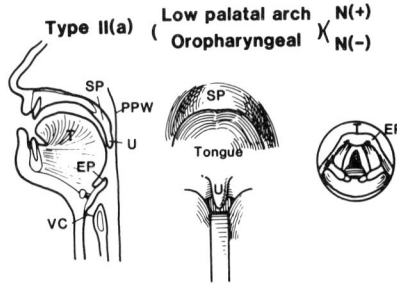

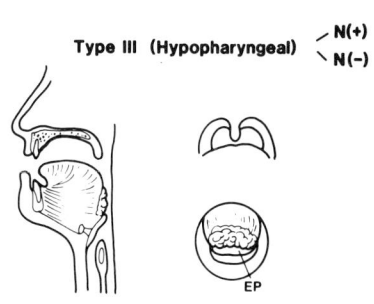

RESUME

On appelle ronflement un bruit respiratoire produit par la vibration du palais mou, causée par une turbulance aérienne provenant d'une obstruction partielle dans les voies de respiration au cours du sommeil. Le ronflement aggravé s'associe souvent aux apnées obstructives au cours du sommeil. On évalue environ 200 ronfleurs aggravés, avec ou sans syndrome d'apnée obstructive au cours du sommeil à la Clinique Oto-Rhino-Laryngologie de l'Hôpital Ford.

On a étudié l'anatomie des voies de respiration supérieures de ces patients au moyen d'examins routiniers otorhinolaryngologiques, nasopharyngolaryngoscopie fibroptique avec manoeuvre Mueller et céphalométrie dynamique (radiographies obtenues à l'inspiration et à l'expiration, debout et couché).

On discutera les méthodes d'évaluation et de classification des anomalies des voies de respiration supérieures responsables des ronflements chroniques.

Mots Clef: apnée au cours du sommeil, anatomie des voies de respiration supérieures, classification, manoeuvre de Mueller, céphalométries dynamiques.

Combined video endoscopy and frequency spectrum analysis of snoring sounds in heavy snorers. A video demonstration

J.W. Schäfer and W. Pirsig

University of Ulm, ENT-Department, 7900 Ulm, FRG

ABSTRACT

The exact identification of the obstructing site in patients with sleep apnea as well as the identification of the sound producing structures in heavy snorers is very difficult in vivo. Conventional diagnostic methods (e.g. Radiocinematography, -fluoroscopy and fiberendoscopy) are connected with the drawbacks of radiation or cannot routinely be performed during night sleep especially in children. An analysis of the frequency spectra of the snoring sounds by FFT (Fast Fourier Transform) can help to identify the anatomical structures concerned without interfering with the sleep state of the patient. Different types of obstruction are demonstrated fiberendoscopically. The frequency spectra of the voluntarily produced snoring sounds are compared to those during night sleep. Additionally a comparison between voluntary snoring and modified Müller Manoeuvre is shown, furthermore snoring in side posture and after advancement manoeuvre of the tongue and mandibula according to Esmarch

KEYWORDS

Videoendoscopy, snoring sound analysis, FFT, voluntary snoring

Methods and results of the diagnostic program developed for heavy snorers and patients with sleep apnea at the ENT-Department of the University of Ulm/FRG are shown.
This program consists of the patient's history and clinical valuation according to the questionaire of Fujita, videoendoscopy with simultaneous sound recording, apnea and sound recording during night sleep, frequency spectral analysis of the recorded snoring sounds and radiocephalometric evaluation.

Videoendoscopy with simultaneous sound recording

Endoscopy is preferably achieved with a 3.7 mm flexible nasopharyngoscope. A Karl Storz Endovision camera system is attached for recording on a U-matic or VHS video cassette recorder. A Sennheiser electret condenser microphone placed about 15 cm from the chin of the patient is used for sound recording on a HiFi video cassette recorder with a frequency response down to at least 20 Hz. During the examination the patient is in a supine position. After topical anaesthesia of the nasal mucosa the flexible endoscope is advanced along the floor of the nose to the supraglottic plane, and the patient is asked to snore and later to perfo-m the modified Müller Manoeuvre (forced inspiratory effort with the mouth and nose closed). This is repeatedly done, and the fiberscope drawn back into the epipharynx. These various steps are repeated while performing a tongue/mandibula advancement manoeuvre (we call Esmarch manoeuvre) to study the influence of this advancement on the anatomical structures in the caudal oropharynx. Finally the patient is asked to bring his head into a side position while snoring.

The video recording is reviewed at normal speed and frame by frame for exact analysis.

Sound recording during night sleep with three different methods
a. Long-term recording up to 8 hours on video tape via HiFi video cassette recorder.
b. Threshold-dependent recording: a high-sensitivity microphone is used to monitor the sound pressure level of the snoring sounds; if the sound pressure level exceeds a preset threshold an electronic circuit is triggered and the sound is recorded on one track of a high quality cassette recorder, the time of the event is encoded on the other track.
c. Apnea-detecting: the cassette tape recorder is started after the patient's breathing ceased for at least 10 seconds; the same electronic circuit as in b. is used. The circuit can be modified for recordings in children by different filters and time constans

a. and b. are used to get high-quality sound recordings for spectral analysis. b. and c. can be used for quantifying severity of disease and control of therapy.

Frequency spectral analysis of the recorded snoring sounds
The recorded snoring sounds are analyzed with a Bruel & Kjaer narrow band FFT spectral analyzer 2033 with a bandwidth of up to 20 kHz and a resolution of 2.5 Hz at 1 kHz bandwidth. The frequency spectra are stored in a Micro computer and can be displayed and plotted in a three-dimensional hidden-line presentation.

Radiocephalometric evaluation
R. is accomplished according to recommendations of Riley and Haase and gives information about the dimensions of the caudal oropharyngeal segment, and the position of hyoid and larynx in relation to the mandibula.

RESUME

Chez les patients souffrant d'un syndrome des apnées du sommeil, l'identification exacte du lieu d'obstruction est in vivo aussi difficile que l'identification, lors de ronflement marqué, des structures anatomiques causant le ronflement. Les méthodes diagnostiques conventionelles, telles que radiocinématographie,

radiofluoroscopie ou endoscopie par fibroscope sont des méthodes relativement invasives. Elles ne peuvent de plus pas être appliquées en routine durant le sommeil du patient. L'analyse spectrale des fréquences du bruit de ronflement par FFT (Fast Fourier Transform) peut permettre par contre d'identifier les structures concernées, sans influencer le sommeil du patient.
A l'aide de la fibroscopie, nous démontrons simultanément les fréquences spectrales des bruits de ronflement lors de ronflement volontaire. Nous comparons cette analyse spectrale avec celle réalisée durant le sommeil. En complément, nous comparons le ronflement volontaire avec la manoeuvre de Müller modifiée et la manoeuvre d'Esmarch.

REFERENCES

Cartwright, R.(1984): Effect of sleep position on sleep apnea severity. Sleep 7, 110-114
Haase, St.(1987): Zum Wachstum des nasomaxillären Komplexes unter Berücksichtigung kongenitaler und traumatischer Einflüsse: eine radiokephalometrische Analyse. Habilitationsschrift
Lugaresi, E.(1975): Snoring. Electroencephalogr. Clin. Neurophysiol. 39, 59-64
Fujita, S.(1986): Snoring and Sleep Apnea Screen Questionaire (personal communication)
Riley, R.W. et al (1986): Maxillary, mandibular, and hyoid advancement: An alternative to tracheotomy in obstructive sleep apnea syndrome. Otolaryngol. Head Neck Surg. 94, 584-588
Sher, A.E. et al(1985): Predictive Value of Müller Maneuver in Selection of Patients for Uvulopalatopharyngoplasty. Laryngoscope 95, 1483-1487
Sher, A.E. et al(1986): Endoscopic observations of obstructive sleep apnea in children with anomalous upper airways: predictive and therapeutic value. Int. J. Ped. Otorhinolaryng.11, 135-146

Polysomnographic study of obstructive sleep dyspnea and snoring

S. Miyazaki, K. Togawa, K. Yamakawa, Y. Itasaka and M. Okawa

Department of Otolaryngology and Neuropsychiatry, Akita University School of Medicine, 1-1-1 Hondo, Akita, 010 Japan

ABSTRACT

For precise analysis of snoring, polysomnography have been done on 50 patients (31 males and 19 females) aged 20 to 73 year-old. Subjects were divided into 4 groups according to their body weight. In the normal-weight group, snoring occurred mainly in the supine position. It was caused by obstruction of the mesopharynx due to the sinking of the pharyngopalatine arch. But the respiratory effort was slight, and sleeping often became normal. In the slight- and moderate-obesity groups, occasional obstructive apnea or hypopnea were observed. Accordingly, frequent changes in the sleep stages were observed on the EEG. Obstructive apnea could be the cause of sleep disturbance. In the marked-obesity group, especially among the cases with tonsillar hypertrophy, severe respiratory disturbance occurred. Sleep disturbance was also remarkable. In the cases with marked obesity alone, respiratory effort was not very hard. Based on these analysis, the surgical ways of treatment were employed. The therapeutic results are presented in another session of this synposium.

KEYWORDS

sleep, breathing disorder, polysomnography, pathophysiology, snoring

INTRODUCTION

The most important factor contributing to snoring, obstructive apnea, or hypopnea is the degree of cross-sectional area opening in the upper airway. Stenosis of the upper airway makes resistance in the airway storonger than normal, thereby causing the patients to exert extra-respiratory effort. For precise analysis of obstructive sleep dyspnea and snoring, such test as polysomnography, multiple sleep laency test, sleep diary and fluoroscopy of the upper airway during sleep were carried out. During the tests, the degree of respiratory disturbance as well as the the site of obstruction were studied.

SUBJECTS AND METHODS

Fifty patients (31 males and 19 females), aged 20 to 73 year-old, who complained of snoring or sleep problems were examined by polysomnography. Parameters such as EEG, EOG, ECG, intraesophageal pressure (EP), transcutaneous pO_2 & pCO_2 ($tc.pO_2$ & pCO_2), expiratory O_2 & CO_2 gas content ($exp.O_2$ & CO_2), tidal volume and respiratory rate were recorded on a data-recorder and analyzed later. Multiple sleep latency test and sleep diary were also recorded to find the daytime somnolence and sleep/wake state. In some cases, fruoroscopy of the upper airway was carried out during sleep in order to determine the site of obstruction.

RESULTS

Obstructive respiratory disturbances and obesity have been thought to be strongly related. Our 50 cases were therefore divided into 4 groups according to the degree of obesity. Eighteen cases (7 male, 11 female) were in the normal group (BWI, body weight index 90-109%), 7 (7 male) were in the slight-obesity group (110-119%), 14 (8 male, 6 female) were in the moderate-obesity group (120-129%) and 11 (9 male, 2 female) were in the marked-obesity group (130-160%).

The followings are generalization about the causes of snoring, the obstructive respiratory patterns and the type of therapy chosen for each group.

In the normal-weight group, the soft palate was abnormally formed. This, along with the unusually low position of the pharyngopalatine arch, was the main cause of the respiratory disturbance. However, this disturbance was slight, and an all-night sleep pattern was usually normal. EP which is helpful in determining the degree of respiratory effort, seldom went below $-20cmH_2O$ (normal value is between -8 and $-12cmH_2O$.). There were few changes in $tc.pO_2$ and $tc.pCO_2$. In these cases, nasal breathing was generally stable, and the degree of snoring was often low enough to be considered as nasal snoring. As a result, uvulopalatopharyngoplasty (UPPP) was recommended for 10 cases (56%). The remaining 8 cases (44%) were treated by conservative therapy (nasal neburizer, vasoconstrictor, etc).

In the slight-obesity group, EP sometimes went as low as $-30cmH_2O$. The type of respiratory disturbance was usually obstructive hypopnea. Obstructive apnea seldom appeared. Changes of $tc.pO_2$ and pCO_2 were mild. In these cases, oral breathing was sometimes unavoidable in the supine position, but nasal breathing was possible in the lateral or prone position. UPPP was recommended for 5 out of 7 cases (71%). The remaining 2 cases, who had slight respiratory effort, were therefore followed up.

In the moderate-obesity group, the majority of the respiratory disturbance was obstructive hypopnea. EP reached $-40cmH_2O$, and $tc.pO_2$ & $tc.pCO_2$ fluctuated according to changes of EP. Occasional awakenings were recorded on the EEG during sleep, but changes of sleep stages were infrequent. In this group, 4 cases (29%) had slight respiratory effort during the night. Any of these cases did not have such deformity as a low-positioned pharyngopalatine arch.

In the marked-obesity group, 3 cases (27%) had tonsillar hypertrophy, and 7 cases (64%) had a low position of the pharyngopalatine arch as a complication which reinforced the stenosis of the pharyngeal space. Chronic inflammation of the pharyngeal mucosa was observed in all cases, but the cause of which was thought to be due to prolonged oral breathing. Three cases with tonsillar hypertrophy had the largest respiratory effort in this group. EP reached $-60cmH_2O$ which was six times more than that of normal people. Obstructive apnea or hypopnea was continuously observed throughout the night. $Tc.pO_2$ variance was as great as 20mmHg. On the ECG, great changes in the R-R interval were observed. The all-night EEG showed frequent alternations of sleep and waking. This indicates difficulty obtaining deep sleep. In one case, no REM sleep was observed all night. Five cases showed the same respiratory disturbances as the cases having tonsillar hypertrophy. This was caused by a narrowing of the mesopharynx due to enlarged palatine and lingual tonsils, as well as swelling of the pharyngeal mucosa due to chronic inflammation. Respiratory disturbances were, however, less severe than that in cases having large tonsils.

Figure (a): A respiratory monitoring in a moderate-obesity case. Obstructive hypopnea and apnea were observed. However, intra-esophageal pressure (E.P.) did not go under $-20\text{cmH}_2\text{O}$.

(b): A monitoring in another moderate-obesity case. Note continuous obstructive hypopnea without obstructive apnea. E.P. went over $-40\text{cmH}_2\text{O}$.

(c): A great respiratory effort in a marked-obesity case. Obstructive apnea appeared every one minute. E.P. went over $-60\text{cmH}_2\text{O}$. He did not show any deep sleep throughout the night.

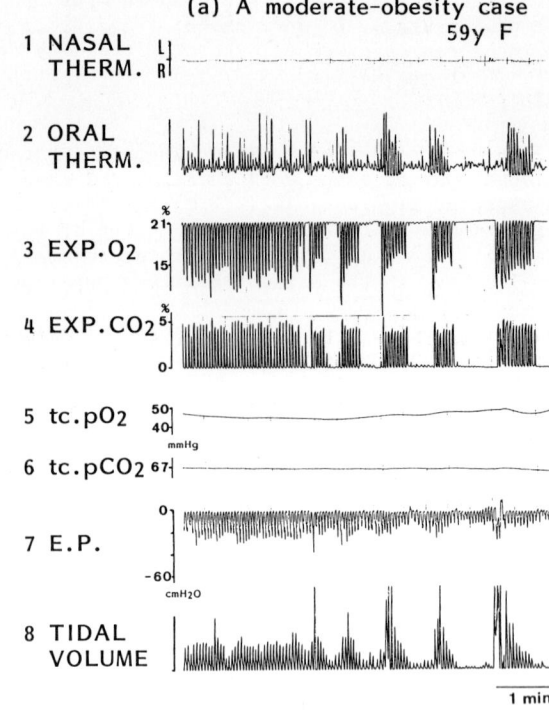

(a) A moderate-obesity case 59y F

1 NASAL THERM. L/R
2 ORAL THERM.
3 EXP.O_2
4 EXP.CO_2
5 tc.pO_2
6 tc.pCO_2
7 E.P.
8 TIDAL VOLUME

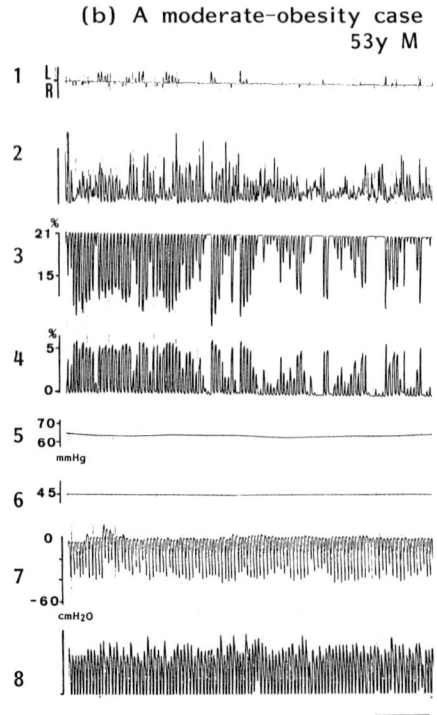

(b) A moderate-obesity case 53y M

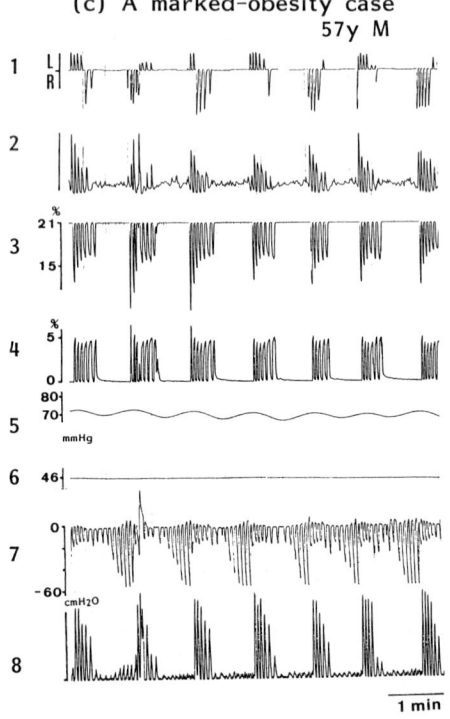

(c) A marked-obesity case 57y M

On the EEG, some cases showed frequent changes of sleep stages, but occasionally deep sleep was observed in spite of obstructive hypopnea. In 2 cases who had no low-positioned pharyngopalatine arch or no stenosis of the pharyngeal space, EP did not go below -30cmH$_2$O, and the snoring sound was mild. However, obstructive apnea appeared more than 200 times during the night. All patients in this group were advised to reduce their body weight as well as to have an operation.

Table 1. Clinical features of patients with snoring or sleep problems

Patient group in weight (BWI %)	Number of subjects (male/female)	Cause of obstruction	Respiratory effort (EP change)	Sleep disturbance	Indication of surgery
Normal weight (100-109)	18 (7/11)	L.P.A.	slight (-20cmH$_2$O)	±	Yes, if required
Slight-obesity (110-119)	7 (7/0)	L.P.A.	mild (-30cmH$_2$O)	+	Yes
Moderate-obesity (120-129)	14 (8/6)	L.P.A.	moderate (-40cmH$_2$O)	++	Yes, desirable
Marked-obesity (130-160)	11 (9/2)	L.P.A.+ T.H.	hard (-60cmH$_2$O)	+++	Yes, absolute

Abbreviation: BWI, body weight index; L.P.A., low position of pharyngopalatine; T.H., tonsillar hypertrophy; EP, intraesophageal pressure.

DISCUSSION AND CONCLUSION

Snoring is one of the signs indicating upper airway obstruction during sleep. The upper airway during sleep becomes narrower than during awake because of relaxation of pharyngeal muscles and falling back of the soft palate. When a patient has palatal tonsillar hypertrophy, a thick and long soft palate and/or uvula, we can easily conjecture that his mesopharynx will be obstructed when he sleeps in the supine position. However, in many cases with complaints about snoring and pharyngeal obstruction during sleep, it is difficult to know whether the obstruction occurs easily or not by simple usual examination. Thus, polysomnography becomes useful to diagnose the grade of sleep dyspnea. However, at present, diagnosis of obstructive apnea places emphasis on the frequency and the duration of apnea, and fails to consider the condition of obstructive hypopnea. Also, patients with snoring due to slight respiratory disturbance are usually placed outside the diagnostic standard. Furthermore, there are various degrees of respiratory effort in obstructive dyspnea. From this polysomnographic study of 50 cases, following conclusions were derived:

(1) Snoring in the normal-weight group occurred mainly in the supine position. It was caused by obstruction of the mesopharynx due to the sinking of the pharyngopalatine arch. It also occurred in women more than in men. An operation was notalways necessary, but such improvements as decreased snoring and decreased intermitent awakenings could be observed after the operation.

(2) In the slight- and moderate-obesity groups, occasional obstructive apnea was

observed. Accordingly, frequent changes of the sleep stages were observed on the EEG. Obstructive apnea could be the cause of slight sleep disturbance. After UPPP, patients who had failed to reduce their weight still had respiratory disturbances.

(3) In the marked-obesity group, especially with tonsillar hypertrophy, severe respiratory disturbance occurred. Sleep disturbance was also remarkable. Respiratory and sleep disturbances were considerably reduced by UPPP. In the cases with marked obesity alone, respiratory effort was not very hard, and improvements after operation was not so satisfactory.

RESUME

Pour l'analyse précise du ronflement, la polysomnographie, le contrôle du sommeil, les tests d'états de sommeil latent, la radioscopie des voies respiratoires supérieures ont été faits sur 50 patients (31 hommens et 19 femmes) agés de 20 à 73 ans. Les données ont été analysées en fonction de l'obésité,de l'hypertrophie amygdalaire et de l'obstruction du nez. Les sujets forment 4 groupes classés selon leur indice de poids (BWI %), normal (BWI 90-109%), léger (110-119), modéré (120-129), lourd (130-160). Dans le groupe des poids normaux, les troubles respiratoires sont bénins. Le changement de pression intra-oesophagienne (EP) reste dans les limites de $-20cmH_2O$, avec des constantes sous-cutanées pO_2 et pCO_2 (tc.pO_2, pCO_2). Les principales causes d'obstruction des voies respiratoires supérieures sont des formes insolites du palais et de l'uvule. Dans le groupe légèrement obèse la respiration fluctue légèrement. L'EP atteint $-30cmH_2O$ avec de légères variations de tc.pO_2 et de tc.pCO_2. Aucune apnée due aux obstructions n'a été observée. Dans le groupe d'obèses moyens, la respiration fluctue en fonction de l'apnée occasionnelle due aux obstructions. L'EP varie et fluctue et dépasse $-40cmH_2O$. Sur l'EEG, la réponse apparait de temps en temps durant le sommeil. Dans le groupe des individus vraiment obeses les efforts respiratoires sont remarquables durant toute la nuit, avec un EP de $-60cmH_2O$. Les intervalles R-R de l'ECG changent en fonction de l'altération de l'apnée et de l'hyperpnée. Sur la polysomnographie les états de sommeil profond apparaissent rarement et les changements d'état de sommeil sont frequents. L'influence de la dyspnée due aux obstructions se développe plus sérieusement chez les obeses avec une hypertrophie amygdalaire ou palaptosis. En se basant sur ces analyses, les traitements adéquats ont été utilisés. Les résultats sont présentés à une autre session de ce symposium.

REFERENCES

Togawa, K. (1974): Snoring -how to manage-. (Japanese) Otolaryngology (Tokyo) 46, 685-690.
Konno, A. (1980): Influence of upper airway obstruction by enlarged tonsils and adenoids upon recurrent infection of the lower airway in childhood. Laryngoscope 90, 1709-1716.
Fujita, S. (1981): Surgical correction of anatomic abnormalities in obstructive sleep apnea syndrome; uvulopalatopharyngoplasty. Otolaryngol Head Neck Surg. 89, 923-934.
Fujita, S. (1984): UPPP for sleep apnea and snoring. Ear Nose Throat Jour. 63, 227-235.
Togawa, K. (1985): Polysomnographic study of snore. Myers, E.N. Ed. New Dimension in Otorhinolaryngology -Head and Neck Surgery- Vol 2, 1112-1113.
Miyazaki, S. (1985): Influence of disordered nasal breathing on sleep in children. Myers, E.N. Ed. New Dimension in Otorhinolaryngology -Head and Neck Surgery- Vol 2 1054-1055.
Miyazaki, S. (1985): The influence of upper airway obstruction on sleep -Pathophysiology, diagnoses and treatment-. (Japanese) The Journal of Japan Rhinologic Society. 24, 302-305.

Do people know about their snoring?

M. Partinen, T. Telakivi*, M. Koshenvuo** and J. Kaprio**

*Departments of Neurology and Public Health**, University of Helsinki, SF-00290 Helsinki, and Ullanlinna Sleep Disorders Centre*, Tarkk'ampujankatu 1 E, SF-00130 Helsinki, Finland*

ABSTRACT

Sixty-two men (median age 46, range 41-50 years) were studied. All-night sleep recordings with monitoring of respiration, body movements, oxygen saturation and snoring sounds were made. There were 26 self reported habitual and 36 non-habitual or never snorers. The sensitivity of the snoring history was 63% and the specificity 80%. The positive and negative predictive values were 77% and 67%, respectively. Habitual snorers usually are true heavy snorers, but 13% of never snorers are not aware of snoring. The estimations, based on questionnaires, of the associations between snoring and disease tend to be underestimations.

KEYWORDS

Snoring, questionnaire methods, validity

INTRODUCTION

Heavy snoring is the most important symptom of obstructive sleep apnea syndrome (OSAS). Epidemiological studies (Lugaresi et al., 1980; Partinen and Palomäki, 1985; Koskenvuo et al., 1987) have indicated that habitual snoring is associated with stroke, arterial hypertension and ischemic heart disease (IHD). We studied a population-based sample of men with known self-report of snoring by doing sleep records to validate the self-reported snoring. Only men were studied because OSAS and snoring are both more prevalent among men than among women.

SUBJECTS AND METHODS

The study base consists of 4388 men of the Finnish Twin Cohort which includes all adult like-sexed twin pairs born in Finland before the year 1958. The population is representative for the adult Finnish population (Kaprio et al., 1979). 62 men aged from 41 to 50 years (median age 46, mean 45.6, SD 2.7) were selected for this study. The subjects were asked, whether they snored "always or almost always", "occasionally" or "never". There were 26 habitual snorers (snoring always or almost always) and 36 non-habitual snorers (20 occasional- and 16 never snorers).

All subjects first underwent medical examination. Subjects with chronic obstructive pulmonary disease, bronchial asthma, severe skull trauma, alcoholism and epilepsy were excluded.

A single whole-night sleep recording was made using the Static Charge Sensitive Bed (Bio-Matt) to record body- and breathing movements. The snoring sound was simultaneously registered with a special microphone suspended 50 cm above the head. The BIOX III oximeter was used to register the blood oxygen saturation from a fingertip. All signals were stored on a cassette recorder (TEAC HR-30) and analyzed by a computer method described earlier (Salmi and Leinonen, 1986; Salmi et al., 1986). A sample of the computerized graphs is shown in the figure below.

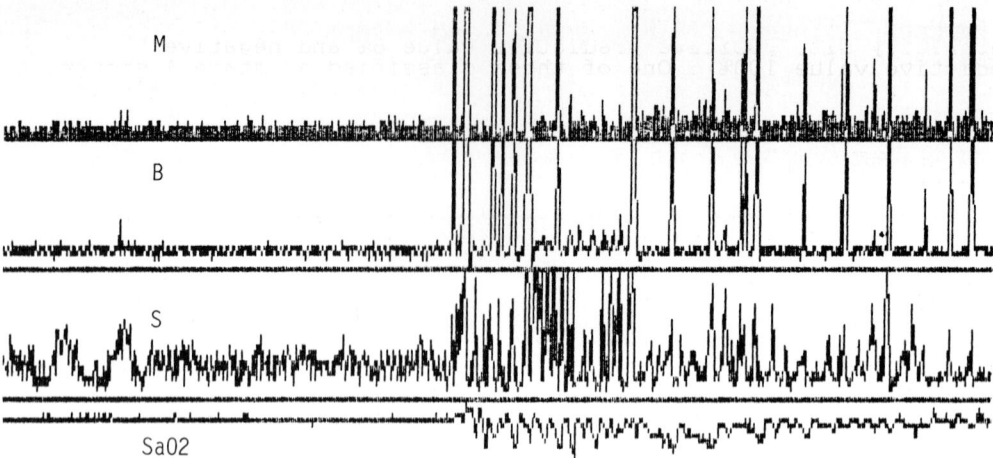

A sample of the graphic representation of a 60-minute recording of the four signals. Read from top to bottom line the graphs represent the SCSB body movement (M), SCSB breathing (B), microphone sound (S), and oximeter (SaO2, range 80-100%). For the first half an hour the subject does not move or snore. Then heavy snoring with periodic breathing, loud snoring sounds and oxygen desaturation events is seen for the remaining part of the hour.

From these graphs, three different indices were calculated manually. The periodic breathing index, PBIf is the mean number of drops to zero level per hour in the respiratory graph. Snoring index, SNI is the mean number of sound spikes per hour exceeding 50% of the graph space height. The oximetric dip index, ODI is the mean number of drops exceeding 4% calculated from the individual baseline level in the oximeter recording per hour.

RESULTS

The mean SNI of the habitual snorers (HabS) group (21.1, SD 16.9, median 14.9) was significantly higher than that (7.5, SD 6.0, median 6.1) of the non-snorers (NonS) ($p < 0.001$). The mean PBIf differed significantly ($p < 0.01$) between the HabS-group (mean 9.6, SD 9.9, median 5.4) and NonS-group (mean 3.1, SD 2.9, median 3.1). The mean ODI-value also was significantly higher in the

HabS-group (mean 5.2, SD 5.9, median 2.9) than in the NonS group (mean 1.3, SD 1.8, median 0.5; $p < 0.01$). Selecting the median (8.4) of the SNI as the limit for "objectively verified" snoring the sensitivity of the questionnaire for self-reported snoring was 63% (20/32) and the specificity 80% (24/30). The positive predictive value was 77% (20/26) and the negative predictive value was 66.7% (24/36). 2 out of 16 (12.5%) never snorers snored during the recording.

Using modified criteria of the heavy snorer's disease presented by Lugaresi et al. (1983), there were 2 subjects classified as stage 2 snorers (obstructive apneas persisting through the whole length of sleep), 13 subjects classified as stage 1 (obstructive apneas persisting during part of the sleep) and the rest of the snorers were classified as stage 0 (sporadic apneas). Both stage 2 snorers were self reported habitual snorers (sensitivity 100%, specificity 51%, positive predictive value 8% and negative predictive value 100%). One of those classified as stage 1 snorer was a self-reported never snorer, 5 were reported occasional- and 7 were reported habitual snorers.

DISCUSSION

The proportion of habitual snorers in the middle-aged Finnish male population is 9% (Koskenvuo et al., 1987). Lavie and coworkers (Lavie et al., 1983) studied industrial workers in Israel and estimated the prevalence of OSAS to be 0.89% on the basis of those results. According to our studies the estimated prevalence of OSAS among middle-aged Finnish men is from 0.4 – 1.4% (Telakivi et al., unpublished).

The validity of self-reported snoring was satisfactory. With this method, 63% of the objectively verified snorers were self reported habitual snorers (sensitivity) and 80% of the objectively verified non-snorers reported of snoring only occasionally or never (specificity).

These results indicate that the risk ratios of cardiovascular disease for snorers in previous studies (Partinen and Palomäki, 1985; Koskenvuo et al., 1987) might be underestimations. From the clinical point of view snoring history is usually reliable. In practice all patients with obstructive sleep apnea report of snoring habitually. In our study both Lugaresi stage 2 snorers also were habitual snorers. On the other hand, about 13% of adult men do not seem to be aware of their snoring. The finding that all habitual snorers did not snore during the recording is explained by our criterion of habitual snoring (i.e. subjects reportedly snore almost always or always).

As a conclusion, questionnaires may be used in epidemiological studies. Questionnaires may also be used in clinical practice when selecting patients for sleep recordings. In the latter case some snorers may escape, but there is practically no risk for clinically significant OSAS patients to escape from the recordings.

REFERENCES

Kaprio J, Koskenvuo M, Artimo M, Sarna S, Rantasalo I (1979): The Finnish Twin Registry: Baseline Characteristics. Section I. Materials, methods, representativeness and results for variables special to twin studies. Publications of the Department of Public Health Science, University of Helsinki, Finland.

Koskenvuo M, Kaprio J, Telakivi T, Partinen M., Heikkila K, Sarna S (1987). Snoring as a risk factor for ischemic heart disease and stroke. <u>Br Med J 294,</u> 16-19.

Lavie P (1983): Sleep apnea in industrial workers. In: Sleep/wake disorders: Natural history, epidemiology and long-term evolution. eds. C Guilleminault, E Lugaresi, pp 127-135. New York: Raven Press.

Lugaresi E, Cirignotta F, Coccagna G, Piana C (1980): Some epidemiological data on snoring and cardiocirculatory disturbances. Sleep 3, 221-224.

Lugaresi E, Mondini S, Zucconi M, Montagna P, Cirignotta F (1983): Staging of heavy snorer's disease. A proposal. Bull Europ Physiopath resp 19, 590-594.

Partinen M, Palomaki H (1985): Snoring and cerebral infarction. Lancet ii, 1325-1326.

Salmi T, Leinonen L (1986): Automatic analysis of Sleep Records with Static Charge Sensitive Bed. Electroenceph Clin Neurophysiol 64, 84-87.

Salmi T, Partinen M, Hyyppa M, Kronholm E (1986): Automatic analysis of static charge sensitive bed (SCSB) recordings in the evaluation of sleep-related apneas. Acta Neurol Scand 74, 360-364.

RESUME

Soixante-deux hommes de 41-50 ans (age median 46) ont eté choisis parmi 4388 hommes du Cohort Finnois de Jumeaux. Ce cohort est formé de tous les jumeaux Finnois de sex identique qui sont né avant 1958. L'histoire de ronflement a eté connu en avant. Il y'avait 26 ronfleurs habituels (toujours ou presque toujours ronfleurs) et 36 ronfleurs non-habituels (20 ronfleurs occasionels et 16 jamais ronfleurs). Les études de sommeil nocturne étaient faites avec monitoring de respiration, mouvements du corps, saturation d'oxygen, et sons du ronflement. Ainsi qui concerne le ronflement, la sensibilité de questionnaire était de 63% (20/32), et la spécificité était de 80% (24/30). La valeur prédictive du résultat positif était de 77% (20/26) et la valeur prédictive du résultat negatif était de 67% (12/36). Ainsi, les ronfleurs habituels dans la questionnaire sont, en générale, de vrais ronfleurs bruyants habituels. Mais en meme temps a peu prés 13% des jamais ronfleurs ne savent pas qu'il sont des ronfleurs. Cela veut dire que les estimations des associations entre ronflement et maladie, basées sur les questionnaires, risquent d'etre des sous-estimations.

Acknowledgements: This study was supported by grants from the Miina Sillanpää Foundation and the Council for Tobacco Research USA-Inc.

The "common" snorer in front of his doctor

F. Langraf-Favre

Steinwiesstrasse 30, CH-8032, Zurich, Switzerland

ABSTRACT

Snoring is mostly considered as a more or less inevitable and normal phenomenon and not as a disease. Now we know, that besides its social importance, it disturbs seriously the economy of respiration and the blood circulation during sleep, especially by its frequent association with periods of obstructive apnea. In this paper we try to describe the possibilities of medical and (or) surgical help, which depends exclusively on the topical origin of the snoring noise, which may be produced in one of the three levels of the upper airways.

KEY WORDS

Snoring, respiration, apnea

INTRODUCTION

When you question your patients about snoring, most of them would answer: "yes, I certainly do, not always, but quite often. Why do you ask?"

This means that snoring is accepted as a harmless and natural phenomenon, creating some trouble, specially for the partner, but without major importance.

SUBJECT

During the last 12 years these ideas have completely changed, and public opinion as much as physiologic and medical sciences are intensely involved with the multiple aspects of the snoring phenomenon and its consequences.

1. Snoring is produced by multiple and versatile factors. There is a slight difference between sexes in favour of the male, more favoured by obesity, alcohol and medication such as tranquillizers and sleeping pills.

2. Snoring is not only a highly disturbing factor concerning bedroom partners, but sometimes a <u>social disaster and a reason for divorce</u>.

3. Snoring is an <u>important hasard to health and well-being at any age.</u>

It is not only a noise problem, but it disturbs seriously and completely the mechanism and the economy of respiration with sometimes disastrous effects on the circulation, especially by the frequent associaiton between heavy snoring and periods of <u>obstructive sleep-apnea</u>. The snorer wakes up in the morning without feeling recovered, tired as before and of bad temper, sometimes with headaches. These facts have been totally confirmed by the sleep-laboratories of the Universities at Freiburg and Marburg (West Germany).

THE SUBJECT

To approach our subject we have to answer 4 questions:

1. Who snores?
2. When does snoring appear?
3. How is the noise produced?
4. Where is the noise produced?

1. <u>Who snores?</u> 45% of all individuals snore occasionally, 25% snore regularly, fat persons more than slim ones, men somewhat more than women. Alcohol and drugs contribute.

2. <u>When does snoring appear?</u> Snoring needs excessive muscular relaxation, so it appears exclusively during the third and fourth, specially when relaxation is at its maximum, during the REM phase of sleep. Here the central control of respiration is out of function and does not depend any more on the CO_2 level of blood. This is also the moment when the periods of apnea may appear.

<u>Some remarks about sleep apnea:</u> Apnea means "no respiration". So when we have to distinguish between the central apnea, a complete stop of the whole activity of respiration, and - what is our actual subject - the <u>obstructive apnea</u> during sleep, the sleep-apnea-syndrome (SAS) the differentiation is easy: during the SAS the respiratory movements of the thorax and abdomen continue, fighting against the obstacle - on the other hand no moving is visible in central apea. SAS is necessarily preceeded and followed by intense snoring; one of its severest consequences is the <u>hypersomnia during daytime</u>, not to be confounded with the similar looking, but pathogenetically completely different narcolepsy. Repeated SAS leads much more than narcolepsy totreat troubles of intelligence, feeble mindedness and character (Hess). Morning headache is quite typical for SAS. The temporary lack of oxygen proved by many recent investigations is not without disastrous effects on the central nervous and circulatory systems.

3. <u>How is the noise produced?</u> Each gas-stream which hurts an obstacle may activate the noise, which in music instruments forms a sound. The loudness of snoring may reach a heroic 80 dB, corresponding to the noise of a middle-sized truck passing in a distance of about 20 feet (Seifert, cit. by Fairbanks), Trachtman (cit by

Fairbanks) reports a case of murder of a snorer by his room-mate!

4. Where is the noise produced? Here we have to consider the three levels of the upper airways.

A. The superior level (nose and pharynx)
It is an absolute rule that in all cases of snoring the physiologic nose breathing has to be checked, and, if necessary, restored. That means that every snorer has to be examined at least once by a rhinologist. Fairbanks reports a success rate of 77% on snoring after surgical correction of disturbed nose-breathing. Nichols, in a recent study, has found a positive relation between nasal resistance and sleep apnea caused by intranasal negative pressure during inspiration. A further reason for consulting a nose-specialist: for children snoring is usually connected with adeno-tonsillar hypertrophy, and SAS is observed in a young age too (Butt). Knowing its disastrous effect on the economy of respiration we consider this an absolute indication for surgery (Grundfast). We all know the salutary effect on school performance in cases of children operated with success. Very often our patients - or their partners - report after nose-surgery, that their snoring, accepted before as something quite natural and inevitable, fortunately disappeared.

B. The inferior level: Tongue and epiglottis may produce noise when slipped backwards. This mechanism occurs principally, but not exclusively in a dorsal sleeping-position, which can easily be avoided by fixing some hard object into the back of the nightgown (walnut, golfball etc). Several devices trying to hold the mandible in the anterior position by external fixation of the chin have been proved as useless. Intraoral fixation by a device which retains the tongue in forward position has given some success, specially in cases of SAS (Cartwright). This author insists once more on the importance of an absolute free respiration at the superior level. It is obvious that such a device brings some problems of acceptance. From 25 persons who have been fitted, 4 reported not wearing it as too uncomfortable, and 16 could wear it every night or almost, except in periods of blocked nose by common cold (Cartwright, Dear). Other cases of this category have been investigated and treated by Continuous Positive Airways Pressure (CPAP) and this with appreciable success (Rühle, Peter).

C. The middle level: Soft palate and uvula are one of the most common sources of snoring noise by fluttering in the respiration air-stream as a sail in the wind. The floppy consistance of the tissues together with the extreme relaxation of the muscular tube contribute to SAS. In these cases exceptionally life-threatening (Pickwick-syndrome). Treatment here is important and promising. First of all we have to make sure, that the snoring is really caused by the fluttering velum. This can easily be demonstrated by an inspection through the half-closed mouth under good illumination. The patient is asked to snore with his tongue only slightly depressed, and the fluttering can be seen directly and confirmed by the listening partner. For more security a tape recorder could help: we use the Olympus C 910, which starts automatically recording in presence of a noise and stops in silence. The sensitivity of the sensor can be regulated between 50 and 70 dB SPL.

All devices which try to awake the snorer by an electric or mechanic stimulation have been proved inefficient, either by non-acceptance or by weakness of the stimulus.

Ikematsu was the first to publish the idea of a surgical resection of the excessive tissues, and Fujita the first to apply this technique to treat SAS. The operation, called uvulo-palato-pharyngo-plasty (UPPP), was then extended to the treatment of heavy snoring (Simmons, Pieyre). As the UPPP is a major operation with all its risks, we believe that a snorer, even with many problems, would be hard to convince if there is another solution possible. Simmons reports 4 cases with "some regurgitation, which shall be permanent after six months". In private practice a single case of this complication would be already too much! For all these reasons we believe that this kind of surgery should be reserved for the very serious cases of SAS, eventually after CPAP. To help the "common" snorer with a floppy palate we were looking out for a simpler and safer method to reach the same target ie to stiffen the floppy tissues without sacrificing mucous membranes (except some partial shortening of a really long uvula). So we came to the idea to create a submucous scar by first injecting some vein-sclerosing agent (we now use Aethoxysclerol Kreussler, first at 2%, later at 4%). The first injection - only a drop and strictly submucously is a test for tolerance. In fact, we had two cases of allergy with excessive swelling and difficulty with talking and swallowing for 3 days, followed by a complete recovery. Usually these injections do not produce more inconvenience than a slight sensation of foreign body for one or two days. After the first injection we start the real treatment with a couple of injections laterally at half distance between the midline and lateral wall, using 0,2 to 0,4 ml each time and repeating the treatment with intervals of 1-3 weeks, five to six times altogether. Sometimes a superficial necrosis appears, which heals after some days and favours the desired shrinking. The success can be estimated after several weeks only. In our cases (approx 40) we had a success rate of about 50%, where snoring was seriously reduced or eliminated. We hope that with more experience the success rate will improve.

The pharmaceutical treatment of heavy snoring is necessarily considered as a measure of only temporary value, destined to offer some help in special situations. Hess recommends the group of tricyclic antidepressants as Clomipramin and in cases of important SAS retarding Theophyllin has proved helpful.

CONCLUSION

Heavy snoring can be treated and should be treated with view to any risks which might be incurred.

RESUME

1. 45% de nos concitoyens ronflent, dont la moitié réguilièrement (les femmes moins).
2. Le ronflement nuit non seulement aux relations de la chambre à coucher, et surtout à la qualité réparatrice du sommeil du ronfleur et de sa (son) partenaire.
3. Le ronflement souvent considéré comme un signe normal d'un sommeil "du juste" n'est souvent pas mentionné lors de l'énumération des

des pliantes.
4. Il appartient donc au médecin de poser la question particulièrement aux patients, qui se plaignent de fatigue avec hypersomnie diurne, aux obèses, aux hypertendus, aux asthmatiques et aux dépressifs.
5. Chaque approche thérapeutique dépend essentiellement d'un <u>diagnostic de localisation</u>, il faut connaître le lieu de l'obstacle qui fait produire au courant aérien le bruit typique. Cet obstacle peut se trouver au niveau de l'un des trois étages des voies respiratoires supérieures: nez et épipharynx, méso-ou oropharynx et hypopharynx avec la base de la langue et l'épiglotte.
6. Le syndrome de l'apnée obstructive accompagne souvent le ronflement et demande un traitement plus ou moins urgent.
7. Le traitement rationnel doit s'orienter du résultat de l'enquête topographique, sans oublier les trois grands facteurs prédisposants, à savoir l'obésité, l'alcool et les somnifères.
8. Les différentes possibilités thérapeutiques sont discutées.

REFERENCES

Bajog M. Medical Tribune 22a,34,1982, Schnarchen
Bailey B. Problematic Snoring, Arch. Otolaryngol. 11o, Aug. 1984
Butt W. Med. J. of Australia, 143, (1985) 33-336
Cartwright R.D. JAMA, 284.705-709, 1982
Cartwright R.S. Arch. Otolaryngol. 111.1985,385
Conway D. Chest, 1985, 88,385 one year follow-up
Cotton R.J. Arch. Otolaryngol. 109.502,183, Uvulopharyngopalatoplasty
Daynal V.S. Nasal Surgery in the Management of Sleep-Apnea, Arch. Otolaryngol 94,1985.550
Dear S.E. Oral Surg. 198o, Sleep-Apnea 534-549
Fairbanks D.N.F. 77th Annual Assembly of Otolaryngol Southern Medical Association, Nov. 1983, Ehe Effect of Nasal Surgery on Snoring
Fujita S. Otolaryngol. Head- and Neck Surg. 89,923,1981 Surgical Corrections of Anatomic Anomalities.
Grundfast K.M. Laryngoscope, 92,65o,1982 Adeno-Tonsillars-Hypertrophy and upper Airways Obstruction.
Guilleminault C. Sleep Apnea Syndromes, Kroc. Foundation Series Vol. 11 Alan R . Liss, New-York 1978
Hess C. Der informierte Arzt, Das Schlaf Apnoe Sendrom, 13,1985,36-44
Ikematsu T.J. Jap. Otolaryngol. 1964, 64,434-435, Study of Snoring
Katsatonis G.P. Respiratory News (Syntex) 6, 3, 1983
Langraf F. Medical Tribune ,32,2,1982 Schnarchbehandlung
Langraf F. Medical Tribune 22a, 34,1982, Gaumensegel und Schnarchen
Langraf F. Ars Medici 7-8, 1983, 338-34o Vom ehezerstörerischen und sauerstoffraubenden Schnarchen.
Lugaresi Neurophysiol. 39,1975, 39-54
Myers N. Internat. Congress Series 68o, Excerpta Medica 1986, 1993-202
Nicolas Am. Rev. Resp. Dis. 126,625-628, 1982 Obstructive Apneas in Seasonal allergic Rhinitis
Orr W.C. Arch.int. Med. 141, 1981 Obstructive Sleep Apnea associated with Tonsillar Hypertrophy in Adults.
Peter J.H. :ed. Trib. 22, 6, 1987
Pieyre J.M. Méd. et Hyg. 41,1983, 3752.3754, le ronflement
Pieyre J.M. Méd. et Hyg. 1984, 42, 769-77o le traitement du reonflement.
Seifert C.M. Southern Med. J. 73, 1035, 1980, Snoring
Willms D, Anatomic Anomalies in obstructive Sleep-Apnea
Zwillich C.M. Arch. Int. Med. 1939, 24,1970, The clinical Significance of Snoring

IV CHRONIC RHONCHOPATHY AND NEUROLOGICAL DISEASES

Chairman: H.P. Cathala

Snoring and occurrence of brain infarction

H. Palomäki, M. Partinen, S. Juvela and M. Kaste

Department of Neurology, University of Helsinki, Haartmaninkatu 4, SF-00290 Helsinki 29, Finland

ABSTRACT

Habitual snoring has been associated with brain infarction. This study included 177 consecutive men (age 16-60 years) admitted to Meilahti University Central Hospital because of brain infarction. For each of them age-matched control was selected. Patients, relatives and controls were interviewed for sleeping habits, snoring, apneas and timing of infarction.
There were together 171 pairs with known history of sleeping habits. Of the brain infarct patients 90 (52.6%) and of the controls 47 (27.5%) snored habitually or often. The risk ratio from the matched series for brain infarction between those who snored and those who did not was 4.1 (95% confidence limits 2.4 - 7.1), McNemar x^2 = 26.0, p<0.0001. Of 166 patients with brain infarction both the snoring history and the exact time of infarction were known. 59 (35.5%) had a nocturnal infarction. Of them 40 (67.8%) snored habitually or often. Of the other patients 48 (44.8%) were snorers. The risk ratio for a nocturnal brain infarction of snoring was 2.6 (95% confidence limits 1.3 - 5.0), x^2 = 8.0, p<0.001.

KEYWORDS

Snoring, sleep apnea, nocturnal brain infarction

INTRODUCTION

There is an accumulating evidence of the interrelationsship between cardiovascular disease and the history of snoring and sleep apnea (Koskenvuo et al., 1985, 1986, Partinen and Palomäki, 1985). Obstructive sleep apnea has many harmful effects on cardiovascular system. Heavy snoring is nearly always present in obstructive sleep apnea syndrome. Habitual snoring has been associated with arterial hypertension and angina pectoris. Snoring has also claimed to be a risk factor for brain infarction. In this age-matched case-control study we have studied if there is any connection between an ischemic brain infarction and the history of snoring and sleep apnea. We also report preliminary results of the diurnal variation of brain infarction related to snoring.

SUBJECTS AND METHODS

We studied 177 consecutive male patients who were admitted to Meilahti Hospital in Helsinki because of brain infarction. The age range of the patients was 16-60 years. Of them, 128 were in the age group of 45-60 years and 49 in the group under 45 years.
177 consecutive male patients admitted with other disease than brain infarction matched by age (+- 6 years) were also selected.
All patients and controls were interviewed by using a standard questionnaire about their sleeping habits and especially about snoring (always or almost always, often, occasionally or never), about possible respiratory pauses when sleeping and about the onset of the symptoms of brain infarction. Snorers were defined as those who snored always or often and habitual snorers those who snoredd always or almost always.
The brain infarct was called nocturnal if it appeared clearly during sleep and the patient noticed it immediately on waking.
Six patients with brain infarction and one of the controls did not know if they snored and the confirmation from a relative was not available. They were deleted from further analyses.

RESULTS

There was no significant difference in the age distribution between the brain infarct group (mean 49.2, SD 9.3, range 16-60, median 52 years) and the control group (mean 48.9, SD 9.8, range 17-65, median 50 years). The mean body mass index of the brain infarct group (26.2, SD 4.1 median 25.7kg/m^2) and that of the control group (25.5, SD 3.9 median 25.1 kg/m^2) did not differ significantly.
63 of the patients with infarction and 38 of the controls had arterial hypertension ($p<0.005$). 51 of the brain infarct patients and 24 of the controls had an ischemic heart disease ($p<0.001$).
There was no significant difference between the groups in the frequency or quantity of alcohol use.
Of the 177 patients and controls we found 171 pairs with known history of sleeping habits. Of the brain infarct patients 90 (52.6%) and of their age-matched controls 47 (27.5%) snored habitually or often. The risk ratio from the matched series for brain infarction between those who snored and those who did not not was 4.1 (95% confidence limits 2.4 - 7.1), McNemar x^2 = 26.0, $p<0.0001$.
Of 166 patients with brain infarction both the snoring history and the exact onset of infarction were known. 59(35.5%) had a nocturnal infarction. Of them 40 (67.8%) snored habitually or often, and the respective number of the other patients was 48 (44.8%)(risk ratio 2.6, 95% confidence limits 1.3 - 5.0, x^2 = 8.0, $p<0.001$).
The association of snoring with nocturnal brain infarction was stronger among the age group 45-60 years (risk ratio 2.9, $p<0.01$) than among the age group 16-44 years (risk ratio 1.5, ns).

Forty (23.4%) of the 171 brain infarct patients with known history of snoring were suspected of having obstructive sleep apnea syndrome (OSAS) because in addition to snoring they also reported to have respiratory pauses when sleeping.
Of the control patients, 13/176 (7.4%) were suspected of having OSAS (RR 3.8, 95% confidence limits 2.0 - 7.2, X^2 = 17.2, p<0.0001.

DISCUSSION

This study confirms our earlier findings that snoring habitually or often is associated with brain infarction. Obstructive sleep apnea is associated with periodic hypoxemia during sleep. Marked hemodynamic changes have also been reported to occur during obstructive apneic periods. Among these are cardiac arrhythmias (Motta and Guilleminault, 1985), decreased cardiac index (Guilleminault et al., 1986) and hypotension (Podszus et al., 1986). These, in turn, can have harmful effects on local cerebral metabolism, being a possible co-factor of nocturnal infarctions. Also alcohol ingestion can have some role behind the association of snoring and nocturnal infarctions by precipitating apneic periods among those who snore habitually or often. Alcohol is reported to be a risk factor for brain infarction (Hillbom and Kaste, 1981, Gill et al., 1986).
In this study snoring is associated especially strongly with nocturnal brain infarction. This is in accordance with earlier suggestions that the association could be explained by the higher frequency of obstructive sleep apnea syndrome among the snorers than among those who report to snore occasionally or never.

REFERENCES

Gill, J.S., Zezulka, A.V., Shipley, M.J., Gill, S.K., Beevers, G. (1986): Stroke and alcohol consumption. The New England Journal of Medicine, 315, 1041-1046.
Guilleminault, C., Motta, J., Mihm, F., Melvin, K. (1986): Obstructive sleep apnea and cardiac index. Chest, 89, 331-334.
Hillbom, M., Kaste, M. (1981): Ethanol intoxication: A risk factor for ischemic brain infarction in adolescents and young adults. Stroke, 12, 422-425.
Koskenvuo, M., Kaprio, J., Partinen, M., Langinvainio, H., Sarna, S., Heikkilä, K. (1985): Snoring as a risk factor for hypertension and angina pectoris. Lancet, i, 893-895.
Koskenvuo, M., Kaprio, J., Telakivi, T., Partinen, M., Heikkilä, K., Sarna, S., (1986): Snoring as a risk factor for ischaemic heart disease and stroke in men. British Medical Journal, 294, 16-19.
Motta, J., Guilleminault, C., (1985): Cardiac dysfunction during sleep. Ann. Clin. Res., 17, 190-198.
Partinen, M., Palomäki, H. (1985): Snoring and cerebral infarction. Lancet, ii, 1325-1326.
Podszus, T., Köhler, U., Mayer, J., Penzel, T., Peter, JH., von Wichert, P. (1986): Systemic arterial blood pressure decreases during obstructive sleep apnea. Sleep res., 15, 155.

RESUME

Roflement habituel est associé avec l'infarctus du cerveau. 177 hommes consecutifs admis dans l'hopital universitaire de Helsinki ont participé dans notre étude. L'age median était de 52 ans (16-60 ans). Un sujet de control de même age (+- 6 ans) sans infarctus du cerveau était choisi pour chacun. L'age median des controls était de 50 ans (17-65 ans). Les malades eux memes, leur relatifs et les controls ont donné leur histoire de ronflement, habitudes de sommeil, apnées du sommeil et le moment de debut de l'infarctus du cerveau.

Il y'vait 171 paires avec l'histoire du sommeil complete. 90 sujets avec l'infarctus (52.6%) et 47 controls (27.5%) ont repondu qu'ils sont des ronfleurs (toujours ou presque toujours ou souvent ronfleurs). Le Risque relatif pour l'infarctus du cerveu entre les ronfleurs et non-ronfleurs était de 4.1 (intervalle de confiance à 95% 2.4 - 7.1, McNemar x^2 = 26.0, p<0.0001).

Dans 166 cas malades avec l'infarctus du cerveau le timing de l'infarctus a éte connu exactement. 59 (35.5%) ont subi un infarctus nocturne. 40 sur 59 (67.8%) ont ronflé habituellement ou souvent. Le Risque relatif pour l'infarctus du cerveau nocturne entre les ronfleurs et non-ronfleurs était de 2.6 (95% IC 1.3 - 5.0, x^2 = 8.0, p<0.001). En somme l'histoire de ronflement est associé avec l'infarctus du cerveau. Il parait aussi, que le risque est particulierment elevé pour l'infarctus nocturne.

Snoring as a risk factor for nocturnal sudden death in spinocerebellar degeneration

Soichi Katayama, Yoshiro Hirano, Seishi Yokoyama, Seiichi Tada and Mari Katayama

Department of Neurology, Dokkyo University School of Medicine, Tochigi 321-02, Japan

ABSTRACT

Spinocerebellar degeneration (SCD) is frequently associated with nocturnal sudden death (NSD) and polysomnographic examinations revealed a significant increase in the variability of respiratory cycles which might be linked with cessation of respiration during nocturnal sleep.

In our series of 40 SCD patients, habitual snoring was observed in 8 out of 9 patients of OPCA group with brainstem dysfunction and in 2 of 31 COA cases with localized lesions in the cerebellum. Six patients among these 10 heavy snorers were cases of nocturnal sudden death. Case records showed loud snoring was only exceptionally observed in other SCD patients. Furthermore, we were able to obtain polysomnograms during the entire course of NSD in a loud snorer with OPCA and catastrophic situations were incidentally recorded during these examinations, and they disclosed that cessation of respiration had preceded cardiac arrest by several minutes.

In the light of our findings, it might be speculated that heavy snoring is to be considered a risk factor for nocturnal sudden death in SCD, when it is associated with instability of generation of respiratory rhythm.

KEYWORDS

Nocturnal sudden death, olivo-ponto-cerebellar atrophy, snoring, spinocerebellar degeneration,

INTRODUCTION

Our previous studies (Katayama et al.,1986) indicated that spinocerebellar degeneration (SCD) is frequently associated with nocturnal sudden death (NSD) and polysomnography (PSG) has revealed a significant increase in the variability of respiratory cycles during sleep and it was suggested that disturbed generation of rhythmicity in the brainstem respiratory center might cause cessation of respiration in patients with NSD.

The present study seeks to determine the incidence of habitual snoring and elucidate the contribution of partial airway obstruction to NSD in these cases.

SUBJECTS AND METHODS

The subjects for this study were 40 SCD patients from whom polysomnograms were obtained. A total of 31 patients were grouped under COA (cerebello-olivary atrophy) with localized lesions of the cerebellum and their average age of onset was 41.0 years with an average duration of illness of 7.6 years. The OPCA (olivo-ponto-cerebellar atrophy) group included 4 Shy-Drager syndrome (SDS) and 5 with olivo-ponto-cerebellar atrophy, whose average age of onset was 54.6 years with an average duration of illness of 3.8 years. Lesions of both brainstem and cerebellum were involved in the latter group.

Polysomnography was performed in these patients and vibration produced by snoring was recorded on the cricothyroid notch using accelerometer in the patients.

RESULTS

Of the 40 SCD patients we studied, ten died. Six of them were cases of NSD. These six patients consisted of 2 of COA and 4 of OPCA groups. Tab. 1 summarizes the diagnosis, history and symptoms of the cases of NSD. Loud snoring was observed in all of these 6 cases of NSD.

Tab. 1 CASES OF NOCTURNAL SUDDEN DEATH IN SCD

No.	Name	Age (yrs)	Sex	Diagnosis	Duration of illness	Cerebellar signs	Extra-pyram- signs	Bulbar signs	Sleep apnea	Heavy snoring
1	T.K.	48	M	OPCA	1.7 yrs	+	+	+	−	+
2	I.N.	54	F	OPCA	4	+	+	+	−	+
3	S.H.	50	F	LCCA	7	+	−	+	−	+
4	B.T.	61	M	LCCA	8	+	−	+	−	+
5	H.N.	53	F	SDS	2	+	+	+	−	+
6	S.M.	71	F	SDS	3.4	−	+	+	+	+

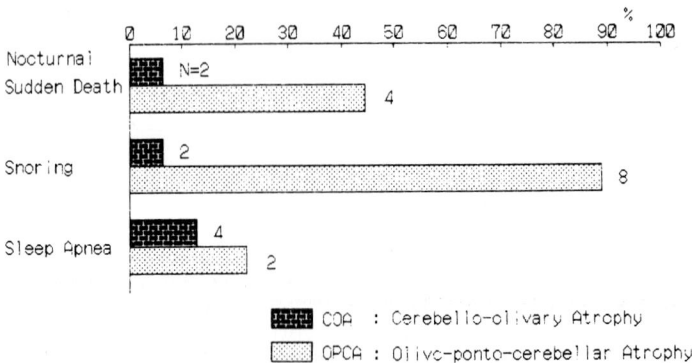

Fig. 1 Incidence of nocturnal sudden death, snoring and sleep apnea in 31 cases with COA and 9 with OPCA

Our case records revealed that habitual snoring was observed exclusively in OPCA group (Fig.1) and two other heavy snorer with COA subsequently became the victims of NSD. There were only 6 cases of sleep apnea among a total of 40 patients with SCD, and the incidence of sleep apnea was not as high as commonly reported.

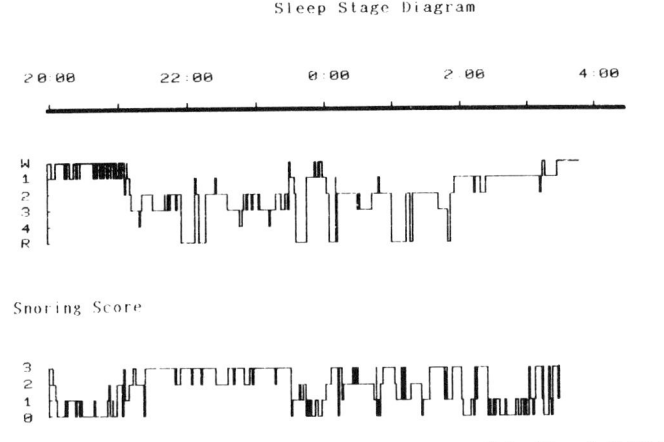

Snoring was usually audible throughout the nocturnal sleep in the patients of NSD,but it was sleep stage dependent. Fig 2 shows correlation between sleep stages and snoring scores. Snoring scores were low in NREM light sleep stages, and increased in NREM deep sleep, remaining high in REM sleep.

Fig. 2 Snoring scores and sleep stages

Fig. 3 demonstrates relationship of snoring to changes in sleep EEG and respiratory pattern.   In the compressed polysomnographic recordings, the upper panel is a power spectral array (PSA) of EEG and the lower two panels indicate respiration and sonogram. Fig. A in the central panel was obtained during the transitional period from drowsy state to deep NREM sleep, which is indicated in the PSA, and Fig. B clearly denotes the periodic occurrence of snoring, which becomes intermittent because of intervening clusters of apneas.

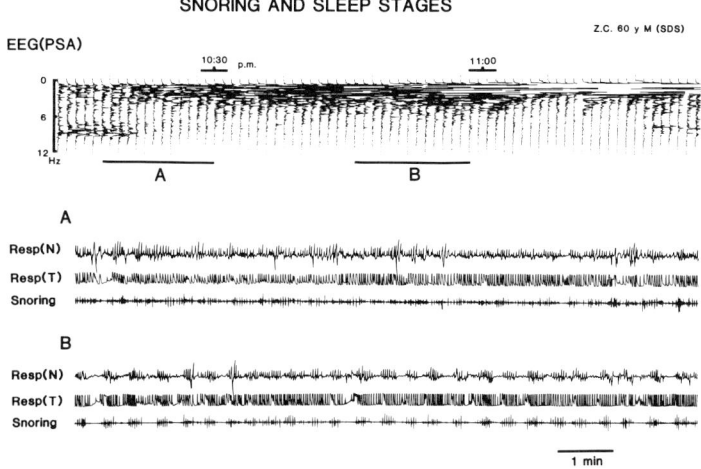

Fig. 3 Correlation between snoring and changes in sleep EEG and respiratory pattern.

111

We were able to obtain polysomnograms recorded during the entire course of nocturnal sudden death in a case with OPCA. The patient was 48 year-old heavy snorer and complained of ataxic gait and dysarthria. Fig. 4 is a polysomnographic recordings of this case. EEG showed slow alpha wave pattern of about 8 Hz. The eye movements persisted and the patient snored profoundly. Fig. A shows irregular periods of respiratory curves during sleep. In Fig.B, rapid eye movements were accompanied by ataxic respiration, and hiccup-like respiration irregularly occurred as seen in Fig. C.

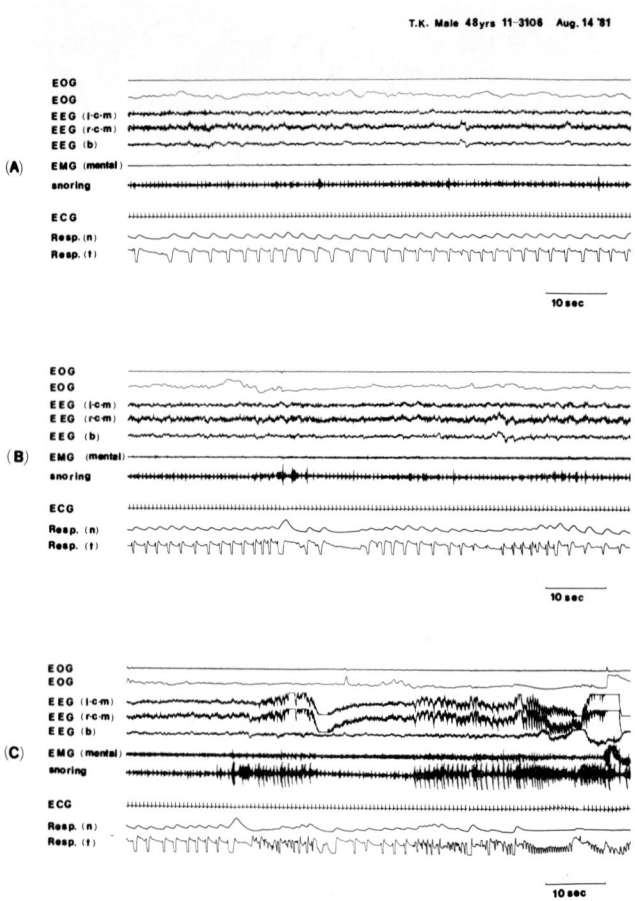

Fig. 4 Polysomnographic records of a case of OPCA who suffered nocturnal sudden death.

The polysomnogram in Fig. 5 were incidentally recorded in the terminal periods in this case. Prominent tachypnea replaced ataxic respiration 3 hours prior to death, leading to the respiratory arrest, which was followed by cessation of heart beat. The autopsy findings revealed depigmentation of the locus coeruleus in the pons, which is believed to be involved in the regulatory mechanism of respiration.

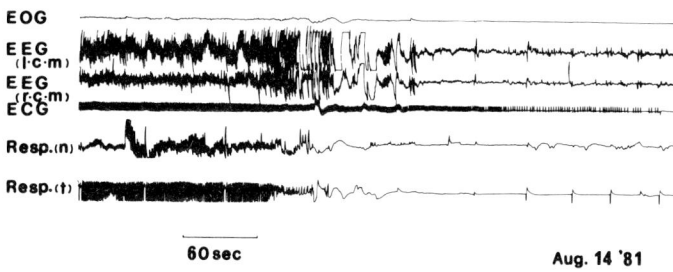

Fig. 5 Polysomnographic records of the same patient at the time of respiratory arrest.

DISCUSSION

Respiratory and circulatory disturbances could be the main causes leading to nocturnal sudden death. Polysomnographic data analysis in SCD patients previously revealed that respiratory instability represents a continuum of cessation of respiration during sleep, which we have demonstrated in a case of NSD.

In this study, we found that 10 out of 40 SCD patients were observed to snore loudly and 6 of them were cases of NSD. The prevalence of snoring was evidently higher in OPCA group, in which brainstem lesions are involved. Snoring is the most obvious sign indicating an obstruction of the upper airway, and appears related to bulbar palsy which was found in all patients of NSD.

In conclusion, we might speculate that snoring is to be considered a risk factor for NSD, when it is associated with instability of respiratory rhythm. We suppose that brainstem dysfunction in SCD might play some role in causing hypotonia in the oropharyngeal muscles which induces snoring.

REFERENCE

Katayama,S., Yokoyama,S., Hirano,Y., Kashima,T and Hirata,K (1986):TRH and sleep abnormalities in SCD. In TRH and Spinocerebellar Degeneration, ed I. Sobue, pp 221-36. Amsterdam: Elsevier Science Publisher BV.

Brainstem dysfunction in sleep apneics as assessed by electrophysiological methods

R.M. Koutlidis*, B. Fleury**, M.C.L. Rousseau* and F. Chabolle***

*Laboratoire d'Explorations Fonctionnelles du Système Nerveux
**Service de Pneumoiogie
***Service d'Oto-rhino-laryngologie, Hôpital Saint-Antoine, 75012 Paris, France

Most of the recent electrophysiological studies dealing with sleep apnea syndrome (SAS) were devoted to define a brainstem lesion or dysfunction, possibly underlying this syndrome. Actually, central structures controlling respiratory rythms are located within the reticular formation of the brainstem (1). The function auditory and trigeminal systems of the brainstem can be tested by electrophysiological methods : brainstem auditory evoked potentials (BAEPs) and blink reflex (BR). A high correlation with anatomical lesions has extensively been demonstrated (2, 3).

However, the results obtained in SAS patients remain controversial.

In a study of 30 patients, Stockard and al.(3) showed that only 2, with central apnea, had abnormal BAEPs, related to intrinsic brainstem tumors : in these cases, SAS was the first or the major manifestation. The other central and obstructive SAS of the latter series, and those of Karnaze and al. (4), Peled and al. (5) had normal BAEPs. In another study (6), the latency of the Vth wave of BAEPs was demonstrated to be statistically delayed in central SAS.

On the other hand, during the drastic decrease of the arterial oxygen saturation which accompanies apneic sleep, there is no significant modifications of BAEPs (7).

In conclusion to these previous studies, the lesion underlying is not yet determined in most of the patients. Furthermore, it is not proved that the incidence of brainstem dysfunction is increased in these patients.

In studying adults snorers suspected of SAS, our purpose was to show a dysfunction of the brainstem at the central (or the peripheral) level.

Actually, we found several abnormalities of BAEPs and BR. Correlation with clinical data was made in an attempt to determine weither or not the observed abnormalities were responsible for SAS.

POPULATION :

Fifty patients were chosen among a snoring population for (I) an excessive daytime sleepiness (II), the absence of well-known uni-or bi-lateral hypoacousia

(III), the absence of other neurological symptom (IV), the absence of any associated pathology known to alter BAEPs (alcoholism, diabetes).

They were first referred to the sleep-EEG laboratory*. SAS was defined as "more than 10 apneas per hour, each one lasting more than 10 seconds". Oxygen saturation during sleep was measured.

The SAS group was composed of 5 patients with predominently central apneas, 16 with predominently obstructive apneas and 9 with pure obstruction apneas. These 30 patients (SAS group) were (mean ± SD) 51.9 ± 9.0 year old (range : 32-71 years) and 90 % were men. The 20 other patients (S group) were 50.9 ± 9.7 year old (range : 32-63 years) and 75 % were men. They were compared to a control group (C group) of 10 healthy, non-snorer subjects (47.4 ± 16.5 year old ; range 31-81 years ; 60 % were men), chosen with the same 5 criteria as the patient groups.

METHODS :

BR and BAEP were performed in the same session in all the subjects (S, SAS and C groups). The latency of the first response of ipsilateral BR was measured. BAEPs were recorded after the measurement of the subjective auditory threshold. The stimulus intensity was adjusted to 70 dB supraliminarly. Auditory threshold, absolute latencies of waves I, III, V, and I-III, III-V interwaves latencies (IL) were calculated. The individual results were compared to the normative data of the laboratory : this confirmed the reliability of our control group (normative values ± 2 SD).

First, statistical analysis by the Student-Fisher t-test compared the results of the 2 patient groups with the control group.

A quotation (0, 1, 2) was established in order to compare clinical and electrophysiological results, as explained in the following tables (A, B).

Clinical data :

	age years	Height-weight index (Wkg-Hcm+200)	Subjective Auditory Thres. dB	Snoring since years	Snoring worsen months	Arterial blood press. cm Hg
mean±SD	45.4±16.5	98.6±8	8.4±3.1	0	0	< 16/9
quotation 0 1 2	45 60	+2SD +3SD	+2SD +3SD	5 15	6 12	16/9 18/11

table A

* Dr. Laffont, Hôpital de la Salpétrière, 75013 Paris.

Electrophysiological data :

	SLEEPING E E G		B A E P			BLINK REFLEX	
	Apnea index N/h	Desaturation index % *	I latency ms	I-III lat ms	III-V lat ms	R1 lat ms	R2 lat ms
mean±SD	0	0	1.68±.13	2.07±.18	1.88±.17	10.2±.6	31.5±2.35
quotation 0 1 2	10 50	10 30	+2SD +3SD	+2SD +3SD	+2SD +3SD	+2SD +3SD	+3SD -

* (O_2 saturation during weakefullness) - (O_2 saturation during sleep)

table B

A statistical multivariate factors analysis was performed for the 60 subjects.

RESULTS :

Clinical and electrophysiological results show that the 2 patient groups differ from the control group (table C, D).

Clinical data (mean ± SD) :

	C group	S group	SAS group
age (years)	47.4±16.5	51.5± 9.0	50.9± 9.7
height-weight index	97.5± 7.5	114.2±15.5	120.8±16.0
Subjection audit. thresh.	8.2± 3.1	15.9± 6.8	21.2±10.3
ABP (quotation)	0	.80± .10	1.10± .20
snoring history (id)	0	1.45± .20	1.65± .20
snoring worsened (id)	0	1.10± .25	1.40± .20

table C

Height-weight index, arterial blood pressure and auditory threshold are significantly increased in the patient groups and this increase is more important in SAS group. R_1 latency of BR (I-III, iL and (III-V) iL of BAEPs are increased in patient groups : 50 % of SAS patients and 42 % of S patients had an increased R_1 latency (> + 2 DS) ; 45 % of SAS patients and 30 % of S patients had an increased (I-III iL) (> + 2 DS) ; prolonged (III-V) iL was found in 18 % of SAS patients and 5 % of S patients (> + 2 SD).

But none of the electrophysiological parameters retained was exclusively impaired in SAS patients.

Electrophysiological data (mean ± SD) :

	C group	S group	SAS group
apnea index (max) (N/h)	0	0	61.3±20.1
desaturation index (%)	0	0	20.2±12.1
I latency (ms)	1.67±.13	1.64±.17	1.70± .20
I-III iL (ms)	2.07±.17	2.22±.17	2.29± .27
III-V iL (ms)	1.88±.17	1.97±.19	2.03± .16
R_1 latency (ms)	10.27±.58	11.1±1.02	11.26± .73

table D

By multivariate factors analysis, we showed that :
- SAS affects predominently fatty men and these patients have noted a recent increase of their snoring. Two electrophysiological parameters (I-III and III-V IL are predominently impaired in these patients.
- None of the electrophysiological parameters correlates with the type of SAS (central or obstructive).
- The (I-III) IL (and no other parameters) is highly correlated with the apnea index. The (III-V) IL and the R_1 latency are correlated with the desaturation index.
- A prolonged (I-III) IL is significantly associated with a prolonged (III-V) IL and a delayed R_1 latency.

DISCUSSION AND CONCLUSION :

The present study, as previous ones, failed to demonstrate a SAS-specific brainstem dysfunction. Furthermore, a unique lesion is unlike to explain the observed abnormalities.

The prolonged (I-III) IL may reflect a cochlear (or a VIIIth cranial nerve) dysfunction (8). It is known that, whereas the circulatory requirements of the cochlea are very low, as compared to those of the brainstem, the cochlea is very sensitive to the alteration of its oxygen blood supply (9). A consequence of repeated decreases of oxygen blood pressure at the level of the cochlea is the occurrence of a dysfunction in the lower part of the cochlea (the more sensitive). This leads to a high frequency hearing loss and to a prolonged (I-III) IL . The latter correlates well with the maximal apnea index.

Prolonged (III-V) IL (and delayed R_1 latencies ?) may underlye a different phenomenon. Brainstem was shown to be relatively resistant to hypoxic conditions (10). However, brainstem abnormalities are observed following asphyxia : these abnormalities may not be due directly to the induced hypoxaemia and hypercapnia, but rather to depressed systemic circulation leading to cerebral ischemia (11). Correlation of prolonged (III-V) IL with the maximal oxygen desaturation may reflect such a mechanism.

Finally, a diffuse demyelination of the cranial nerves (12) has been described in apneic neonates. Such a mechanism is not excluded in our patient groups. It would explain delayed R_1 latency and prolonged (I-III) IL. This may occur in S patients as in SAS patients. Its mechanism remains unclear.

Further anatomical investigations of brainstem with MRI, for instance, are required to support these hypothesis.

REFERENCES :

1. Cohen, M.I. : Neurogenesis of respiratory rythm in the mammal.
   Physiol. Rev., 1968, 59 : 1105-1173.

2. Starr, A., Hamilton, A.E. : Correlation between confirmed sites of neurologic lesions and abnormalities of far-fields auditory brainstem responses.
   EEG Clin. Neurophysiol., 1976, 41 : 595-608.

3. Bender, L.F., Maynard, F.M., Hastings, S.V. : The blink reflex as a diagnostic procedure.
   1969, Arch. Phys. Med. Rehabil., 50 : 27-31.

4. Stockard, J.J., Sharbrough, F.W., Staats, B.A., Westbrook, P.R. :
   Brainstem auditory evoked potentials (BAEPs) in sleep apnea.
   American EEG Society, 1979, meeting.

5. Karnaze, D., Gott, P., Mitchell, F., Loftin, J. : Brainstem auditory evoked potentials are normal in idiopathic sleep apnea.
   Ann. Neurol., 1984, 15, 4, 406.

6. Peled, R., Pratt, H., Scharf, B., Lavie, P. : Auditory brainstem evoked potentials during sleep apnea.
   Neurology, 1983, 33, 4, 419-423.

7. Snyderman, N., Johnson, J., Moller, M., Thearle, P. : Brainstem evoked potentials in adults sleep apnea.
   Ann. Otol. Rhinol. Laryngol., 1982, 91, 597-598.

8. Mosko, S.S., Pierce, S., Holowach, J., Sussin, J.F. : Normal brainstem auditory evoked potentials recorded in sleep apneics waking and as a function of arterial oxygen saturation during sleep.
   EEG Clin. Neurophysiol., 1981, 51, 477-482.

9. Eggermont, J.J., Don, M. : Mechanisms of central conduction time prolongation in brainstem auditory evoked potentials.
   Neurology, 1986, 43, 116-120.

10. Perlman, H.B., Kimura, R., Fernandez, C. : Experiments on temporary obstruction of the internal auditory artery.
    Laryngoscope, 1959, 69, 591-613.

11. Sohmer, M., Gafni, M., Chisin, R. : Auditory nerve-brainstem potentials in man and cat under hypoxic and hypercapnic conditions.
    EEG Clin. Neurophysiol., 1982, 53, 506-511.

12. Sohmer, H., Gafni, M., Havatselet, G. : Persistence of auditory nerve response and absence of brainstem responses in severe cerebral ischemia.
EEG Clin. Neurophysiol., 1984, 58, 65-72.

13. Johnson, L.G., Hawkins, J.E. Jr. : Perivascular demyelinization of cochlear neurons in two neonates.
Acta Otolaryngol. (suppl.), 1985, 423, 73-80.

KEYWORDS :

BRAINSTEM ; SLEEP-APNEA ; AUDITORY EVOKED POTENTIALS ; BLINK REFLEX.

SUMMARY :

A prospective electrophysiological study of 50 patients suffering of severe snoring was conducted to evaluate their brainstem function. Among them, 30 patients had sleep-apnea syndrom (SAS), as defined by polygraphic EEG recordings. The others were defined as snoring (S) group.

As compared with an age-matched control group of 10 healthy, non-snorer subjects, (SAS) and (S) groups showed several abnormalities which were worsened in SAS group :

In brainstem auditory evoked potentials, (I-III) and (III-V) interwave latency were statistically prolonged ; in blink reflex, the latency of the first response was delayed. But none of the electrophysiological abnormalities was specific of SAS.

Several vascular hypothesis may underlye the observed abnormalities. These are discussed with a particular reference to the cochlea and to the brainstem itself.

Brainstem structure and function in patients with sleep apnea syndrome

B. Fleury, R. Morizot-Koutlidis, M.C. Lavallard-Rousseau, F. Chabolle, E. Cabanis and J. Ph. Derenne

*Hôpital Saint-Antoine, 184 rue du faubourg Saint-Antoine, 75012 Paris, France

Central and obstructive apneas are always intricated (with the exception of the rare exclusively central apnea Syndromes) in the sleep apnea Syndrome (SAS) patients. The central component seems to be the consequence of an increase in the pysiological ventilatory instability during sleep onset period. Decrease in inspiratory effort prior to the onset of occlusive apnea as well as continued decreasing inspiratory efforts subsequent to the onset of occlusion suggest a fundamental alteration in neural regulation of breathing and in reflexes responses to occlusion of the airway in SAS.

Then, respiratory centers dysfunction may be responsible for a part of the abnormalities observed in SAS patients.

Respiratory centers are located in the reticular formation of the brainstem.

Brainstem auditory evoked potentials (BAEPs) have been proved useful in detecting structural and/or functional damage of the brainstem (STARR et Al, 1976).

Chemical stimulation (CO_2) is a classical method to test the respiratory centers function.

Magnetic resonance imaging (MRI) is the best radiological technic to appreciate the brainstem anatomical structure.

The aim of our study was, using the combination of these three methods, to detect functional and/or structural changes in the brainstem of SAS patients.

MATERIAL - METHODS

POPULATION : We have studied 10 patients with a SAS confirmed by polysomnographic recording.
SAS was defined as "more than 10 apneas per hour, each one lasting more than 10 seconds"
The group was composed of 8 patients with predominently obstructive apneas and 2 patients with predominently central apneas.
The patients characteristics are summarized in the table 1.

SEX	Age (Yr)	Ideal Body Weight (%)	Apnea Index NREM	Apnea Index REM	PaO2 mmHg	PaCO2 mmHg
9 ♂	50,6	149	56,5	35,2	85,6	37,4
1 ♀	± 2,6	± 5,6	± 5,1	± 2,31	± 2,9	± 0,95

VALUES ARE MEAN + SD
IDEAL BODY WEIGHT : Height cm - 100 - (Height cm - 150) / 2 FOR MAN
                                                          4 FOR WOMAN

METHODS

ELECTROPHYSIOLOGICAL STUDY

BAEPs were recorded in the 10 SAS patients after the measurement of the subjective auditory threshold. The stimulus intensity was adjuted to 70 dB supraliminary.
I-III and III-V interwaves latencies (IL) were calculated. The individual results were compared to the normative values of the laboratory and with these of a control group of 10 healthy non snorers subjects (47,5 + 16.5 years old, 60 % men). This confirmed the reliability of our control group (normative values + 2 SD)
Statistical analysis using student t test was performed.

PHYSIOLOGICAL STUDY

Respiratory response to CO2 was elicited according to the method of Read, 1967 the ventilatory response was expressed in terms of slope $\Delta VE/\Delta PACO2$) and ventilation at a PACO2 of 55mmHg.

BRAINSTEM ANATOMY was studied using 1500 G Resistive Magnet (MAGNISCAN). Sagittal, axial and coronal jointive images were obtained at 9 mm intervals.

RESULTS

BRAINSTEM FUNCTION

a) ELECTROPHYSIOLOGICAL STUDY

BAEPs were abnormal in 8/10 SAS (7 O, 1 C).
Significant prolongation of I-III and III-V interwave latency was observed, as expressed in the table 2.

	I-III MSEC	III-V MSEC
SAS GROUP	2.59 ± 0.07	2.07 ± 0.05
CONTROL GROUP	2.07 ± 0.04	1.883 ± 0.03
	$p < 0.001$	$p < 0.05$

Table 2

RESPIRATORY RESPONSE TO CO2

It was tested in 7/10 SAS with BAEPs abnormalities (6 O, 1 C).
6/7 (5 O, 1 C) had a normal ventilatory response, both in terms of slope
(m + SE : 1.78 +)
0,24 l/min/mmHg), and ventilation measured at PACO2 55 mmHg (m + SE : 42,2 + 3,9 l/min/mmHg)
1/7 (O) had a decrease in slope (0,70 l/min/mmHg)

C) BRAINSTEM ANATOMY, was normal in all the 10 patients. No lesion was observed in the respiratory centers area

DISCUSSION AND CONCLUSION

The results of BAEPs recording in SAS patients remain controversial in the litterative (Karnage et al, 1984 ; Peled et al, 1983).In this report it has been shown that nervous conduction at the brainstem level can be abnormal in SAS patients. Similarly snyderman et al (1982) have previously reported that the Vth wave of BAEPs was stastically delayed in Central SAS. Then a brainstem dysfunction can be evocated in some SAS patients.In our study these BAEPs abnormalities are isolated. In all the patients the respiratory centers are responders to chemical stimulation. Only one of the obstructive SAS had a decrease in the ventilatory response to CO_2.Morever the anatomical structure of the brainstem was normal in all the patients. With the limits due to the MRI discriminative possibility, an anatomical lesion of the respiratory centers area in the brainstem can be eliminated.
Then, further investigations are needed to determine the exact nature of the lesions responsible of the BAEPs abnormalities.

BIBLIOGRAPHY

KARNAZE D., GOTT P., MITCHELL F., LOFTIN J.,
Brainstem auditory evoked potentials are normal in indipathic sleep apnea
Ann Neurol. 1984, 15, 4-406

PELED R., PRATT H., SCHARL B., LAVIC P.,
Auditory brainstem evoked potentials during sleep apnea
Neurology, 1983, 33, 419-423

READ D.J.C.,
A Clinical method for assessing the ventilatory response to carbon dioxide
Australian Ann Med. 1967, 16, 20-32

SNYDERMAN N., JOHNSON J., MOLLER M., THEARLE P.,
Brainstem evoked potentials in adults sleep apnea
Ann. Otol. Rhinol. laryngol. 1982, 91, 597-598

STARR A., HAMILTON A.E.,
Correlation between confirmed sites of neurologic lesions
and abnormalities of far-fields auditory brainstem responses
EEG. Clin. Neurophysiol., 1976, 41, 595-608

Chronic rhonchopathy. Ed. C.H. Chouard. © 1988, John Libbey Eurotext Ltd. pp.125-131.

Etude du sommeil chez les patients améliorés après uvulopalatopharyngoplastie (UPPP)

F. Laffont, M.O. Josse, M. Minz, P. Waisbord, B. Fleury and F. Chabolle

Service du Professeur HP, CATHALA, Explorations Fonctionnelles, Neurologie, Hôpital de la Salpétrière, 75651 Paris Cedex 13, France

RESUME

Le sommeil a été étudié avant et 3 mois après UPPP, chez 22 patients présentant un syndrome d'apnées du sommeil (SAS).
Seize patients sont considérés comme améliorés après l'intervention (diminution de plus de 50 % de l'indice d'apnées).
L'aspect séquentiel du sommeil est considérablement modifié ; après intervention le pourcentage de sommeil fragmenté, par les éveils de fin d'apnées, est significativement diminué dans tous les stades de sommeil et on observe le plus souvent un sommeil continu.
La saturation de l'oxyhemoglobine est significativement plus élevée après l'intervention dans tous les stades de sommeil.

MOTS CLEF

Sommeil   -   UPPP   -   SAS

INTRODUCTION

Le syndrome d'apnées du sommeil (SAS) est bien défini (Guilleminault et coll ,1978). Aux désordres respiratoires nocturnes,(apnées essentiellement obstructives et mixtes) est associée une pathologie diurne.
Les symptômes qui amènent les patients à consulter sont essentiellement un ronflement important et une somnolence diurne.

On a proposé de traiter chirurgicalement ces apnées obstructives par uvulopalatopharyngoplastie (UPPP)(Fujita et coll,1981).

Il existe actuellement dans la littérature peu de séries de patients présentant un syndrome d'apnées du sommeil traités par UPPP et contrôlés polygraphiquement.

Fujita et coll (1981) et Hernandez(1982) ont publié les premiers résultats sur un nombre peu important de cas (8 améliorés sur 12 dans la première série, un seul dont l'amélioraton est confirmée polygraphiquement dans la deuxième série.

Guilleminault et coll (1983) ont publié une série importante : 69 patients opérés avec un contrôle polygraphique post opératoire chez 35 d'entre eux.

Une amélioration des troubles respiratoires nocturnes est constatée sur l'ensemble des patients contrôlés, avec toutefois d'importantes variations inter- individuelles.

Une autre série plus récente est celle publiée par Fujita et coll (1985) sur 66 patients dont 33 sont désignés comme "répondeurs" et sont améliorés après UPPP.

Le but de cette étude est,sur une population de patients adressés à une consultation d'O.R.L. pour ronflement, de voir ,chez les patients présentant un syndrome d'apnées du sommeil ,quel est le pourcentage de patients dont l'amélioration est vérifiée polygraphiquement, et de décrire dans ce groupe les modifications du sommeil et de la somnolence diurne par comparaison des enregistrements polysomnographiques pratiqués avant et après l'intervention.

POPULATION

22 patients présentant un syndrome d'apnées du sommeil ont subit une UPPP.

Un enregistrement polysomnographique de 24 heures permet de diagnostiquer un syndrome d'apnées du sommeil ;tous les patients retenus dans cette étude ont un index d'apnées (nombre de pauses respiratoires supérieures à 10 secondes par heure de sommeil) supérieur à 10 (l'index le plus bas ,dans notre série ,est égal à 17).

Un deuxième enregistrement 3 mois après l'intervention permet de contrôler les résultats.

16 patients sur 22 ont une diminution de l'index d'apnées de plus de 50 %, et sont considérés comme améliorés conformément au critère proposé par Conway et coll(1985). L'étude porte sur ces 16 patients (15 hommes et 1 femme), moyenne d'âge 53 ans. Ces patients présentaient tous une somnolence diurne et une obésité, avec un poids supérieur à 123 % du poids théorique.

MATERIEL ET METHODE

Les patients ont deux enregistrements polysomnographiques de 24 heures, avant et 3 mois après l'intervention.
L'enregistrement comprend : un Electroencéphalogramme (E.E.G.), un Electrooculogramme (E.O.G.) des mouvements oculaires horizontaux et verticaux, un Electromyogramme (E.M.G.) des muscles sus-hyoïdiens et du menton, un Electrocardiogramme (E.C.G.) ; les flux aériens buccal et nasal sont enregistrés par des thermistances, les mouvements respiratoires thoraciques et abdominaux par des jauges de contrainte.
La saturation de l'oxyhémoglobine est enregistrée en continu par un oxymètre (Ohmeda).
L'enregistrement de nuit est analysé suivant les critères de Rechtschaffen et Kales (1968). En fait les microéveils, ou les allègements brefs du sommeil, survenant en fin d'apnée ou d'hypopnée ne sont pas comptabilisés ; le stade de sommeil retenu est celui pendant lequel survient l'apnée. Le sommeil est donc fragmenté par ces éveils périodiques de fin d'apnée ou d'hypopnée et le pourcentage de la durée de sommeil fragmenté est calculé par rapport à la durée du stade considéré.
L'apnée est un arrêt respiratoire supérieur à 10 secondes : l'index d'apnée est le nombre d'apnées par heure, défini pour chaque stade de sommeil.
Enfin la saturation minimale de l'oxyhémoglobine dans le sommeil lent et le sommeil paradoxal est mesurée.
Un test de t apparié permet la comparaison des valeurs des différents paramètres avant et après UPPP.

RESULTATS

6 patients sont considérés comme non améliorés. Il faut signaler que leur poids moyen est supérieur à celui du groupe de patients améliorés. Les gaz du sang montrent une Pa O2 plus faible et une Pa CO2 plus élevée.

La saturation de l'oxyhémoglobine pendant le sommeil lors de apnées est également plus importante .Pour deux d'entre eux, bien que l'indice d'apnées ne soit pas diminué, la désaturation nocturne est beaucoup moins importante.(Cf.Communication du Docteur Chabolle et Coll).

Dans le groupe de patients améliorés si l'on ne tient pas compte de la fragmentation des stades de sommeil , nous n'observons aucune différence dans les aspects quantitatifs et séquentiels du sommeil (tab.I).

Tableau 1. Etude des aspects quantitatifs et séquentiels du sommeil chez les patients améliorés par UPPP.

	Avant Intervention	3 mois après intervention
Temps de sommeil nocturne	485 ± 60	446 ± 80
Durée du stade I	44 ± 30	50 ± 35
Durée du stade 2	316 ± 72	257 ± 64
Durée des stades 3 et 4	41 ± 34	53 ± 32
Durée du sommeil pardoxal	76 ± 46	76 ± 24
% du SP/ TST	17 ± 7	24 ± 7
Temps de sommeil diurne	135 ± 92	87 ± 69
Latence d'endormissement	12 ± 12	14 ± 17
Latence de sommeil paradoxal	122 ± 67	116 ± 64
Nombre de phase de S.P.	4 ± 1,3	4 ± 1,2
Nombre d'éveils nocturnes	6 ± 4	8 ± 6
Durée totale des éveils nocturnes	56 ± 51	97 ± 68

Les durées sont exprimés en minutes . Aucune différence significative n'est observée avant et après UPPP).

Par contre l'aspect morphologique du sommeil est considérablement modifié après l'intervention : on observe un sommeil continu ,en effet les pourcentages de sommeil fragmenté des différents stades sont significativement diminués (Fig.1).
Les indices d'apnées sont diminués significativement (Fig.2) dans tous les stades ; l'indice après intervention est égal à 11 dans le stade 1 et à 12 dans le sommeil paradoxal , mais est inférieur à 10 dans les stades 2,3 et 4 du sommeil lent.

Fig. I   POURCENTAGE DE SOMMEIL FRAGMENTE

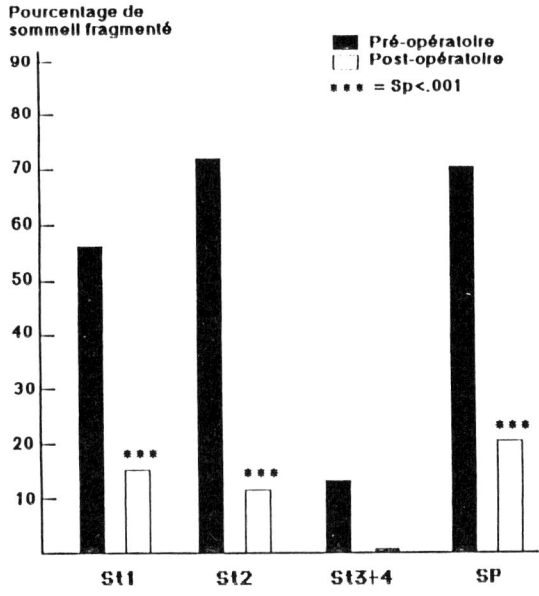

Fig. II   INDICES D'APNEES DANS LES DIFFERENTS STADES DE SOMMEIL

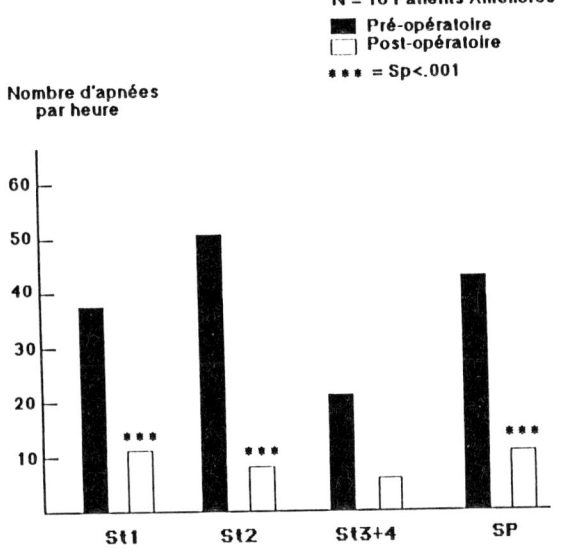

Enfin la saturation minimale de l'oxyhémoglobine dans le sommeil lent est de 80 % avant l'intervention et de 89 % après l'intervention (Sp <.001) et dans le sommeil paradoxal elle est de 70 % avant intervention et de 85 % après(Sp<.001).

Quant à la somnolence diurne, bien que les patients améliorés affirment qu'elle a disparue, la durée du temps de sommeil diurne, mesurée au laboratoire, chez les patients couchés après l'intervention, n'est pas diminuée de façon significative.

CONCLUSION

Chez les patients améliorés les indices d'apnées sont très bas après UPPP, la saturation de l'oxyhémoglobine nocturne est correcte et le sommeil est continu pendant un pourcentage de temps important.
Les problèmes qui se posent sont : tout d'abord de savoir de façon plus précises qu'elles sont les patients qui peuvent bénéficier de l'intervention. Il semble que les syndromes d'apnées du sommeil sévères, chez les patients à un stade d'obésité très important, avec une hypoventilation alvéolaire, ne soient pas améliorés.
Il faudra ensuite vérifier si les améliorations constatées après 3 mois se maintiennent ultérieurement.

REFERENCES BIBLIOGRAPHIQUES

Conway,W. Fujita,M.D. Zorick, F. Sicklesteel, B.A. Roehrs PhD. Wittig,M.D. and Roth, PhD.(1985) :Uvulopalatopharyngoplasty, Chest,88,3 385-387.

Fujita, S. Conway,WA. Zorick,F. et al (1981) : Surgical correction of anatomic abnormalities in obstructive sleep syndrome; uvulopalatopharyngoplasty. Otolaryngol Head Neck Surg;89:923-34.

Fujita,S. Conway,W. Zorick,F. et al. (1985) :Evaluation of the effectiveness of uvulopalatopharyngoplasty.Laryngoscope;95:70-4.

Guilleminault C. Hayes B. Smith L. et al. (1983) : Palatopharyngoplasty and obstructive sleep apnea syndrome. Bull Europ Physiopath Resp;19:595-99.

Rechtschaffen A. Kales(eds). (1968)A manual of standardized terminology, techniques and scoring system for sleep stages of human subjects. Brain Information Service/Brain Research Institute, University of California at Los Angeles

SUMMARY

SLEEP WAS STUDIED IN 22 PATIENTS WITH SLEEP APNEA SYNDROME (SAS), BEFORE AND 3 MONTHS AFTER UVULOPALATOPHARYNGOPLASTIE (UPPP). SIXTEEN WERE IMPROVED (I.E. DECREASE OP APNEA INDEX >50%). SEQUENTIAL COURSE OF SLEEP WAS DEEPLY MODIFIED : PERCENTAGE OF SLEEP INTERRUPTED BY END OF APNEA AWAKENINGS WAS SIGNIFICANTLY DECEASED,FOR ALL SLEEP STAGES, AND SLEEP WAS MOSTLY UNINTERRUPTED.
OXYHEMOGLOBIN SATURATION WAS SIGNIFICANTLY HIGHER IN 22 ALL SLEEP STAGES.

V. CHRONIC RHONCHOPATHY AND CARDIO VASCULAR DISEASES

Chairman: P. Valty

Prevalence and correlates of snoring in an adult population

W.W. Schmidt-Nowara, D.B. Coultas, C. Wiggins, B.E. Skipper and J.M. Samet

Departments of Medicine and of Family, Community and Emergency Medicine; and the New Mexico Tumor Registry; University of New Mexico, Albuquerque, New Mexico 87131, USA

ABSTRACT

Snoring was investigated as part of a health survey in a population-based sample of 1,219 Hispanic-American adults (40% male, median age 39 years). The data consisted of a questionnaire, which included an item for the frequency of loud snoring, and measurements of blood pressure, height, and weight. The age-adjusted prevalence of regular loud snoring was 11.2% in men and 6.9% in women. Logistic regression was used to assess the determinants of snoring. Significant independent predictors of regular loud snoring included male sex, middle age, obesity, and smoking. In a univariate analysis, snoring was also associated with hypertension. However, when examined in a multiple logistic model which adjusted for the effects of age, sex, obesity, and smoking, snoring showed no independent association with hypertension. Using the same model, frequent loud snoring was associated with doctor-diagnosed myocardial infarction but not with angina. The prevalence of snoring in this survey and its correlates are similar to previous reports with the exceptions of hypertension, which was not related in this study.

KEY WORDS

Snoring, prevalence, sleep apnea, hypertension

INTRODUCTION

Snoring indicates a partial upper airway obstruction (Lugaresi). Because it is the most common symptom in sleep apnea syndrome, and because snoring has been associated with male sex, increasing age, obesity, and hypertension (Lugaresi, Mondini, Koskenvuo), snoring may be a useful indicator of sleep apnea syndrome in population surveys. Accordingly, snoring was investigated as part of a comprehensive health survey of Hispanic-American adults.

METHODS

A community based sample of Hispanic-American families in a New Mexico town were surveyed by questionnaire and with a limited examination. The sample included

1,219 adults, median age 39 years, 40% male. The interviewer-administered questionnaire classified the frequency of loud snoring as always, often, infrequent, or never. In addition, symptoms of respiratory disease, smoking habits, history of doctor-diagnosed hypertension, angina, and heart disease, and medication use were defined; and blood pressure, height, and weight were measured.

For this analysis, a response of "always" was considered positive, a response of "infrequent" or "never" was considered negative for regular loud snoring and a response of "often" was excluded. In a separate study of 50 patients with sleep apnea syndrome and 129 normal subjects, this dichotomy produced a sensitivity of 83% and a specificity of 96% for sleep apnea syndrome. Crude prevalence rates were standardized for age by reference to United States census data. The data were stratified by sex, age, and body mass index, Kg/m^2 (Table 1). Smoking was classified as never, former, or current use of cigarettes. Lung disease was defined as chronic bronchitis, emphysema, or chronic obstructive lung disease. Hypertension was defined as an average measurement of 140/90 or greater or current use of antihypertensive medication. Angina was defined as "chest pain from the heart," and myocardial infarction as "heart attack." Logistic regression was used to evaluate predictors of snoring. Variables were examined singly and also together in a multiple logistic model. In addition, snoring was examined as a predictor of hypertension, angina, and myocardial infarction by univariate logistic regression with snoring as the independent variable; and by a multiple logistic model which also included age, sex, weight, and smoking. Differences in proportions were examined with the Chi-square test.

RESULTS

Of the 1,139 subjects who could describe their snoring, 11.4% of men and 6.8% of women were regular loud snorers; the respective age-adjusted rates were 11.2 and 6.9 percent. The difference was significant (by Chi-square, $p<.01$ for male versus female). When examined separately, snoring was more prevalent in men in each age group, but only the difference in young subjects was significant ($p<.05$) (Table 1). When examined by weight group, snoring was more prevalent in non-obese men ($p<.001$), but in obese subjects sex differences were not significant.

Table 1. Prevalence of regular loud snoring by sex, age, and body mass index.

Body Mass Index	Men				%(n)	Women			
	<27	27-29	≥30	All		<27	27-29	≥30	All
Age									
<40	5.2	11.6	24.1	9.2* (19)		3.3	2.6	6.2	3.6 (12)
40-64	17.2	8.9	12.9	14.1 (23)		2.5	12.2	23.5	9.5 (20)
≥65	13.6	5.6	12.5	11.4 (8)		3.8	0	21.4	6.3 (5)
All	10.6	9.4	14.7	11.4† (50)		3.2	6.6	15.9	6.0 (37)

* P<.05 men vs. women   † P<.01 men vs. women

By univariate logistic regression, the significant predictors of regular loud snoring included middle age, male sex, substantial obesity (BMI≥30), and current smoking (Table 2). When examined by multiple logistic regression in a model using the same variables, the same significant effects remained. Lung disease was not associated with snoring.

Table 2. Predictors of regular loud snoring by univariate and multiple logistic regression.

Variable		Univariate Odds Ratio	95% CI*	Multiple Variable Odds Ratio	95% CI
Age	<40†	1.0	-	1.0	-
	40-64	2.6	1.6-4.2	2.2	1.3-3.7
	≥65	1.9	1.0-3.6	1.6	0.8-3.3
Sex	Female†	1.0	-	1.0	-
	Male	2.2	1.4-3.4	2.2	1.3-3.5
Body Mass Index	<27†	1.0	-	1.0	-
	27-29.99	1.5	0.8-2.7	1.3	0.7-2.4
	≥30	3.4	2.1-5.7	3.6	2.1-6.2
Lung Disease	No†	1.0	-	1.0	-
	Yes	1.1	0.5-2.6	1.2	0.5-2.8
Smoking	Never†	1.0	-	1.0	-
	Former	2.2	1.2-3.9	1.9	1.0-3.5
	Current	2.5	1.5-4.0	2.5	1.5-4.3

* CI = confidence interval † Reference group

Regular loud snoring was significantly more prevalent in hypertensive compared to normotensive women (Table 3). In men, however, no difference was observed. With univariate logistic regression, regular loud snoring was a significant predictor of hypertension (odds ratio 1.8, 95% confidence interval 1.3-2.5). However, when examined in a multiple logistic model which also included the effects of age, sex, weight, and smoking, the effect of snoring disappeared (Table 4). In a similar analysis, doctor-diagnosed angina was not but doctor-diagnosed myocardial infarction was significantly associated with snoring.

Table 3. Prevalence of regular loud snoring by hypertension*, sex, and age.

	Men Hypertension		%(n)	Women Hypertension	
	Yes	No		Yes	No
Age					
<40	8.3	9.2		5.3	3.5
40-64	11.5	15.2		15.6†	6.7
≥65	8.8	12.9		11.1	2.9
All	9.8 (12)	11.7 (38)		12.8 (18)‡	4.3 (21)

* Hypertension = BP≥140/90 or current use of antihypertensive medication
Hypertension yes vs. no: † P<.05;   ‡ P<.01

Table 4. Regular loud snoring and other predictors of hypertension, angina, and myocardial infarction by multiple logistic regression.

Variable*		Hypertension Odds Ratio	95% CI†	Angina Odds Ratio	95% CI	Myocardial Infarction Odds Ratio	95% CI
Snore (+:-)		1.0	0.6-1.7	1.2	0.4-3.4	2.5	1.0-6.2
Age	<40	1.0	-	1.0	-	1.0	-
	40-64	4.8	3.1-7.3	3.5	1.3-9.5	25.7	3.2-187
	≥65	14.3	8.6-23.8	9.9	3.7-26.7	39.3	4.8-321
BMI	<27	1.0	-	1.0	-	1.0	-
	27-29	2.8	1.8-4.4	0.4	0.1-1.3	0.4	0.1-1.9
	≥30	6.2	3.9-9.8	1.2	0.5-2.9	4.0	1.6-9.9
Sex (M:F)		1.2	0.8-1.7	1.3	0.6-2.8	2.4	1.0-5.8
Smoking	Never	1.0	-	1.0	-	1.0	-
	Former	1.3	0.8-2.1	1.5	0.6-3.7	2.6	0.9-7.4
	Current	0.9	0.6-1.4	1.1	0.5-2.7	2.4	0.9-6.7

* reference groups same as Table 2 † CI = confidence interval

DISCUSSION

In this survey of adults, regular loud snoring was found to be more frequent in men and was significantly associated with middle age, obesity, smoking, and heart disease. Hypertension was more frequent in regular loud snorers, but the association was attributable to the confounding effects of age and obesity.

Because the sample was population-based, our results reflect the prevalence of regular snoring in the population of Hispanic adults in a New Mexico community. It remains to be determined whether racial factors or altitude (1500 m) affect snoring and whether these observations can be extended to the general population. Two other surveys provide data on the prevalence of snoring in the general population. In 5,713 residents of San Marino, habitual snoring was reported by 24.1% of men and 13.8% of women (Mondini). In 7,511 Finnish adults, age 40-69, habitual snoring was reported by 9.0% of men and 3.6% of women (Koskenvuo). The frequency of snoring in this survey is similar to the Finnish data and lower than the San Marino survey. The difference may be attributable to the definition of snoring and its frequency. All three studies find an approximately two-fold greater frequency of regular snoring in men, document an increased frequency in middle age, and demonstrate an association with obesity.

The lack of significant association between hypertension and snoring in this study conflicts with the finding of an association in other surveys (Mondini, Koskenvuo). In this study an increased prevalence of hypertension was observed only in female snorers, and when the data were corrected for sex, age and obesity, no association remained. Definitions of hypertension may account for these differences. In this study hypertension was defined by measurement, and systolic and diastolic criteria were used. The other studies used self-report, and the Italian study focused on systolic hypertension. It is noteworthy that in the Finnish study, when the data were adjusted for age and obesity, the effect of snoring on hypertension was larger in women than in men, and the effect in men, although significant, was small (odds ratio 1.51). Thus age and obesity are the principal reasons for the association between snoring and hypertension, and a separate contribution from snoring alone is small, or absent as in this study.

In addition to hypertension, ischemic heart disease has been associated with snoring (Koskenvuo). Angina, but not myocardial infarction, was significantly more prevalent among habitual snorers in the Finnish study. In this study, snoring was associated with myocardial infarction but not with angina. In both studies the effect of ischemic heart disease was separate from the effects of age and weight.

Smoking was associated with regular snoring, current smoking producing a greater effect than former smoking and both significantly different from never smoking. The mechanism for this effect is unknown, but chronic lung disease, as defined in this study, does not explain it.

These findings confirm the concept that regular loud snoring is associated with morbidity. The clinical significance of this morbidity remains uncertain. Confounding effects, such as age and obesity with hypertension, may explain some of this morbidity. Alternatively, regular loud snoring may identify previously unrecognized cases of sleep apnea syndrome, and morbidity may be due to that condition.

RESUME

PRÉVALENCE ET CORRÉLATIONS DU RONFLEMENT DANS UNE POPULATION ADULTE

Le ronflement a été étudié dans le cadre d'une enquête de santé portant sur un échantillon de population composé de 1,219 adultes Hispano-américains (40% de sexe masculin, âge moyen 39 ans). Les observations consistaient en un questionnaire qui comprenait une rubrique portant sur la fréquence du ronflement sonore, ainsi que sur la mesure de la tension artérielle, la taille et le poids. La prévalence, ajusté à l'âge, du ronflement sonoré regulier (se produisant "toujours") était de 11.2% pour les hommes et de 6.9% pour les femmes. La régression logistique fut utilisée afin d'identifier les associations significatives. Les facteurs indépendants indicatifs du ronflement sonore régulier incluaient le sexe masculin, l'âge mûr, l'obésité et l'usage du tabac. Le ronflement était aussi associé à l'hypertension, définie comme tension artérielle égale ou supérieure a 140/90, ou à un traitement antihypertensif en cours. Néanmoins, éxaminé à l'aide d'un modèle logistique multiple corrigeant les effets de l'âge, du sexe, de l'obésité et de l'usage du tabac, le ronflement ne montrait pas d'association séparée à l'hypertension. En utilisant le même modèle, le ronflement sonore fréquent fut lié à l'infarctus du myocarde diagnostiqué par un médecin, mais non pas associé à l'angine.

La prévalence du ronflement dans cette étude et son association au vieillissement, au sexe masculin et à l'obésité sont similaires aux rapports précédents. La corrélation avec l'usage de la cigarette n'a pas été constatée dans les études antérieures. Dans cette étude, l'association du ronflement à l'hypertension peut être seulement attribuée à l'âge et à l'obésité. On a constaté une corrélation entre le ronflement et la cardiopathie ischémique en présence d'infarctus du myocarde mais non pas en présence d'angine.

REFERENCES

Lugaresi, E., Coccagna, G., Farneti, P., Mantovani, M., Cirignotta, F. (1975): Snoring. Electroenceph. Clin. Neuro-physiol. 39, 59-64.
Koskenvuo, M., Partinen, M., Seppo, S., Kaprio, J., Heimo, L., Kauko, H. (1985): Snoring as a risk factor for hypertension and angina pectoris. Lancet i, 893-895.
Mondini, S., Zucroni, M., Cirignotta, F., Aguglia, U., Leuzi, P.L., Zauli, C., Lugaresi, E. (1983): Snoring as a risk factor for cardiac and circulatory problems: an epidemiological study. In Sleep/Wake Disorders: Natural History, Epidemiology, and Long-Term Evolution, eds C. Guilleminault, E. Lugaresi, pp 99-105. New York: Raven Press.

Apport de l'enregistrement holter au diagnostic du syndrome d'apnées du sommeil

J.Y. Le Heuzey*, P. Romejko*, B. Fleury**, J. Ph. Derenne**, C.H. Chouard*** and J. Valty*

Services de Cardiologie, Pneumologie**, Otorhinolaryngologie***, Hôpital Saint-Antoine, 75012 Paris, France*

RESUME

Afin de préciser si l'enregistrement Holter pourrait aider au diagnostic de syndrome d'apnées du sommeil (SAS), nous avons étudié 39 patients ayant tous le symptome ronflement et suspects de SAS. L'analyse des fréquences cardiaques nocturnes montre que les patients considérés comme SAS (+) par l'enregistrement polygraphique ont un écart entre fréquence maxima et minima significativement plus important que les patients SAS (-) (63,1 ± 3,6 contre 45,4 ± 3,9 battements par mn, $p < 0,05$). L'enregistrement Holter peut apporter des arguments pour différencier le ronflement simple du SAS. Il n'apporte que des éléments de présomption mais a l'avantage de sa simplicité par rapport à la polygraphie, examen lourd et plus difficile à réaliser en routine.

MOTS CLEFS

Syndrome d'apnées du sommeil, enregistrement Holter, enregistrement polygraphique du sommeil, ronflement.

INTRODUCTION

Sleep apnea syndrome is known to be associated with cardiac arrhythmias. Several data of the literature reported the occurrence, in this syndrome, of sinus bradycardia, sino-atrial or atrio-ventricular blocks, atrial fibrillation, supraventricular or ventricular premature beats (2, 8, 9). The aim of our study was to assess the ability of Holter monitoring to contribute to the diagnosis of sleep apnea syndrome (SAS).

MATERIAL AND METHODS

We studied 39 patients, aged 34 to 75 (mean 54.2 ± 8.8). All these patients (34 males, 5 females) exhibited snoring. We performed, in each patient, a 24 hours Holter monitoring (Anatec, ELA Medical Co) and a polygraphic recording of sleep. The results of Holter monitoring were analysed as a function of the polygraphic recordings results.

RESULTS

Polygraphic recording of sleep allowed to affirm the diagnosis of sleep apnea syndrome in 32 patients. On the contrary this recording remained negative in 7 patients. The mean ages of the two groups were not significantly different (53.8 ± 9.0 versus 55.9 ± 8.1, respectively).

The analysis of Holter monitoring recordings allowed to show in the SAS (+) patients, the occurrence of sino-atrial blocks (n = 6) and/or atrial pauses longer than 2.5 seconds (n = 10). These conduction disturbances were observed during the nocturnal period (0 AM - 5 AM). Such abnormalities were not observed in the SAS (-) patients. We also observed that, during this nocturnal period, the mean number of supraventricular premature beats was higher in the SAS (+) group (89.9 ± 28.6 versus 9.6 ± 5.2). The results were similar for premature ventricular beats (34.1 ± 14.1 versus 2.0 ± 0.8). No difference was observed during the diurnal period. The analysis of nocturnal cardiac rates in the two groups showed that in the SAS (+) patients the discrepancy between maximal and minimal rates was significantly higher than in the SAS (-) patients : 63.1 ± 3.6 beats per mn versus 45.4 ± 3.9 beats per mn, $p < 0.05$.

DISCUSSION

Cardiac arrhythmias and conduction disturbances have been described in the sleep apnea syndrome but their frequency has been diversely evaluated (6), reaching 60 to 70 % in some series (1,5). Data of the literature reported the occurrence, as in our series, of sino-atrial blocks, atrial pauses, supraventricular or ventricular premature beats, but also of atrial fibrillations and ventricular tachycardias. Apneas are accompanied by a bradycardia often in association with premature ventricular beats followed by a tachycardia when ventilatory resumption takes place (10). The repetition of these apneas confers a cyclical aspect to the heart rate (3).

In our study this type of heart rate disturbance can be assessed by the measurement of the discrepancy between maximal and minimal nocturnal rates, though computeriezed analysis provided by the Anatec devices was calculated by averaging of 5 mn R-R interval. However, the use of a beat to beat R-R interval plotting system (4,7) would allow a best analysis of these cyclical changes in heart rate during the sleep apnea syndrome.

The mechanism of these cyclical variations of the heart rate has been attributed to a stimulation of carotid chemoreceptors by hypoxaemia, bringing into play vagal afferences (10).

CONCLUSION

In conclusion, Holter monitoring can contribute to the diagnosis of the sleep apnea syndrome. It can bring evidences to differenciate a single snoring and a sleep apnea syndrome. It brings only a presumption but is more easy to perform in routine than polygraphic recordings during sleep.

REFERENCES

1- BURACK B. (1984) : The hypersomnia-sleep apnea syndrome : its recognition in clinical cardiology. Am. Heart J. 107, 543 - 548

2- GUILLEMINAULT C., CONNOLLY S.J., WINKLE R.A. (1983) : Cardiac arrhythmia and conduction disturbances during sleep in 400 patients with sleep apnea syndrome. Am. J. Cardiol. 52, 490 - 494

3- GUILLEMINAULT C., CONNOLLY S., WINKLE R.A., MELVIN K., TILKIAN A. (1984) : Cyclical variation of the heart rate in sleep apnea syndrome. Lancet i, 126 - 131

4- GUILLEMINAULT C., MONDINI S. (1983) : Need for multi-diagnostic approaches before considering treatment in obstructive sleep apnea. Bull. Europ. Physiopath. Resp. 19, 583 - 589

5- GUILLEMINAULT C., SIMMONS F.B., MOTTA J., CUMMISKEY J., ROSEKIND M., SCHROEDER J.S., DEMENT W.C. (1981) : Obstructive sleep apnea syndrome and tracheostomy. Long-term follow up experience. Arch. Int. Med 141, 985 - 989

6- KRIEGER J. (1986) : Les syndromes d'apnées du sommeil de l'adulte. Bull. Europ. Physiopath. Resp. 22, 147 - 189

7- LOPES M.G., FITZGERALD J., HARRISON D.C., SCHROEDER J.S. (1975) : Diagnosis and quantification of arrhythmias in ambulatory patients using an improved R-R interval plotting system. Am. J. Cardiol. 35, 816 - 823

8- MILLER W.P. (1982) : Cardiac arrhythmias and conduction disturbances in the sleep apnea syndrome. Prevalence and significance. Am. J. Med. 73, 317 - 321

9- TILKIAN A.G., GUILLEMINAULT C., SCHROEDER J.S., LEHRMAN K.L., SIMMONS F.B., DEMENT W.C. (1977) : Sleep induced apnea syndrome : prevalence of cardiac arrhythmias and their reversal after tracheostomy. Am. J. Med. 63, 348 - 358

10- ZWILLICH C., DELVIN T., WHITE D., DOUGLAS N., NEIL J., MARTIN R. (1982) : Bradycardia during sleep apnea. Characteristics and mechanism. J. Clin. Invest 69, 1286 - 1292

RESUME

In order to assess the ability of Holter monitoring to contribute to the diagnosis of sleep apnea syndrome (SAS), we studied 39 patients exhibiting snoring. Polygraphic recordings during sleep were positive in 32 patients, negative in 7. The analysis of Holter monitoring showed, in SAS (+) patients, the occurrence during the nocturnal period, of sino-atrial blocks (n = 6) and/or atrial pauses longer than 2.5 seconds (n = 10). Such abnormalities did not occur in SAS (-) patients. The mean number of supraventricular and ventricular premature beats, during this nocturnal period, was higher in the SAS (+) group (89.9 $\pm$ 28.6 and 34.1 $\pm$ 14.1 versus 9.6 $\pm$ 5.2 and 2.0 $\pm$ 0.8). The analysis of nocturnal heart rates showed, in SAS (+) patients significantly higher discrepancy between minimal and maximal heart rate (63.1 $\pm$ 3.6 versus 45.4 $\pm$ 3.9 beats/mn, $p < 0.05$). In conclusion Holter monitoring can bring evidences to differenciate a single snoring and a SAS. It brings only a presumption but is more easy to perform in routine than polygraphic recordings.

Snoring and cardiovascular diseases

Jean Valty*, Claude Henri Chouard**, Jean Yves le Heuzey* and Antoine Buoncuore*

Departments of Cardiology and Otorhinolaryngology**, Hôpital Saint-Antoine, 75012 Paris, France*

SUMMARY

Epidemiologic studies suggested that habitual snoring was an indépendant risk factor for cardiovascular diseases. Significant relations were observed between snoring and hypertension, angina pectoris (in men only), stroke (associated with ischemic heart disease) and arrhythmias.

Frequent snoring is likely revealing sleep apneas. Repeated and prolonged apneas are accompagnied by an increase of arterial pressures.

The reversibility of hypertension is suggested. It is proposed to question patients about snoring, and in some cases to discuss uvulopalatoplasty.

KEY WORDS – MOTS CLES.

Ronchopathy. Sleep apnea syndrome. Hypertension. Risk factor. Coronary heart disease. Arrhythmias. Snoring.
Ronchopathie. Apnée du sommeil. Hypertension artérielle. Facteur de risque coronaire. Troubles du rythme. Ronflement.

INTRODUCTION

Snoring is more frequent among men than women. Its incidence increases with age and weight, but is often underestimated. Frequent snoring is suggestive of the sleep apnea syndrome (SAS) described by Guilleminault (6). Obesity, sleepiness and cor pulmonale described in the Pickwickian syndrome 30 years ago, are not necessary to establish the diagnosis of SAS.

Catheterization during sleep was done in 12 patients by Tilkian (16). During apneic episodes 9 patients had cyclic elevations of systemic arterial pressure; pulmonary artery pressures increased in 10 and 8 had arterial $po_2 < 50$ mm.Hg with hypercapnia.

SYSTEMIC HYPERTENSION

Koskenvuo (8) made an epidemiologic inquiry by 7501 postal questionnaires. The relative risk of hypertension between habitual snorers and never snorers was 1.94 in men and 3.19 in women.

Norton (12) questionned the family of 2001 subjects; snoring prevalence was 85 p.cent among husbands with an incidence of hypertension twice that of non-snorers. This relationship persists when corrected for smoking and obesity.

The clinical study of Burack (2) founded 10 hypertensions among 25 SAS. Inversely Fletcher (4) among 46 essential hypertensions founded 14 SAS. In both studies systemic pressure usually lowered after treatment of SAS.

CORONARY HEART DISEASE

In the study of Koskenvuo there was a significant association between angina pectoris and habitual snoring, with a relative risk of 2.22, (2.01 after adjusting for hypertension and body mass index). In women the relative risk was not significant.

There was no significant relation between snoring and myocardial infarction.

The same author made a prospective study (9) in 4388 men. The age adjusted relative risk of ischaemic heart disease between habitual + frequent snorers and non-snorers was 1.91; it did not significantly decrease after adjustment for age, body mass index, history of hypertension, smoking and alcohol use.

The relationship of sleep disorders to coronary heart disease was discussed by Partinen (14) who opposed extreme sleepers among 5419 men: Those who slept more than 9 hours with a higher prevalence of myocardial infarction and those who slept less than 6 hours with more chest pain as compared with intermediate sleepers.

Influence of breath disorders in 13 patients among 17 with coronary artery disease demonstrated by coronarography was studied by de Olabazal (13). Ten oxygen desaturations occurred without angina or myocardial infarction and were not significantly related to cardiac arrhythmias observed in 12 patients.

ARRHYTHMIAS

Guilleminault (7) founded 31 nocturnal cardiac arrythmias by polygraphic records in 50 patients with SAS. Apneas usually corresponded to bradycardia. Transient auricular fibrillation was observed. Abnormal stimulation of autonomic nervous system is possible.

Burack (2) observed 17 arrythmias among 25 patients with SAS (68 %).

Flick (5) selected 10 patients with chronic obstructive pulmonary disease and frequent nocturnal desaturation; 9 of them had ventricular premature beats prevailing during the night on continuous electrocardiograms. Oxygenotherapy significantly reduced the ventricular arrhythmia in 4 patients.

Tirlapur (17) studied by the same method 7 patients with arterial desaturation and premature ventricular contractions; in 4 of them the ectopic activity rate decreased with oxygen therapy.

Zwillich (18) founded an highly significant relation between SAS, bradycardia and hemoglobin desaturation in 6 patients; in 4 of them bradycardia was improved by oxygenotherapy.

STROKE

In the Koskenvuo study (9) the age ajusted relative risk of stroke and ischemic heart disease between habitual + frequent snorers and non-snorers was 2.38. It was 2.08 after adjustment for other risk factors.

Among 1260 Holter recordings with ventricular arrythmias, Rosenberg (15) compared 50 patients who had significant increase in sleep related ectopy to a matched control group. There was no significant difference regarding organic heart disease or hypertension. Neurologic abnormalities, particularly cerebrovascular disease, were significantly more common in the study group.

Krieger (10) collecting 458 references reported sudden death possibly related to cardiac arrythmias.

MANAGEMENT

The diagnosis of SAS is difficult and would need polygraphic records. Snoring is an indirect witness of SAS. A sufficient number of patients is required to found significant relations.

Among 288 patients consecutively hospitalised in the service of cardiology at hospital Saint Antoine in Paris, the incidence of hypertension is 46 % among 57 frequent snorers and 31 % among 134 non-snorers. This difference is statiscally significant ($p<0.05$).

The reversibility of hypertension after correction of SAS is suggested by some studies. Medical treatments by respiratory stimulants or oxygenotherapy does not seems to be very effective for a long period. Surgical treatment like tracheostomy mentioned by Moran (11) does not apply to every snorer. Uvulopalatoplasty is probably more widely indicated. Chouard (3) suggests to select high-risk patients, with diurnal symptoms or cardiovascular pathology. He observes an improvement of respiratory diseases and general troubles after uvopalatoplasty.

There is a need for further studies since the degree of reversibility of cardiovascular disorders is still unknown.

REFERENCES

1 - Bradley T.D., Phillipson E.A. (1985): Pathogenesis and pathophysiology of the obstructive sleep apnea syndrome. Med Clin. North Am. 69, 1169-85.
2 - Burack B. (1984): The hypersomnia sleep apnea syndrome : its recognition in clinical cardiology. Am. Heart J. 107,543-548.
3 - Chouard C.H., Valty J., Meyer B., Chabolle F., Fleury B., Véricel R., Laccoureye O., Josset P. (1986): La ronchopathie chronique ou ronflement. Aspects cliniques et indications thérapeutiques. Ann.Oto-Laryng. 103, 319-327.
4 - Fletcher E.C., DeBehnke R.D., Lovoi M.S., Gorin A.B. (1985): Undiagnosed sleep apnea in patients with essential hypertension. Ann.Intern.Med. 103,190-195.
5 - Flick M.R., Block A.J. (1979): Nocturnal vs diurnal cardiac arrhythmias in patients with chronic obstructive pulmonary disease. Chest 75,8-11.
6 - Guilleminault C., Tilkian A., Dement W.C. (1976): The sleep apnea syndrome. Ann. Rev. Med. 27, 465-484.
7 - Guilleminault C., Mondini S. (1983): Need for multi-diagnostic approaches before considering treatment in obstructive sleep apnea. Bull.europ.Physiopath. 19,583-589.
8 - Koskenvuo M., Kaprio J., Partinen M., Langinvainio H., Sarna S., Heikkila K. (1985): Snoring as a risk factor for hypertension and angina pectoris. Lancet 8434,893-96.
9 - Koskenvuo M., Kaprio J., Telakivi T., Partinen M., Heikkila K., Sarna S.: Snoring as a risk factor for ischaemic heart disease and stroke in men. Br. Med. J. 294,16-19.
10- Krieger J. (1986): Les syndromes d'apnées du sommeil de l'adulte.Bull. Eur. Physiopathol. Respir. 22,147-18.
11- Moran W.B., Orr W.C. (1985): Diagnosis and management of obstructive sleep apnea.P.II. Arch.Otolaryngol. 111,650-58.
12- Norton P.G., Dunn E.V. 1985): Snoring as a risk factor for disease: an epidemiological survey: Br. Med. J. 291,630-2.
13- De Olazabal J.R., Miller M.J., Cook W.R., Mithoefer J.C. (1982): Disordered breathing and hypoxia during sleep in coronary artery disease. Chest 82 ,548-552.
14- Partinen M., Putkonen P.T.S., Kaprio J., Koskenvuo M., Hilakivi I. (1982): Sleep disorders in relation to coronary heart disease. Acta. Med. Scand. 660, 69-83.
15- Rosenberg M.J., Uretz E., Denes P. (1983): Sleep and ventricular arythmias. Am.Heart J. 106, 703-709.
16- Tilkian A.G., Guilleminault C., Schroeder J.S., Lehrman K.L., Blair Simmons F., Dement W.C. (1976): Hemodynamics in sleep-induced apnea: Ann.Intern. Med. 85,714-719.
17- Tirlapur V.G., Mir M.A. (1982): Nocturnal hypoxemia and associated electrocardiographic changes in patients with chronic obstructive airways disease. N.Eng J.Med. 306,125-130
18 Zwillich C., Devlin T., White D., Douglas N., Weil J., Martin R. (1982): Bradycardia during sleep apnea: J.Clin.Invest. 69, 1286-92.

RESUME

Des enquêtes épidémiologiques suggèrent que le ronflement habituel est un facteur de risque cardio-vasculaire indépendant. Il existe une relation significative entre le ronflement et l'hypertension artérielle, l'angine de poitrine (chez l'homme uniquement), les accidents vasculaires cérébraux (associés aux cardiopathies ischémiques) et certains troubles du rythme.

Le ronflement intense est volontiers révélateur du syndrome d'apnées du sommeil (SAS). Les apnéés répétées et prolongées s'accompagnent d'une élévation des pressions artérielles systémique et pulmonaire.

La réversibilité de l'hypertension est suggérée. Ce fait incite à s'enquérir du ronflement chez certains patients et le cas échéant à discuter une uvulopalatoplastie.

A battery-operated device for home monitoring of oximetry, heart rate, respiration, eye movements, sleeping position, and body movement in patients with snoring and sleep apnea

Laughton E. Miles

Clinical Monitoring Center, 900 Welch Road, Palo Alto, California 94304, USA

ABSTRACT

The Vitalog cardio-respiratory monitor has been reassembled together with its sensor interface unit, a battery-operated oximeter, an LCD electrical multimeter, a multi-sensor cable, and new sensors for body sleeping position, eye movements, and respiration (VIP), in a small (30 cm x 22 cm x 12 cm) case. The data are recovered using an IBM-pc compatible computer, but the device also provides real-time analog and digital outputs which can be directly interfaced with a polygraph or other recorder. The system utilizes new data collection and data analysis software (VITACORE V4.0 and VITARESP V4.1) from Vitalog Corporation; and the final clinical report is prepared using a medical information system based on the PARADOX Relational Data Base Program (Version 1.1). The system has been used to evaluate patients with loud and disruptive snoring and obstructive sleep apnea. It has proved to be especially suitable for home calibration of Nasal-CPAP treatment, and for evaluating the effect of sleeping position on airway obstruction.

KEY WORDS

Respiration-Oximetry-Sleep-Apnea-Computer-Monitoring-Analysis

INTRODUCTION

The Vitalog HMS-2000 home cardio-respiratory monitoring system (Vitalog Corporation, Redwood City, California, USA) was originally designed to measure continuous tidal volume, paradoxical breathing, heart rate, oximetry, and body movement (Miles and Rule, 1982). Recently, this array has been extended by the development and application of a new type of inductive plethysmography respiration sensor (the VIP sensor) (Miles et al., 1986), a new infra-red sensor for measuring eye movements, and a new sensor which distinquishes supine, prone, right or left sleeping positions. The data are recovered from the portable monitor by using an IBM-pc compatible computer, and analysed with the aid of special software.

However, the commercially available system requires the patient to cope with several devices (including a separate oximeter). Furthermore, unreliable electrical connections between these devices are the most common cause of unsatisfactory recordings.

A NEW CONFIGURATION OF THE VITALOG CARDIORESPIRATORY MONITOR

The Vitalog cardio-respiratory monitor has now been reassembled together with its sensor interface unit, a battery-operated oximeter, an LCD electrical multimeter, and a multi-sensor cable, in one small (30 cm x 22 cm x 12 cm) case. The oximeter is a modified version of the 501+ model manufactured by Criticare Systems Inc., Milwaukee, Wisconsin. Although data are still recovered using an IBM-pc compatible computer, the device also provides real-time analog and digital outputs which can be directly interfaced with a polygraph or other recorder. In addition, a more effective and simple respiration sensor calibration procedure incorporating a hand-held spirometer, now includes screening pulmonary function tests (Vital Capacity and FEV-1). The system utilizes new data collection and data analysis software (VITACORE V4.0 and VITARESP V4.1) developed by Vitalog Corporation.

Because non-invasive respiration recordings are commonly distorted and uncalibrated by movement artefact, physical displacement of the sensors and changes in body position, computerized analyses (including apnea detection) of an overnight respiration record are often unreliable or misleading. The VITARESP V4.1 computer program (written in "C") addresses this problem by utilizing the concept of a local inspiratory reference amplitude (IRA), against which changes in the respiration signal can be compared. The preliminary IRA values allotted by the computer are manually reviewed on a video screen in a first editing pass which also allows specification of wake, sleep, REM, artefact, and brief arousals. The computer then scores the record for apneas and hypopneas, paradoxical breathing, oximetry, heart rate, body position, and body movement. The scored record is displayed on a video screen for final editing. The events are identified by a bar code, and numerically characterized in a continuously updated screen window according to the position of a moveable cursor. The program can randomly access and display the longest event in each category, or any location in the record, in a detail which can vary from 5 minutes to 180 minutes per screen. The data is then summarized numerically; and histograms, compressed plots, and examples from the record are automatically generated. The final clinical report, with interpretation and conclusions, is prepared using a medical information system based on the PARADOX Relational Data Base Program (Version 1.1) from Ansa Software, Belmont, California.

The new system has been used to evaluate people with loud and disruptive snoring, and patients with obstructive sleep apnea. It has proved to be especially suitable for a new protocol which allows home calibration of Nasal-CPAP treatment (Miles, 1987), and for evaluating the effect of sleeping position on airway obstruction.

REFERENCES

Miles, L.E., Rule, R.B., (1982): Long term monitoring of multiple physiological parameters using a programmable portable microcomputer. In ISAM-GENT-1981, ed F.D. Stott et al. pp 249-257. London: Academic Press Inc.

Miles, L.E., Herekar, B.V., Rule, R.B., (1986): An improved sensor for recording respiration by inductive plethysmography. Sleep Research, 15,249.

Miles, L.E. (1987): Optimization of nasal-CPAP airflow pressure by use of home oximetry recordings. Sleep Research, (in press).

RESUME

Le moniteur cardio-vasculaire Vitalog a ete reassemble avec un reseau capteurs accouple, un oximetre a piles, un LCD electric multimetre, un cable a plusieurs reseau capteurs, et des nouveax reseaux sensoriels pour la position du corps en etat de sommeil, les mouvements des yeux, et la' respiration (VIP), dans une petite trousse de 30 x 22 x 12 cm. Les donnees sont recuperees a l'aide d'un ordinateur compatible IBM pc mais l' appareil fournit aussi un analog a temps veritable et des resultats digital qui peuvent etre directement accouple a un polygraphe ou autre appareil enregistreur. Le systeme se sert de la collection des nouvelles donnees et de l'analyse des donnees du programme (VITACORE V4.0 et VITARESP V4.1) de Vitalog Corporation, et le rapport final clinique est prepare en se servant du systeme medical d'informations base sur le PARADOX Relational Database Program (Version 1.1).

Le system a ete employe pour faire l'evaluation des malades avec ronflement sonore et disruptif et apnea de sommeil obstructif. Il convient particulierement bien pour un nouveau protocol pour le calibrage a domicile du traitement nasal CPAP et pour l'evaluation des effets de la position de sommeil sur l'obstruction des conduits respiratoires.

Sleep apnea syndrome without apnea

C. Aubert-Tulkens, D.O. Rodenstein, C. Culée and D.C. Stanescu

Cliniques Universitaires St Luc, 10 avenue Hippocrate, B-1200 Bruxelles, Belgium

ABSTRACT

A 38 years old lady presented with obesity (146 kg), loud snoring, restless sleep, hypersomnia, personality changes and systemic hypertension. A full night polysomnography disclosed a tachypnea of 35 breaths/min, continuous loud snoring, but only 2 apneas for the whole night. Stage IV sleep was absent and movement arousals were numerous. Transcutaneous oxygen saturation showed periodic oscillations between 95% and 70% in NREM sleep and between 95% and 60% in REM sleep. A second polygraphic study while continuous positive airway pressure was administered through the nose (nCPAP) revealed disappearance of snoring, movement arousals and desaturations, slowing of rate of breathing (26 min) and reappearance of stage IV sleep. Home treatment with nCPAP has resulted in complete abolition of all symptoms. We conclude that snoring without apnea may induce the full tableau of the obstructive sleep apnea syndrome and responds remarkably well to nCPAP therapy.

KEYWORDS

Snoring, nCPAP, Obstructive Sleep Apnea Syndrome, oxygen desaturation, obesity, systemic hypertension.

INTRODUCTION

The natural history of sleep-related respiratory disturbances remains unclear. The idea that prevails is that there would be a continuum of clinical conditions between so-called simple or trivial snoring and the severest pickwickian form of the obstructive sleep apnea syndrome (OSAS) ; a staging of heavy snorer's disease has been proposed by Lugaresi et al (1983). We present here a patient with upper airway obstruction during sleep who does not fit in the proposed classification.

METHODS

All-night polygraphic study was performed according to standard techniques (Rechtschaffen and Kales, 1968). Continuous oxygen saturation was measured by pulse oxymetry (Nelcor pulse oxymeter N-100). Airflow was qualitatively assessed by thermocouples placed in front of nose and mouth. Respiratory movements were qualitatively estimated by a Volucapt Alvar strain gauge. Breathing sounds were recorded by a microphone glued on the neck. Sleep staging was performed by epochs of 40 seconds.

CASE HISTORY

A 38 years old woman was admitted for sleep study. She weighted 146 kg for a height of 165 cm. She complained of loud snoring, restless sleep, nocturnal sweating, morning headache and sleep drunkenness. Persistent daytime tiredness interfered with housework. Mild effort dyspnea was noted. The patient felt depressed and irritable. Systemic hypertension was present for six years. An extra-uterine pregnancy, in 1976 had resulted in secondary sterility ; various pregnancy induction attempts were fruitless.

Clinical examination disclosed a systemic tension of 16/10 cm Hg and ankle edema. The nose and throat were normal on clinical examination. Static and dynamic lung volume were within normal limits according to our laboratory standards. Arterial blood gas levels determined while the patient was resting, awake and breathing room air were as follows : PaO_2 75 mm Hg ; $PaCO_2$ 41 mm Hg, arterial oxygen saturation (SaO_2), 95 %. Electrocardiography and echocardiography were normal. Chest Xray showed a borderline cardio-thoracic ratio. Hormonal screening at 7th day of cycle disclosed borderline low progesterone and elevated testosterone levels. The polysomnographic data are summarized in Table I.

Table I. SLEEP DATA

	Baseline	nCPAP
Total Sleep Time (TST ; min)	589	384
Stage I (% of TST)	18.51	7.81
II (% of TST)	58.91	29.69
III (% of TST)	4.92	9.90
IV (% of TST)	0	28.91
REM (% of TST)	16.81	22.92

There was a clear hypersomnia with numerous awakenings and short movements during sleep period. Stage IV was absent. Respiratory frequency was irregular, abnormally high (30-36 breaths/min), and increased with deepening of sleep. Loud snoring was continuous. There were no overt periodic variations in respiratory movements amplitude or aiflow ; for the whole night only 2 apneas were noted. SaO_2 recording was stable at 95-96 % when awake. In NREM sleep it fluctuated irregularly between 70 and 90 % and in REM sleep was as low as 60 %. Continuous positive airway pressure through the nose (nCPAP) was proposed. After 3 habituation nights, a control polysomnography was performed. Although shorter, sleep was stable and stage IV was abundant (Table 1). Breathing was now regular with a frequency of 26-27/min. Twelve isolated central apneas were noted. SaO2 was stable at 95 % when awake, 90-95 % in NREM sleep and 91-99 % in REM sleep. Home treatment was then began instituted. Follow-up at 1 and 4 months disclosed abolition of daytime sleepiness, quiet and recuperative sleep without snoring and excellent psychological. However when sleeping without nCPAP, snoring is still present. No significant weight loss or reduction of hypertension have been obtained until now.

DISCUSSION

We present a young, morbidly obese woman without cardio-pulmonary disease and with a clinical tableau of OSAS. Polysomnography disclosed polypnea with snoring, severe desaturation and multiple arousals but only 2 apneas, with no evidence of periodic hypopneas. All these sleep abnormalities were completely reversed by nCPAP.

In a thorough search of the literature on sleep-related respiratory disturbances in adults we did not find any similar observation. Indeed, in all cases of heavy snoring, clinical evidence of OSAS was associated with the presence of repeated apneas (Berry and Block, 1984, Lugaresi et al, 1983). The accepted criteria for the diagnosis of OSAS require the finding of more than 5 apneas per hour of sleep (Guilleminault et al, 1978). However, this definition of OSAS does not take into account the age-related changes in breathing during sleep (Berry et al, 1984) or the presence of incomplete airway obstruction episodes, i.e. hypopneas. Unfortunately, the definition of hypopneas varies widely among authors (Bliwise et al, 1984, Berry and Block, 1984). But even if hypopneas are taken into account our patient could not fit into this classification.
Snoring indicates some degree of decreased airway size and increased upper airway resistance. The passage from "simple" snoring to OSAS could be partly triggered, as suggested recently by Onal et al (1986), by periodic breathing with periodic changes in upper airway muscle tone. Our patient represents most probably a different mechanism, since snoring per se resulted in profound desaturations and hypoxia-induced arousals, leading to the same daytime consequences as true apneas or hypopneas. The unusal tachypnea might represent vagally-mediated rapid shallow breathing.
Snoring, apnea, hypopnea and oxygen desaturations show a strong male predominance, even in morbidly obese subjects (Block et al, 1979, Harman et al, 1981, Guilleminault et al, 1978). Interestingly, this woman had a borderline low progesterone and a high testosterone levels, that could have favored the appearance of snoring.

Berry and Block (1984) demonstrated that nCPAP eliminates snoring as well as obstructive sleep apnea. Complete reversal of sleep-related respiratory disturbance was also achieved in our patient.

CONCLUSION

Snoring without apnea can lead to a severe clinical condition, very similar to OSAS and completely reversible by nCPAP.

ACKNOWLEDGMENTS

The authors wish to acknowledge the expert technical and secreterial assistance of Mrs V. Franche.

REFERENCES

Berry, R.B, Block, A.J. (1984) : Positive nasal airway pressure eliminates snoring as well as obstructive sleep apnea. Chest 85, 15-20.
Berry, D.T.R., Webb, W.B., Block, A.J. (1984) : Sleep apnea syndrome. A critical review of the apnea index as a diagnostic criterion. Chest 86, 529-531.
Bliwise, D., Carskadon, M., Carey, E., Dement, W. (1984) : Longitudinal development of sleep-related respiratory disturbance in adult humans. J. Gerontol. 39, 290-293.
Block, A.J., Boysen, P.G., Wynne, J.W., Hunt, L.A. (1979) : Sleep apnea, hypopnea and oxygen desaturation in normal subjects. A strong male predominance. N. Engl. J. Med. 300, 513-517.
Guilleminault, C., van den Hoed, J., Mitler, M.M. : Clinical overview of sleep apnea syndrome. In Sleep Apnea Syndromes, eds Guilleminault C, Dement W.C : Alan R Liss, New-York, pp 1-12.
Harman, E, Wynne, J.W., Block, A.J., Malloy-Fisher, L. (1981) : Sleep disordered breathing and oxygen desaturation in obese patients. Chest 79, 256-260.
Lugaresi, E., Mondini, S., Zucconi, M., Montagna, P., Cirrignotta, F. (1983) : Staging of heavy snorers' disease. A proposal. Buil. Europ. Physiopath. Resp. 19, 590-594.
Onal, E., Burrows, D.L., Hart, R.H. and Lopata, M. (1986) : Induction of periodic breathing during sleep causes upper airway obstruction in humans. J. Appl. Physiol. 61, 1438-1443.
Rechtschaffen, A., Kales, A : A manual of standardized terminology, techniques and scoring system for sleep stages of human subjects. Los Angeles, UCLA, 1968.

RESUME : SYNDROME DES APNEES LIEES AU SOMMEIL SANS APNEE.

Une femme de 38 ans présente un syndrome évocateur d'apnées liées au sommeil (OSAS) : obésité (146 kg), ronflement bruyant, sommeil agité, somnolence diurne, modification de la personnalité et hypertension systémique. Une polysomnographie nocturne met en évidence une fréquence respiratoire de 35 respirations/min, un ronflement continu, mais seulement deux apnées pour l'ensemble de la nuit. Le stade IV est absent et les mouvements brefs sont nombreux. La saturation oxyhémoglobinique nocturne oscille de façon périodique entre 95 % et 70 % en sommeil NREM et entre 95 % et 60 % en sommeil REM. Une deuxième étude polygraphique, réalisée alors que la patiente reçoit de l'air sous pression positive continue par voie nasale (nCPAP) montre la disparition du ronflement, des désaturations, et de la fragmentation du sommeil ; le stade IV de sommeil est présent de façon abondante et la fréquence respiratoire est ralentie (26 respirations/min). Après un mois de traitement à domicile par nCPAP, la vigilance diurne est normalisée et les troubles de l'humeur ont disparu sans modification de l'obésité ni de l'hypertension artérielle. En conclusion, le ronflement sans apnée peut induire un tableau clinique en tous points identique à celui du OSAS ; la réponse au traitement par nCPAP est excellente. La place d'une telle observation dans la classification des troubles du sommeil est discutée.

The effects of alcohol on snoring-induced hypoxic events in males during the first 3 hours of sleep

P.G. Hartman, L. Scrima, D. Stedman and F.C. Hiller

Sleep Disorders Center – 594, University of Arkansas for Medical Sciences, 4301 W Markham Street, Little Rock, AR 72205, USA

Sixteen non-obese male snorers and 16 non-obese male non-snorers, all 30-50 years old, received trace amount, 0.4, 0.8, and 1.0 gm/kg of alcohol on non-consecutive nights in a Latin-square repeated-measures design. The alcohol was divided into 3 doses given within 1 hour, with ingestion completed 1/2 - 1 hr prior to bedtime. The table shows the number of hypoxic events ($SaO_2 \leq 92\%$) during the first 3 hrs of sleep at the 4 alcohol dose levels. The effect of alcohol dose on the frequency of hypoxic events during these 3 hrs was not significant for the snorers or non-snorers. Over the entire 3 hr period, snorers had significantly more hypoxic events (mean = 21.9) than non-snorers (mean = 8.2; $p < .02$). The snorers had significantly more hypoxic events than the non-snorers in the first and third hrs ($p < .02$, $p < .05$, respectively), and there was a trend for snorers to have more hypoxic events during the second hour ($p < .10$). The interaction between subject group (snorers versus non-snorers) and alcohol dose was not significant. Further analysis is underway to determine the effects of alcohol on hypoxic events and other respiration variables during each hr of sleep in these subjects. In addition, the experimental protocol is being performed on older males and obese males, who are at higher risk for snoring and hypoxic events during sleep.

HYPOXIC EVENTS ($SaO_2 \leq 92$) DURING SLEEP (MEANS $\pm$ SDs)

NON-SNORERS

Time Alcohol Dose:	trace	0.4 gm/kg	0.8 gm/kg	1.0 gm/kg
1st hour	2.1 ± 3.4	2.5 ± 5.5	0.6 ± 1.0	2.9 ± 4.4
2nd hour	3.3 ± 11.2	4.2 ± 11.8	1.3 ± 2.9	4.2 ± 8.0
3rd hour	4.9 ± 8.1	1.8 ± 5.7	2.7 ± 4.5	2.1 ± 3.3
1st three hours	10.4 ± 20.9	8.5 ± 18.5	4.6 ± 4.9	9.2 ± 11.3

SNORERS

Time Alcohol Dose:	trace	0.4 gm/kg	0.8 gm/kg	1.0 gm/kg
1st hour	4.4 ± 8.6	7.1 ± 9.4	10.5 ± 16.0	9.8 ± 13.9
2nd hour	7.4 ± 17.8	6.6 ± 6.9	10.1 ± 15.8	6.2 ± 9.0
3rd hour	4.9 ± 10.5	9.4 ± 11.9	5.9 ± 8.8	5.2 ± 7.4
1st three hours	16.8 ± 35.4	23.1 ± 24.6	26.5 ± 33.8	21.1 ± 26.0

Supported by grant AA06700 from the National Institute on Alcohol Abuse and Alcoholism

Effects of alcohol on snoring in men ages 30-50

L. Scrima, P. Hartman, F. Johnson, D. Stedman and F.C. Hiller

Sleep Disorders Center – 594, University of Arkansas for Medical Sciences, 4301 W Markham Street, Little Rock, AR 72205, USA

Snoring may reflect the degree of obstruction in the upper airway and can help in identifying those who have obstructive sleep apnea (OSA) or who are at risk of developing OSA. Using a repeated measures design, we are evaluating the effects of 4 doses of evening-ingested alcohol (trace, .4, .8, & 1.0 gm/kg body wt) on respiration and arterial oxygen saturation during polygraphically recorded sleep in 128 male snorers and non-snorers between the ages of 30 and 70. One hypothesis that we are testing is that alcohol increases snoring quantity and loudness as a function of dose and age.

To objectively differentiate snorers from non-snorers (classification was based on a screen PSG) and measure loudness and frequency of snoring, we used a wideband AC preamplifier and an integrator with DC driver amplifier to convert magnetic microphone output (suspended 18" over the bed) to a pen tracing on a Grass polygraph, calibrated in decibles (1).

The table shows the number of minutes of snoring at the 4 alcohol doses for 11 non-obese snorers and 4 non-obese non-snorers, all 30-49 years old. The effect of alcohol dose on snoring was not significant in these subjects. The experiment is continuing with testing of subjects at higher risk for snoring and hypoxic events, namely, obese males and males 50 to 70 years of age.

SNORING IN MINUTES

SNORERS

Alcohol dose:	TRACE	0.4	0.8	1.0
S#				
1	70.0	44.0	32.3	74.7
2	55.3	0.0	0.0	13.7
3	69.0	102.3	105.3	5.0
4	75.3	48.7	63.3	56.0
5	36.3	34.3	201.0	43.3
6	58.3	1.3	0.0	85.3
7	0.0	0.0	22.7	58.7
8	110.7	*	107.3	130.7
9	4.3	37.7	67.3	97.7
10	199.3	156.3	131.7	244.0
11	61.3	1.0	94.0	75.7
MEAN	67.3	42.6	75.0	80.4
SD	53.9	51.3	61.2	65.0

NON-SNORERS

Alcohol dose:	TRACE	0.4	0.8	1.0
S#				
1	51.0	81.0	20.7	70.3
2	0.0	0.0	5.3	0.0
3	4.3	17.0	0.0	0.3
4	34.7	19.0	75.0	22.0
MEAN	22.5	29.2	25.2	23.2
SD	24.5	35.5	34.3	33.1

* On this night, snoring was not recorded

1. Johnson, F.H. Jr., Scrima, L., Thomas, E. E., Stedman, D., & Hiller, F.C. (1986). Calibrated snoring polysomnogram system. Sleep Res 15: 132.

Research supported by grant AA6700 from the National Institute of Alcohol Abuse and Alcoholism.

The velo-impedancemetry — a new technique for dynamic study of soft palate

C.H. Chouard, B. Meyer and F. Chabolle

Hôpital Saint-Antoine, Service ORL, 184 rue du faubourg Saint-Antoine, 75012 Paris, France

SUMMARY :

We designed a device for soft palate movements registration, using a slightly modified electro-glottograph. Correlating such curves with corresponding phonogram and physio-pathogical data, we have been able to define an iconographic semiology, which may be useful in the functional pathology of the soft palate and indications of uvulo-pharyngo-plasty for snoring.

KEYWORDS :

Soft Palate - Registration - Impedance -

The soft palate is the main cause of chronic snoring whatever would be the stage of the chronic rhonchopathy (Chouard et al 1986). Trying to understand how does the soft palate vibrate during snoring whatever would be the mouth aperture, we designed a system which uses a slightly modified electro glottograph, allowing to obtain a curve, that we called velo-impedance-gram (VIG). It represents some features of the morphological modalities of the rhino-pharyngeal isthmus closure.

As an illustration of th possibilities and limits of this technic, we shall expose the results which we have yet described (CHOUARD et al 1987) and which we obtained in the field of snoring which we specially studied. But VIG may be currently obtained and worthwile in most cases of the various pathology of the soft palate.

MATERIAL AND METHOD

A - THE DEVICE The goal of the system is to study the tissues impedance variations when closing the rhinopharyngeal isthmus. It directly derives from the electoglottograph. It consists in a source of 0.5 volt, 10 milliamperes, 300 kilohertz current which is delivered between two electrodes. These two electrodes (auto adhesives standard electroencephalography electrodes) are pasted on the skin of the medial part of hyoid bone and forehead. These impedance variations do not greatly overpass 300 ohms. They are stored and plotted as a function of time. During the test the emitted sound - which we call sonogram - is simultaneously registrated owing to a microphone placed at 30 cm before the patient's lips. This position allows to estimate that there is a delay between the sound signal and the registration of the VIG. This delay is of about 1,5 msec in case of laryngeal sound, and 1,3 msec in case of pharyngeal sound. Sonogram and VIG are monitorized on a scope and stored on magnetic tape before graphic representation (Fig. 1).

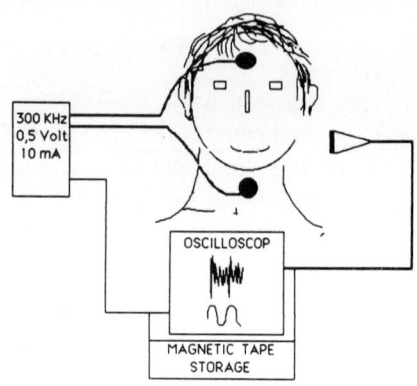

Fig. 1 - Schema of the velo-impedance-graph.

B - THE TEST PROCEDURE A registration of snoring during sleep, or in recumbent position, can be performed. But usually the patient is awake. Sitting on a chair he is asked either trying to perform a voluntary snoring (owing to a noisy inspiratory sniffing), or to precisely articulate a series of quickly pronounced nasal syllabs. The quality of the curves is overseen on the scope during storage.

Using this procedure we have performed 259 VIG in various circumstances (Table I).

TABLE I. *Origins of the 259 studied VIG UPPP = Uvulopharyngoplasty (M = Male ; F = Female)*

	SNORER N = 171				NON SNORER N = 88			
	effective registration		impossible registration		effective registration		impossible registration	
	M	F	M	F	M	F	M	F
Voluntary snoring	63	17	6	12	25	20	4	8
Sleeping snoring	9	2						
Post UPP voluntary snoring	3		21	5				
Nasal syllab	24	7			7	6		
soft palate various pathogy voluntary snoring	1				1	1	4	3
nasal syllab	1				1	1	4	3
TOTAL	101	26	27	17	34	28	12	14

TABLE II. *Correlation of the VIG types and various data in case of voluntary snoring in snorer group.*
Pharynx : Hertz = VIG frequency ; left column : < 30 Hertz ; middle column : <=30 Hertz and > =50 Hertz ; right column : > 50 Hertz. Corp = corpulence (see in text) Neck : N = normal ; S = shortness. Retrog : retrognathia absent (0) or present (+) Tongue : N = normal ; / = hypertrophied. Tonsil : 0 + absent or very small ; / = present and hypertrophied PP : posterior pillars ; 0 = small and thin ; / = large and or thick SP = soft palate ; 0 = normal ; / hypertrophied in size or thickness U = Uvula ; 0 = normal ; / hypertrophied in length and or in thickness. VIG : R = round shape ; M = multipeak ; D = double peak.

Pharynx	Sex		Hertz			Corp		Neck		Retrog	
VIG (N=80)	M	F	<30	<=>	>50	-	+	N	S	0	+
R (N=26) 32%	21	5	2	14	10	8	18	14	12	18	8
M (N=14) 18%	13	1	5	8	1	7	7	13	1	12	2
D (N=40) 50%	29	11	4	25	11	38	2	39	1	37	3
TOTAL	63	17	15	40	25	53	27	66	14	67	13
%	79	21	19	50	31	67	33	82	18	84	16

TABLE II (Suite)

Tongue		Tonsil.		PP		SP		U	
N	/	0	/	0	/	0	/	0	/
14	12	17	9	13	13	20	6	18	8
7	7	11	3	6	8	6	8	4	10
37	3	35	5	10	30	12	28	32	8
58	22	63	17	2	5	38	42	54	26
72%	28%	79%	21%	36%	64%	48%	52%	68%	33%

TABLE III. *Correlation of the VIG types and various data in case of voluntary snoring in snorer group.*
Pharynx ; Hertz = VIG frequency ; left column : < 30 Hertz ; middle column : <=30 Hertz and > =50 Hertz ; right column : > 50 Hertz. Corp = corpulence (see in text) Neck : N = normal ; S = shortness. Retrog : retrognathia absent (0) or present (+) Tongue : N = normal ; / = hypertrophied. Tonsil : 0 + absent or very small ; / = present and hypertrophied PP ; posterior pillars ; 0 = small and thin ; / = large and or thick SP = soft palate ; 0 = normal ; / hypertrophied in size or thickness U = Uvula ; 0 = normal ; / hypertrophied in length and or in thickness. VIG : R = round shape ; M = multipeak ; D = double peak.

Pharynx	Sex		Hertz			Corp		Neck		Retrog		Tongue		Tonsil.		PP		SP		U	
VIG (N=45)	M	F	<30	<=>50		−	+	N	S	0	+	N	/	0	/	0	/	0	/	0	/
R (N=11) 24%	4	7	1	7	3	5	6	7	4	9	2	5	6	5	6	10	1	11	0	11	0
M (N=10) 22%	5	5	2	5	3	8	2	9	1	9	1	8	2	8	2	8	2	9	1	10	0
D (N=24) 45%	16	8	6	12	6	22	2	23	1	24	0	23	1	20	4	22	2	22	2	23	1
TOTAL	25	20	9	24	12	35	10	39	6	42	3	36	9	33	12	40	5	42	3	44	1
%	56	44	20	53	27	78	22	87	13	93	7	80%	20%	71%	27%	89%	11%	93%	7%	98%	2%

Snorer group consists in patients pre operatively examined before uvulo palato plasty for severe snoring. Non-snorer group consists in normal and married voluntary patients whithout any complain of snoring from spouse. The anatomical features of the rhino pharyngeal isthmus of each patient have been clinically assessed by the approximative measurement (binary quoted) of the main factors of snoring : corpulence, retrognathia, neck shortness, size of tonsills, size of tonsills posterior pillars, size of soft palate, and size of uvula. Corpulence (C) has been quantified using the Ducimetiere's formula : if P = size in cm, and T = weight in gram, $C = 1000 \times \text{Log } P/T$. The value of C may be considered as normal if $C = 404 +/- 51$. In our assessment C has been considered as positive when it was $>= 455$.

Artificial snoring and nasal syllab have been also registrated after uvulo palato plasty in order to verify the efficacy of the operation. Sound of singing vowell A, of various frequencies, have been also studied in order to detect the eventual simultaneous registration of the glottogram.

RESULTS

A - THE VIG DURING SNORING

One must underline that in about 20 % of cases the voluntary snoring is impossible ; this percentage is approximatively the same in snorer and non snorer groups. The males competences in the achievement of this artificial symptom is very much better than the females possibilities. There is no other correlation between this competence and any data concerning age or anatomical features. In these cases the registration of uneffective attempts for snoring supplied us with only anarchic and insignificant diagram.

In its typical aspects the VIG of spontaneous or voluntary snoring consists in a succession of regular curves oscillating between high and low parts of the diagram, which correspond with the high and low impedance values. These values do not greatly vary from one test or one patient to the other; they are generally in scale of 300 -100 Ohms.

The shape of this curve greatly varies from one patient to another, but it is always the same for one patient as far as soring is correctly performed. One may describe 3 types of VIG: a) the type R (Round) is in sinusoidal and almost symetric shape; b) the type M (Multipeak) is less regular ans presents several and soft inflexions; c) the type D (Double peak) presents one or two acute peaks; its curve frequently consists in almost horizontal then almost vertical portions; its amplitude is generally more important than in case of type R.

The correlation between these 3 types and frequency of VIG, sex, corpulence and anatomical features of the rhinoparyngeal isthmus allows to consider the type M as an intermediar aspect between type R and type D. On may note that there is no difference in the type of the VIG between the snorer ans non-snorer status (respectively R = 32%, 24%, ; M = 18%, 22% ; D = 50%, 45%). In the snorer group, high frequency of D-type curve is found when corpulence and pharyngeal morphology are normal (D between 55% and 71%) except if we consider the normal size of posterior pillars, and soft palate (respectively 34% and 32%). In this case, R-typer curver are a little more frequent.

But in cases of anormal corpulence and pharyngeal morphology, we may notice a reverse of frequency. However in consideration of the too poor population we could not statistically correlate the association of different items. In the other hand the size of posterior pillars, soft palate and uvula appears to be responsible for the difference between snorer and non-snorer groups.

The VIG is generally accompanyed with parallel oscillations of the sonogram, the peaks of which appear approximatively 1,5 msec later than the VIG low impedance value peaks. However the features of these oscillations vary with the VIG types. In type R and type M the sound is more continuous than in type D, and sometimes it is not easy to identify the sonogram peaks. In type D the sonogram peaks are evident; moreover accessory peaks frequently accompagn the VIG low impedance peak or accessory peak, specially in snorer group.

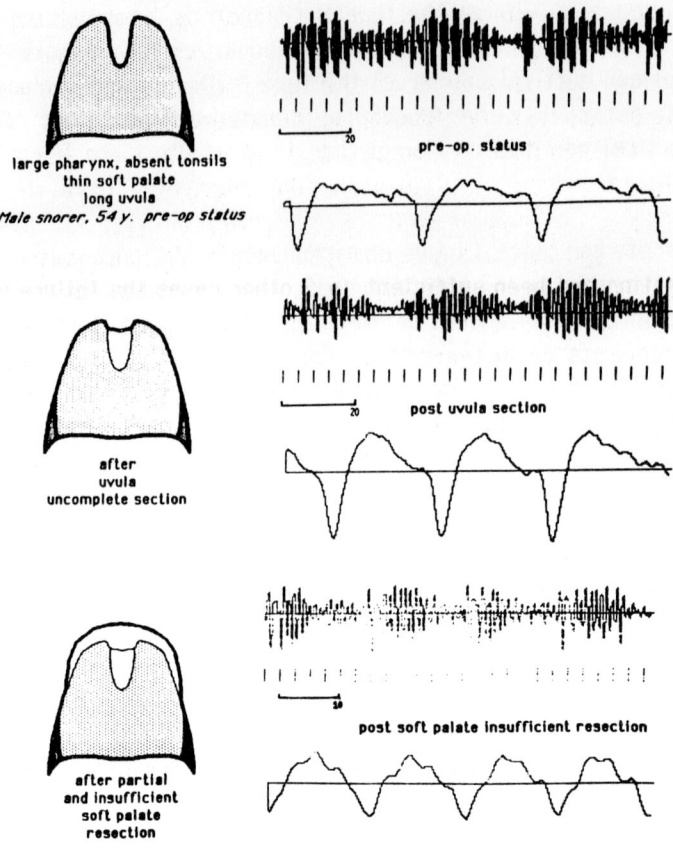

Fig. 2. Successive VIG of voluntary snoring of a snorer male, 54 y. Who supported two unsuccessful operations for snoring.
Bar = 20 msec ; upper lign = sonogram ; lower lign = VIG ; the upper part of the VIG corresponds with high impedance values, it means rhinopharyngeal isthmus aperture. The magnitude of these impedance variations is approximatively 300 ohms, but cannot be precisely determined in ordinate.
A = pre-operative ; B = after uncomplete uvulectomy ; C = after partial uvulo palato plasty.

One may underline that the features of the VIG only slightly vary with the recumbent position. During sleep the frequency increases, but the type of the VIG does not really change. On the contrary these features are greatly modified after uvulo pharyngo plasty. In most case artificial snoring is impossible; the irregular noise of the inspiratory sniffing and the small irregularities of an almost linear VIG may only be registrated. In few cases the surgery has not been totally successful. In 3 of them the voluntary snoring could not be registrated because the relative failure of the operation - it means the residual sleeping respiratory noise - was due to the presence of retrognathia and tongue hypertrophia: in these cases the soft palate resection had been sufficient. In 2 other cases the failure was due to the unsufficient resection of the soft palate, and the voluntary snoring and its specific aspect on VIG could be obtained. One of these 2 cases is particularly demonstrative, which is the case of a patient who feared the consequences of a too resection.

He successively supported a partial uvula section (whithout any improvement of his sleeping snoring), then a too partial and uncomplete uvulo palato plasty, which uncompletely improved his spontaneous snoring. The different aspects of the corresponding succession of VIG illustrate (Fig. 2) the anatomical changes of his rhino pharyngeal isthmus.

This patients had a large and normal pharynx ; his pre-operative VIG was type D. The partial uvulectomia changed slightly the shape of the peaks, without changing his VIG type. The partial uvula palato plasty results in several in several and soft inflexions (type M), as a consequence of the suppression of the uvula and of the medial and hypertrophied part of the soft palate, but the diagram amplitude remained large. For this patient the anatomical and complete closure of the isthmus is always possible, but necessitates now a more important participation of the whole set of the nasa pharyngeal isthmus organs. That explains the large amplitude of his VIG, but explains also why his wife stil describes a slight and intermittent residual sleeping snoring.

The VIG of a non snorer female could be registrated prior and after tonsillectomy. The differences between the 2 diagrams consists in a change of the type of the VIG (Fig. 3).

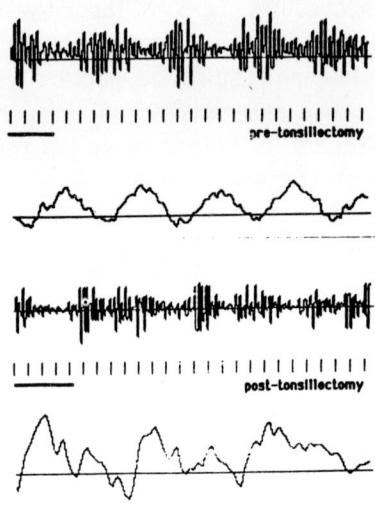

Fig. 3. Non snorer female VIG prior (type R) and after tonsillectomy (type M). Same legend as Fig. 2. Singing of phonem A at hight frequency (upper VIG) and low frequency (lower VIG). Same legend as Fig. 2.

B - THE VIG DURING PHONEMS PRONOUNCIATION

In case of nasal syllabe, a single and large oscillation appears on the VIG on the begining of the phonem emission. Despite its duration is longer, its general shape is approximatively the same than in case of snoring. The particular features of some phonems may be described Fig. 4 et 5.

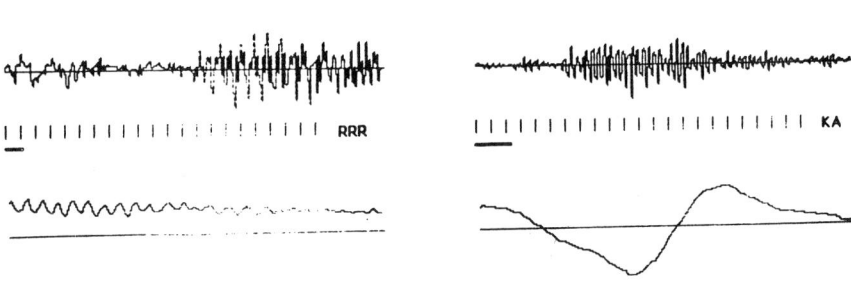

Fig. 4. VIG of phonems RRR, without any laryngeal emission. Same legends as Fig. 2. After the large initial inflexion (no represented on the picture), a succession of small oscillations on the same frequency than the emitted rolling sound.

Fig. 5. VIG of phonems KA. Same legend as Fig. 2. Only one principal oscillation is obtained presenting or not small oscillations on approximatively the same rythm as the sonogram all along the duration of the emission of the phonem A following the phonem K.

In case of nasal phonems pronounciation after uvulo palato plasty, the first large oscillation of the VIG preceding the small variation is in round shape which could be described as type R.

In case of vowells pronounciation the VIG. Becomes almost linear, or it presents very small variations. The study of the VIG successively obtained through the emission of singing phonem A at low then high frequency demonstrates that these small variations are generally without correlation with the frequency of the laryngeal sound. However, during some ten milliseconds the rythm of the 2 phenomenons may be the same (Fig. 6).

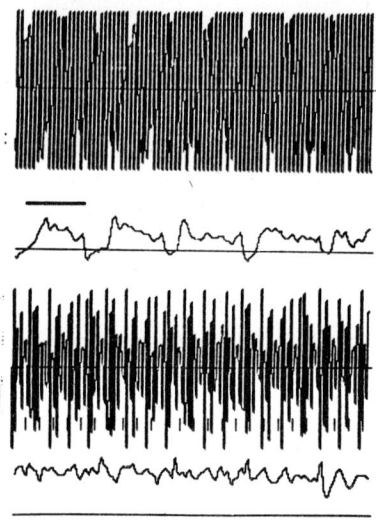

Fig. 6. Singing of phonem A at high frequency (upper VIG) and low frequency (lower VIG). Same legend as Fig. 2.

DISCUSSION AND COMMENTARIES

1) The position of the electrodes does not seem perfect, because the naso pharyngeal isthmus is not directly in the the field designed by the electrodes position we described. We tried several variable - lateral or sagittal - set placements. Hyoid and bregma location is the only set which allowed to obtain VIG of approximatively the same quality; but we must underline that this bregma position frequently prohibits the easy use of auto adhesive electrodes.

2) Does VIG represent the glottogram variations, too ? The general amplitude of the glottogram we currently obtain owing to the same device is due to an impedance variation the scale of which is very narrower (5-10 Ohms). Moreover the electric field designed by these forhead and hyoid electrodes does not anatomically contain the vocal cords. Nevertheless one may ask if the VIG small oscillations we described during the pronounciation of phonem containing laryngeal sound are not the expression of additional glottogram. In fact these oscillations are not constant, and they may be considered as the expression of a passive vibration of the soft palate due to the pressure variations of the supra laryngeal and pharyngeal air column.

3) Regarding the correlation of morphological data and various types of VIG, one may criticize the subjective appreciation of most of the anatomical measurements of the pharynx. However a numerical and pseudo precize measurement of these data would have contained a large risk of errors. Moreover the binary measurement we used decreases the importance of this objection.

4) An other important problem is to exactly know what the VIG represents. First of all it seems logical to consider that low and high impedance values of the VIG correspond with closure and aperture of the naso pharyngeal isthmus. But if the VIG variations represent the movements of the rhino-pharyngeal isthmus, it is not evident that they represent only the soft palate movements. In case of narrow pharynx (burgundish pharynx) the generally round aspect of the curve (type R) may be interpreted as the fact that closure and aperture of the isthmus are progressively and regularly obtained owing to a simultaneous action of all its components ; this fact

suggests that not only the soft palate movements, but also the pharynx diameter changes, and perhaps the hypertrophied tongue shifting are responsible for the VIG design.

The narrowness of the pharynx and of the isthmus is probably objectived by the relative low amplitude of the VIG type R. On the contrary in case of large and normal pharynx, the presence in the VIG of a succession of almost horizontal then almost vertical portions suggests that the movements of the different hypertrophied parts of the soft palate are responsible for these irregular changes of the impedance. The study of the successive VIG of some patients who have been registrated prior then after pharynx surgery (uvulo palato pharyngoplasty or tonsillectomy) seems to confirm this hypothesis. That is especially the case of our almost experimental patient, who supported two unsuccessful operations for snoring. This patients had a large and normal pharynx; his pre-operative VIG was type D.

The partial uvulectomia changed slightly the shape of the peaks, without changing his VIG type. The partial uvula palato plasty made his VIG almost round, but the diagram amplitude remained large. The peaks disappearance is probably due to the suppression of the posterior pilars, of the uvula and of the medial and hypertrophied part of the soft palate. For this patient the anatomical and complete closure of the isthmus is always possible, but necessitates now a more important participation of the whole set of the nasa pharyngeal isthmus organs. That explains the large amplitude of his VIG, but explains also why his wife still describes a slight and intermittent residual sleeping snoring.

5) We cannot take in count the types of curves in relation with each pharyngeal morphology. The association of two or more abnormalities would be statistically studied and need a more numerous population. However by comparing normal clinical examination and type of curve, it appears that D-type is very frequent. So, VIG can contribute to determine the importance of the surgical resection for caring snoring.

In cases of D-type VIG, the surgical resection can remove the sole soft palate and superior part of posterior pillar. On the contrary in cases of R-type VIG, very often associated with hypertrophy of the pharyngeal walls, the surgical procedure must be larger, too concerning the lateral part of pharynx (tonsillis and muscular constrictors) and perhaps the tongue in some cases of sleep apnea syndrome.

But VIG does not help us to know what is the correct height of soft palate to be removed. The flexion point of soft palate when pronouncing vowell A as the upper limit of the resection was suggested by M.F. Colman. We totaly agree with his proposition.

6) When a pre operative registration of the voluntary snoring has been possible, the post-operative feature of the VIG must be also discussed and commented. In the first post operative weeks no voluntary snoring is possible, and in most cases this impossibility is definitive. These cases correspond with a successful operation; clinically one may observ that the isthmus closure is obtained by a thin and linear contact of the residual soft palate on the pharyngeal posterior wall. But in a few cases a very slight snoring reappears after 3 or 4 months, and voluntary snoring and its registration become again possible; in these cases the isthmus closure is obtained through a large surface contact of the soft palate and pharyngeal wall. The post operative tissues stiffness explains this initial success of this unsufficient soft palate resection. But when after some months the tissues become again perfectly flexible, one may understand why a slight snoring may be sometimes achieved. In the other hand a non negligeable percentage of these residual respiratory sleeping noise - post operatively described by by about 20 % of our patients - is due to a nasal obstruction, the etiology of which could not have been surgically suppressed (especially allergic rhinitis). In these cases the impossibility for the patient to realize a voluntary snoring VIG may be worthwile to demonstrate that this relative failure is not due to an unsufficient soft palate resection.

CONCLUSION

Regarding the velo impedancemetry applications in case of surgery for chronic snoring one must not forget that about 20 % of patients are unable to perform this voluntary snoring. Presently this impossibility decreases the interest of this method in the daily practice of uvulo palato plasty for snoring, because it makes necessary a sleeping registration.

However the velo impedancemetry is able to supply the physician with a graphic representation of the rhinopharyngeal isthmus movements which will be perhaps interesting in some particular circumstances, mainly in case of phoniatric troubles. Indeed a lot of complementary studies are necessary, especially for improving the registration of the fast and non repetitive displacements of the soft palate during speech. But in the next future one may think that the possibilties of this new technic will be usefull for the E.N.T. specialists or speech therapists.

REFERENCES

1) CHOUARD C.H., VALTY J., MEYER B., CHABOLLE F., FLEURY B., VERICEL R., LACCOURREYE O. and JOSSET P. - La Rhonchopathie Chronique ou ronflement: aspects cliniques et indications thérapeutiques. Ann.Oto.Laryng. (Paris) - 1986 - 103; 319-327.

2) CHOUARD C.H., MEYER B., CHABOLLE F.
The velo impedancemetry.
Acta Otolaryngol. 1987 - 103; 537-545

3) COLMAN M.F. and RICE D.H. - A method of determining the correct amount of palatal resection in palatopharyngoplasty - Laryngoscope - 1985 - 95; 609-610.

4) DEJEAN Y., CRAMPETTE L., BILLIARD M. and GROSS F. - Intérêt de l'examen ORL dans le syndrome des apnées du sommeil. Traitement chirurgical et indications. Les Cahiers Français d'ORL (Montpellier) - 1985 - 20; 571-584

5) DUCIMETIERE P., RICHARD J., CLAUDE J.R. and WARNET J.M. - Les cardiopathies ischémiques: incidence et facteurs de risque. INSERM Edit. Paris - 1981 - 235p.

Snoring of nasal origin by vibrations of the salpingoseptal fold

Vincent Bouton

CMC Les Fontaines, 77007 Melun Cedex, France

SUMMARY

Relatively unknown, the salpingo-septal fold participates in the anatomy of the choana, stretched from the external wall of the nasal fossa to the posterior region of the septum.
In low position or ptosis, this fold receives the turbinal air-flow, which makes it vibrate, creating a nasal snoring. The author describes the subject with a short video projection.

KEYWORDS

Salpingo-septal fold, nasal snoring.

INTRODUCTION

The salpingo-nasal fold or, more precisely, the salpingo-septal fold, is absent from classic anatomical descriptions.
It is however present in the descriptive anatomy of the naso-pharynx, written by LEGENT, PERLEMUTER and VAN DEN BROUCKE.
"The upper wall of the naso-pharynx corresponds with the occipital bone or the base of the occiput, and the adjacent part of the sphenoid bone, hollowed out by the sphenoid sinuses.
Towards the front, the superior wall continues, either side of the nasal septum with the roof of the nasal fossae, separated from it by the salpingo-nasal fold".

DESCRIPTION

The salpingo-nasal fold is a mucous falciform band, stretched from either side of the nasal septum to the external border of the choana, at the level of the tubal orifices.
This fold, by its internal insertion, takes part in the dynamics of the soft palate.
It is fastened to the postero-superior face of the soft palate aponevrosis, contributing to the formation of the median raphe of the soft palate with the internal fibers of the petrostaphylinus.
Two tracts are discovered, one anterior, the other posterior. The external insertions of these two tracts diverge inside, with a maximum at the top of the fold convexity. Then, the two tracts come closer and join in the nasal septum.

These two tracts, falciform, are brought together by a loose mucous pons.
In a high that is to say normal position, this fold does not receive the turbinal air-flow but the olfactory sulcus air-flow in a minimal amount.

CONNECTIONS

We are essentially going to describe the connections with the naso-pharynx walls.
Above : - the occipital corps or base of occiput and the adjacent part of the sphenoide bone hollowed out by the sphenoid sinuses.
Outward : - the naso-pharynx lateral wall in its upper part on top of the pharyngal superior constrictor muscle and the peristaphyline muscle aponevrosis. The relation zone of the salpingo-septal fold internal insertions is, at this level, the supra tubal fossa.
Behind : - the gland of LUSCHKA.
Inside : - the posterior boundary of the nasal septum delimited by the vomer bone pressed on the horizontal lamina of the palatine where the soft palate is inserted.
In the free boundary of the fold is a salpingo-septal pedicle, anastomosis between the external and internal branches of the naso-palatin pedicle.

PHYSIOLOGY

The physiology of the salpingo-septal fold is, of course, as rarely described as its anatomy. Owing to its anatomic position, and its orientation in the nasal fossa, and according to the observed disorders, it seems that this fold could act on the Eustachian tube in synchronism with the petrostaphylinus.
In a high or normal position, it participates accessorily in the opening of the Eustachian tube at the top and to the front when the petrostaphylinus dilates the Eustachian tube, deporting behind and inside the posterior tubal labium. Thus, it works as a passive elevator of the palate ; or more exactly : it participes in palate elevation by the intermediary of its soft palate fastening close to the median raphe petrostaphylinus insertions.
In a low position or ptasis and in its bifid configuration (in two tracts), the salpingo-septal fold receives a part of the turbinal air-flow which makes it vibrate. It well seems to appear out of our observations, that the production of snoring must be due, not only to the fold ptosis, but principally to the disposition of its two tracts.
These two conditions have to be brought together : the two mucosa bands are made to vibrate one against the other, creating the nasal snoring when the turbinal air flow passes through.
In a low position or ptosis, the salpingo-septal fold no longer plays a part in the opening of the Eustachian tube, which may explain a certain degree of tubal pathology among some of our patients.
Or, on the contrary, because of a strong nocturnal sollicitation of the fold, a permanent opening of the Eustachian tube can sometimes inconvenience the patients (one case).

STUDY MATERIAL

We report five cases of snoring of nasal origin with bilateral ptosis of the salpingo-septal fold, and four cases with unilateral ptosis, once on the right side and three times on the left side. These numbers are still not very high because of the recent discovery in the snoring disease of this etiopathogeny on the one hand and that it seemed otherwise preferable to us to put aside all the documents in which another nasal cause of snoring had been found :
- septal deviation
- turbinal pathology...

In three cases a buccal cause of snoring was found (indicating an associated surgery).
The patients's origin is variable, one of the men is Canadian, one of the women is from the south of France. The seven others live in the Paris region.
The average age is thirty five years, no tobacco intoxication, neither ethylism no general disorders associated.

MEANS OF STUDY

To make the role of the salpingo-septal fold obvious in the snoring genesis of these patients, beyond the usual anamnestic information, the usual clinic data and the phonic nocturnal registration, we used the endonasal fibroscopy with video-camera coupled, fixed on the optic fibre. We asked our patients, during this video, to have a forced nasal breathing in a supine position or Andral's decubitus.

RESULTS

These patients consulted on their own initiative or on the family's request, for snoring with, most often, the mouth closed and not ceasing in Andral's decubitus or in ventral decubitus as is the case in other snoring causes.
A phonic record on cassette is requested to confirm the patient's assertions and verify the abscence of nocturnal respiratory pauses, lately tested by oxymetry and the way snoring commences.
The pharyngeal disease on waking is the second functional sign of which the patients complain, predominant sign with three of them with the sensation of a dry throat posterior pharyngeal scraping, with short hacking cough, dry cough, dysphagia, thus justifying consultation.
Often, these signs disappear in the morning mostly after the first morning drink. This pharyngeal symptomatology is often associated with a tubal symptomatology : sensation of deafness or scratching or crackling in one or both ears. Sometimes a real otalgia (two cases) may exist with the notion of nocturnal or morning recrudescence.
Clinical examination shows a clean throat, a clean pharynx without infection, no tumor. If the soft palate seems to be heavy with a big uvula, even if it is evocative of a snoring disease, this must not satisfy the examiner too quickly.
Ear-drums are examined with the microscope researching a peripheric inflammation, a retraction (five cases) but never serous effusion. Sometimes, the tympanogram is abnormal (one case) showing ear-drum hyperlaxity. No real deafness is found.

Finally, we did not find any permanent dysphagia, or disphonia or chronic dyspnea in our observations.
The fibroscopic examination of nasal fossa shows the salpingo-septal fold ptosis uni or bilaterally.
This fibroscopic examination must systematically be carried out in any case of snoring disease, especially if it occurs with a closed mouth.
We also noticed during this fibroscopic examination abundant secretions on the salpingo-septal fold which receives the flow of secreted substances from the superior meatus. With the film study, one can see the vibrations of both tracts, appearing in supine position or Andral's decubitus.
An evaluation of the ptosis degree is made with the tailend of the concha nasalis media used as a mark. These vibrations are essentially produced by an inspiratory movement. With it a certain degree of vibration on the dorsal side of the soft palate can be observed.

DISCUSSION

In view of such a pathology, the question is : what kind of treatment to prescribe.
Which kind of attitude to have knowing that uvulo palato plasty will not modify
the rhinologic causes of the snoring disease.
Theoretically, the aim is the stretching of salpingo-septal fold.
The most easy way to reach in this goal is to do a simple vertical section to stop
the vibrations.
But my aim is not to discuss the treatment, it is to submit to your proficiency
this new etiopathogeny of snoring disease.

CONCLUSION

Each of us must know the possibility of a ptosis of the salpingo-septal fold when
faced with a nasal snoring disease, and must check the soft palate mobility by
fiberendoscopy each such case. During this fibroscopic examination we must think
to analyse the fold, appreciate its position, normal or ptosis, its particular
aspect with both tracts and their vibrations during nasalforced inspiratory in
supine position.

RESUME

Relativement méconnu, le ligament salpingo-septal participe à la formation de
la choane. Tendu de la paroi externe de la fosse nasale à la zone postérieure
du septum, il sépare vers le haut la partie supérieure de la fosse nasale et
la paroi supérieure du cavum. En situation basse, ptosé ou distendu, ce
ligament reçoit une partie du flux turbinal inspiratoire qui le met en vibration, créant un ronflement nasal dont l'auteur fait une description étayée par
une projection vidéo, après un bref rappel anatomique.

Chronic rhonchopathy. Ed. C.H. Chouard. © 1988, John Libbey Eurotext Ltd. pp.181-184.

The endoscopic examination of voluntary snoring

E. Truffer

Special ENT, N-D des Marais 1, CH-3960 Sierre, Switzerland

SUMMARY

Endoscopic examination of voluntary snoring permits direct visualisation of vibrating structures which are at the origin of this sound phenomenon. The description of the instrumentation and methods shows that this procedure does not need any special preparation and can be effected with routine ENT equipment. It enables the pre-operatory assessment of the amount of tissular resection necessary to the suppression of the snore, thus preventing such sequellae as open rhinolalia and nasal regurgitation. Finally, it enhances our understanding of physiological snoring in sleep inducing original hypothesis, not yet verified, on possible cardio-pulmonary and cerebral repercussions and on the origin of the apnea sleep syndrom.

KEYWORDS

Endoscopy, snoring, vibrations, voluntary, velic, pharnygeal.

INTRODUCTION

In this age of ecological triumph, it is almost inevitable that at some point attention should begin to focus on that major, though admittedly intimate, source of acoustic pollution, the snore. A breaker-up of couples and families and, to boot, the root of cardio-pulmonary disorders and brain deterioration, it is cause for wonder that snoring has for so long escaped the vigilant scrutiny of the medical sciences. Over the last few years, however, things have begun to change and this phenomenon has now become a terrain visited by explorers from every walk of medical life: cadiologists, pneumologists, sleep and brain physiologists, and, we hardly need add, the otorhinolaryngologists. For the latter speciality, whose prime focus of activity is none other than the very seat of the phenomenon itself, makes possible the visual exploration of snoring, thanks to the equipment employed in rhino-sinusal endoscopy.

It should be understood that the object of this paper is not the physiological act of spontaneous snoring during sleep but the active, deliberate and voluntary version of that act in the waking state. Admittedly voluntary snoring fails to reproduc all the conditions present during physiological snoring: there is a difference in the moistness of the mucous membranes which may modify the kinetic behaviour of the structures responsible for snoring, and an absence of the apnea syndrom which it is impossible to reproduce in the waking state, etc... It is nonetheless true that a study of induced snoring does provide a clear view of the action of the structures whose vibration gives rise to the sound in question. This study is in fact the study of the voluntary velic snoring.

EQUIPMENT

In this exercise we make use of Hopkins telescopic stems as manufactured by Storz. sinuscopical purposes. These are 3 and 4 mms in diameter, 23 cms long and are connected by a fibre-glass cord to a cold-light source. The optical axes employed are: $0°$, $/0°$ and $120°$. An anti-mist and antispetic solution is used to keep the optical equipment clean. (dia 1)

A contact anesthetic with an added constrictor facilitates introduction of the stems into the nasal fossae and the back of the mouth. With very nervous patients an oral tranquiliser may be used and should be administered 20 minutes before commencement of the examination.

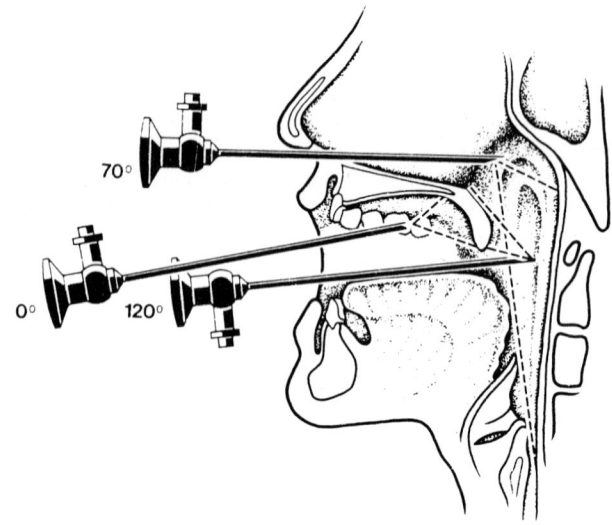

Fig. : Field of vision of optical instruments. (dia 2)

METHOD

The patient is seated in the normal position in the ENT examination chair. After anaesthetizing the nasale fossae, a $70°$ telescopic stem is introduced into the nasale fossae and pushed into position above the velo-pharyngeal orifice whence the latter can be examined at leisure.

1) With spontaenous breathing, this orifice is wide open and provides a clear view of the hypo-pharynx, the laryngeal margella, and of the epiglottis (dia 3)
2) Active, voluntary snoring causes this orifice to contract to one fifth its size on inhaling and its anterior and lateral edges (soft-palate, uvula and posterior pillars) to vibrate. (dia 4)
3) During swallowing, the orifice closes hermetically like a diaphragm. (dia 5)

A $0°$ or direct optical device is then placed in the mouth to examine the forward surface of the soft-palate, uvula and posterior pillars.
1) During spontaneous breathing, the fineness and flexibility of these tissues can be observed.
2) During voluntary snoring, all these structures begin to vibrate violently. Thus it is possible to ascertain the amount of tissue to be removed in order to relieve these vibrations to the greatest possible extent without in any way reducing the firmness of the closure of the velo-uvalo-pharyngeal valve during swallowing.

Finally a $120°$ retrograde optical device enables us to examine the posterior surface of the structures in question (dia 6 - 7)

Video film (4' 30'')

DISCUSSION

The visual examination of the velo-pharyngeal orifice and of its contraction to one fifth its normal size during induced snoring provides, when applied to prolonged spontaneous snoring during sleep, evidence of the part played by this contraction in producing cardio-pulmonary and cerebral complications. Indeed, anyone who cares to do so, can verify this for him or herself deliberately imitating the act of snoring and observing the effort this involves and the increase in chest expansion it occasions.

The sight of velic vibrations suggests another hypothesis: couldn't these vibrations, which are propagated to the brain via the LCR and skull, provoque microtraumatisms which could explain morning headache in the snorer and which could possibly even induce at long term, chronic and diffuse cerebral lesions. Furthermore, could the apnea - at least the apnea of central origin - be caused once a certain quantity of vibrations is transmitted to the cerebral bulb, seat of the respiratory center and very close to the source of vibrations.

At least and above all, the endoscopic study of voluntary and velic snoring enables to understand the mechanism of physiological snoring, and therefore to put the indication to operate, because it makes possible the distinction between:
1) pure velic snoring which responds extremely well to the UPPP.
2) pure pharyngeal snoring (or rattle), leading to pharyngeal apnea, which does not respond or responds only partly to the UPPP.
3) the most frequent case, mixt velo-pharyngeal snoring, which responds only partially - through its velic component - to the UPPP.

We should add that at the epiglottis plays no part in velic induced snoring.

CONCLUSION

What we have here is a straightforward endoscopical examination which requires no special preparation and can be carried out during any normal consultation with the basic equipment to be found in any ordinary ENT surgery.
It enables us to observe and examine the mechanics of the act of snoring, to locate them with precision, to assess the extent of the activity by observing the vibrations of the tissues concerned and, consequently, prior to operating, to assess the extent of tissues resection required and thus to avoid post-operative complications like open rhinolalia and nasal regurgitation.

Finally, a study of induced snoring provides an uncomplicated and reliable approach to a spontaneous physiological phenomenon and improves our understanding of that phenomenon and of its consequences.

L'EXAMEN ENDOSCOPIQUE DANS LE RONFLEMENT VOLONTAIRE.

L'examen endoscopique du ronflement volontaire, permet la vision directe des structures en vibration qui sont à l'origine du phénomène sonore. La description de l'instrumentation et de la méthode, démontre que cet examen ne nécessite pas de préparation particulière et se satisfait de l'instrumentation ORL ordinaire. Il permet d'estimer, pré-opératoirement, l'importance de la résection tissulaire nécessaire à la suppression du ronflement et d'éviter ainsi des séquelles de rhinolalie ouverte ou de régurgitation nasale. Enfin il facilite la compréhension du ronflement physiologique à l'état de sommeil et induit des hypothèses originales, quoique non encore vérifiées, sur ses éventuelles conséquences cardio-pulmonaires, cérébrales et sur l'apnea sleep syndrom.

Chronic rhonchopathy. Ed. C.H. Chouard. © 1988, John Libbey Eurotext Ltd. pp.185-189.

Studies of snoring disease by videofiberscope, X-rays and xerography – 23 cases

Jean Abitol* and P. Katz**

*ORL Ancien Chef de Clinique-Assistant à la Faculté de Médecine de Paris, 1 rue Largillière, 75016 Paris, France
**Radiologue Paris, 7 rue Théodore de Banville, 75017 Paris, France

RESUME

Snoring needs before any surgical treatment a complete screening.
In this paper, we study the objective explorations to quantify the most responsable reasons of the snoring.

The fiberscope gives a dynamic exploration of the nose-pharyngeal tract. It studies the uvula, the velum, the shape of the posterior third of the septum, the turbinates and the supraglottic air tract.

x-rays and tomography precise the position of the septum and maxillary sinus infection.

Xerography gives the real dimension of the uvula length and thickness. We found out that for 22 patients uvula was superior at 4 cm length and 0,8 mm thickness. Normal dimensions are 2,2 cm and 0,6 mm.

On 23 cases, uvula and hyperflaccidity velum seem to be the main reasons of snoring, 22 cases were pathogical, 1 normal.

INTRODUCTION

The main reasons of snoring are the hyperflaccidity of the velo-uvula system. The vibrations are increased by the vortex air flue in these anatomical locations. A best understanding of that pathology is given by videofiberscopy, x-rays and xerography.

MATERIALS AND METHODS

In the last three years, we planified these explorations for 23 patients :
22 men and 1 woman, 44 to 73 years old, 20 people were obese.

VIDEOFIBERSCOPY

It explores the anatomical structures of nasal fossa, cavum, velum and oropharynx and allows us to explore the shape of the naso-pharyngeal tract.

- **On nasal fossa**
    : 9 septum deseases
    : 11 hypertrophies of turbinates
    : 1 polyposis

- **In the cavum**
    : 2 adenoïtis (47 and 55 years old)

- **In oral-pharynx**
    * tonsils : 2 hypertrophic tonsils and 3 removed tonsils, and 18 cases normal.
    * lingual tonsils : 1 hypertrophied

- **In the uvula**

    1) the fiberscope is located on the floor of the nasal fossa. The patient says "A" and the nasal sound "IN". We can observe the move of the valum, it is an hyperflaccidity in 22 cases.

    2) The fiberscope is located on the roof of the cavum :
    We ask to the patient to breath very fast.
    We observe the move of the uvula.
    It slaps the tongue and sometimes the epiglottis.

    3) The fiberscope is located just behind the uvula and we observe, when the mouth is closed :
        : 19 cases uvula touches the posterior third of the tongue.
        : 4 cases uvula touches the epiglottis.
    We also did observe 3 cases of cervical arthrosis which gives a very narrow space for the air tract.

X-RAYS

Tomographies are indispensable :

* Front tomography will precise the shape of the septum, of the turbinates we found 14 asymptomatic maxillary sinus cysts.

* The profile brings us less than xerography

NASO-PHARYNGO-LARYNGEAL XEROGRAPHY

- Front-views are less intersting than x-rays
- Profiles will precise the real length of the uvula : 22 cases were more than 4 cm (the normal length is around 2,2 cm).
The maximum thickness of the uvula for all them was more than 0,8 mm.
We observe the hyperflaccidity of the valum on "A" and "IN" in 2 views.

RESULTS

* 22 long uvula
* 9 pathological septum
* 14 asmptomatic maxillary sinus cysts
* 23 hyperflaccidities of velum
* 19 cases = mouth closed, uvula touches the posterior third of the tongue.
* 4 cases = the uvula touches the epiglottis
* 2 cases of hypertrophic tonsils
* 2 cases of adenoïtis (47 and 55 years old)

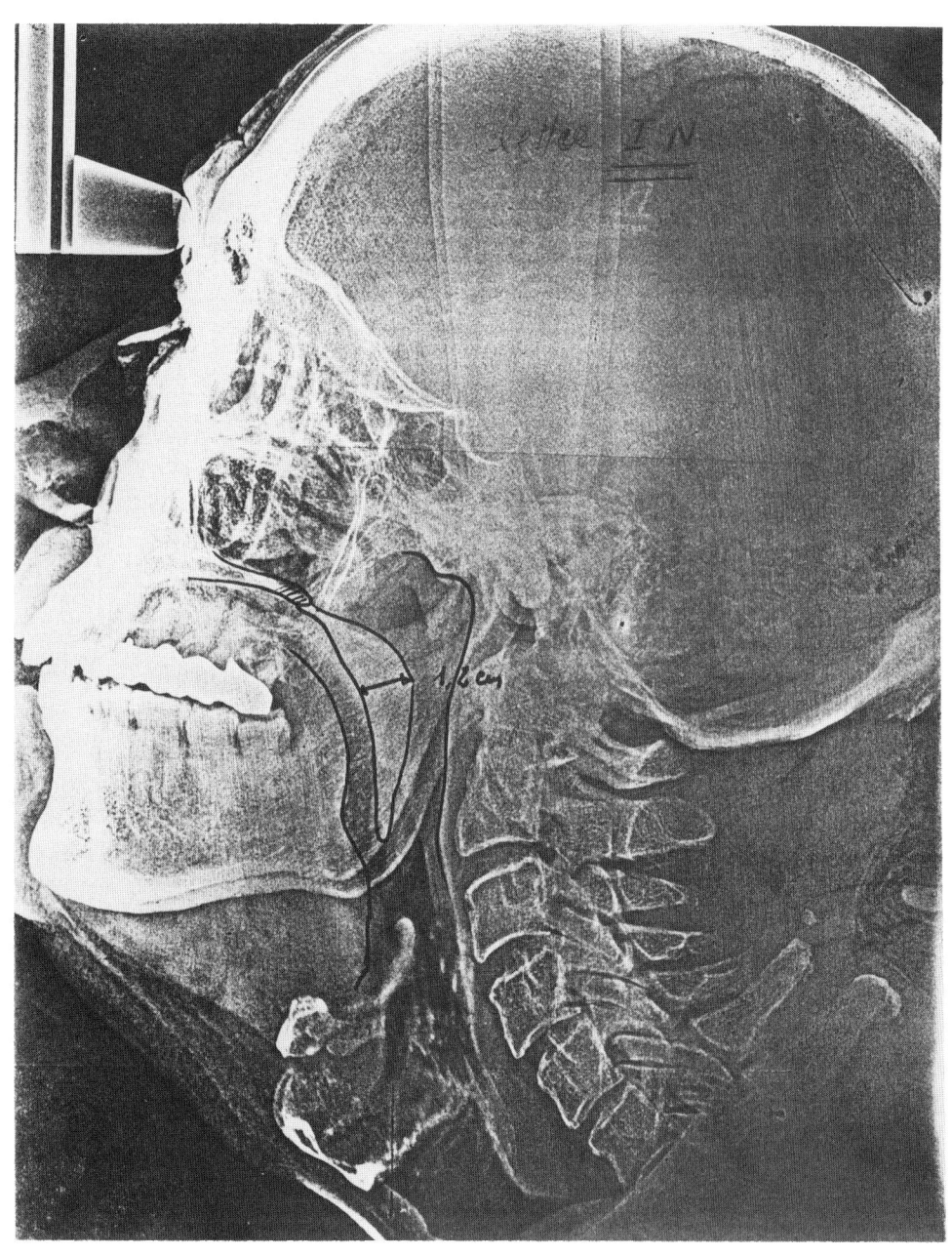

XEROGRAPHY : Phonem IN.

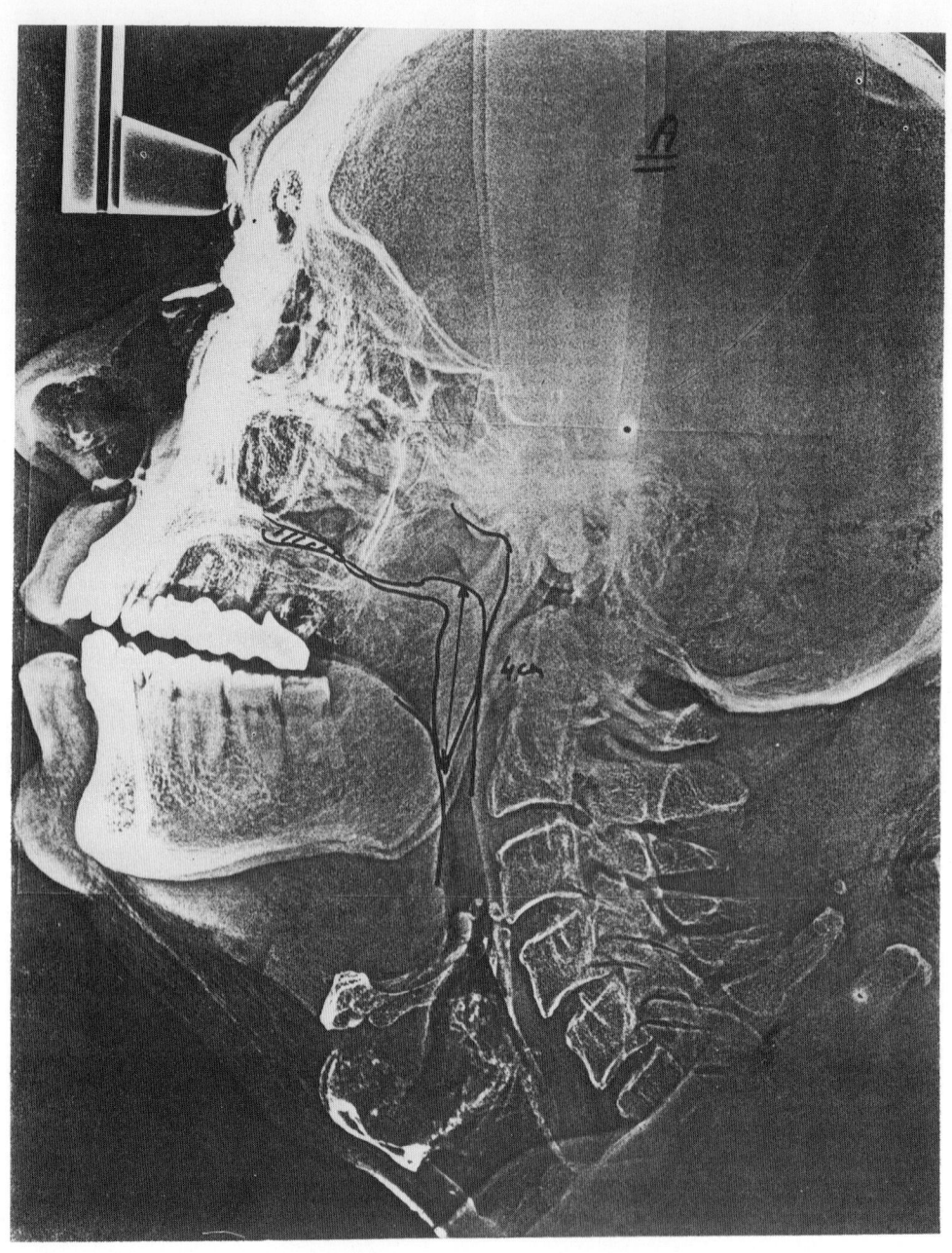

XEROGRAPHY phonem A

CONCLUSION

All these methods had allowed us to conclude that, to value the snoring desease we must care about septum, turbinates and chiefly uvula.
The shape of the oro-pharynx ogive is also very important.

On 23 cases, by uvula and hyperflaccidity velum seem to be the main reason of snoring, 22 cases were pathogical.
Deviation of the septum is not involve in 14 cases and turbinate desease in 12 cases.
We may conclude that with these explorations we must first treat the uvula and hyperflaccidity, velum and than, in a second time, if necessary, treated the others parameters.

RESUME

L'étude du ronflement demande avant tout traitement chirurgical une exploration complète.
Dans cet article, nous étudions les explorations objectives pour quantifier les principales étiologies du ronflement.
Le fibroscope donne une exploration dynamique du tractus naso-pharyngé. Il étudie la luette, le voile du palais, la forme du 1/3 postérieur du septum, les cornets et le conduit aérien supraglottic.
Les radiographies et tomographies précisent la position du septum et l'infection des sinus maxillaires.
La xérographie donne la vraie dimension de la longueur et de l'épaisseur de la luette.
Nous avons relevé que chez 22 patients souffrant de ronflement, la luette était supérieure à 4 cm de long et 0,8 cm d'épaisseur.
Les dimensions normales étant respectivement 2,2 cm et 0,6 cm. Sur 23 cas, l'hyperfalaccidité de la luette et du voile semblent les principales étiologies du ronflement.

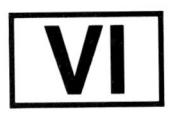# CLINICAL ASPECTS OF SLEEP APNEAS SYNDROME
Chairman: J.F. Derenne

Cardio-respiratory investigations during sleep in subjects with chronic rhonchopathy: the use of the static charge sensitive bed method

M. Billiard, L. Brissaud, B. Sales and O. Polo

Sleep Disorders Unit, Gui de Chauliac Center, 34059 Montpellier Cedex, France

RESUME

Le traitement de la ronchopathie chronique repose sur une identification précise de la pathologie sous-jacente, ronflement avec ou sans perturbation respiratoire, syndrome d'apnées récurrentes au cours du sommeil. L'examen le plus fiable est l'enregistrement polysomnographique associé à un contrôle de la fonction cardio-respiratoire à l'aide de différents capteurs. Il s'agit toutefois d'une technique réservée à quelques centres spécialisés. L'enregistrement sur matelas électro-statique permet de se passer des contraintes représentées par les différents capteurs attachés au sujet. 50 sujets atteints de ronchopathie chronique ont été étudiés par cette technique et répartis en trois groupes différents : ronfleurs sans anomalies respiratoires (11), ronfleurs avec anomalies respiratoires (16), ronfleurs atteints du syndrome d'apnées au cours du sommeil (23).

MOTS CLEFS

Chronic ronchopathy, Static charge sensitive bed.

Snoring and obstructive or mixed sleep apneas are, at a different degree, potential sources or contributing factors of morning fatigue and/or headache, daytime somnolence, systemic and pulmonary hypertension, cardiac arrhytmias, cardio-circulatory insufficiency and cerebro-vascular disease. Thus treatment of these conditions is warranted. However there is a wide range of disorders including simple snoring without any alteration of the respiratory function, snoring with various modifications of the respiratory function, obstructive sleep apnea syndrome and obstructive sleep apneas associated with permanent alveolar hypoventilation.

Symptomatology including snoring, occasional or habitual, light or heavy, recent or long lasting, isolated or associated with respiratory pauses during sleep, agitated sleep, morning fatigue and/or headache, daytime somnolence, may help in recognizing the different conditions.

Also of interest are the morphological aspect of the subject, body-mass index, upper airway structure, blood pressure, cardio-circulatory and pulmonary functions, intellectual and psychological status.

Anyhow cardio-respiratory investigations during sleep are indicated in all subjects showing some evidence of organic repercussion.

Today's best method is polysomnography which enables the concomitant evaluation of the states of alertness, wakefulness, NREM sleep, and REM sleep, and of related abnormal cardio-respiratory events by means of a variety of devices measuring airflow, respiratory efforts, oxygen saturation, electrical activity of the heart, endooesophageal pressure, etc. The only drawback of this method is the need of well-equipped specialized centers which are still rather rare in comparison with demand.

We were interested in a new technique, the Static Charge Sensitive Bed Method, based upon the use of a very sensitive sensor of mechanical movements. The Static Charge Sensitive Bed (SCSB) consists of "active" layers in which the subjects movements generate a static charge distribution. These changes induce potential differences between two large metal sheets located under the SCSB and isolated from each other by a stiff insulating plate. The potential difference between the metal sheets is amplified by a conventional differential AC or DC amplifier and recorded on a tape recorder or an EEG recorder. This method enables the recording of body movements, respiratory movements and ballistocardiographic movements (BCG) reflecting the mechanical activity of the heart (Alihanka et al. 1981). It does not require any electrode attached to the subject and can be used in an ordinary bed at a hospital ward. It seems of special interest in the evaluation of sleep-related disturbances such as heavy snoring or the sleep apnea syndrome. It makes it possible to record different abnormal respiratory or cardio-respiratory patterns of increasing severity (Alihanka 1987) : periodic breathing (P.B.) ; central periodic apneas (C.P.A.) ; obstructive apneas with normal or slightly increased respiratory variation of the BCG during the apnea period (o II) ; periodic breathing with decreasing and increasing amplitude of the BCG (PB + abn. BCG) ; obstructive apnea with decreasing and increasing amplitude of the BCG and/or cardiac arrhythmia during the apnea period (o III) ; and two yet poorly defined cardio-respiratory patterns : gradually increasing large amplitude respiratory movements and markedly increased respiratory variation of the BCG amplitude (IRR) ; isolated decreasing and increasing BCG amplitude (BCG $\pm$).

Despite the limitations of this method, hight sensitivity but only relative specificity (Salmi et al. 1986, Polo et al. submitted), we used it in a population of 50 subjects (44 males, 6 females), median age 54, range 31 to 80, referred to our clinic for a complaint of chronic ronchopathy, in comparison with 7 controls (all males) median age 44, range 32 to 66.

11 subjects did not differ from normal controls in terms of the types of recorded cardio-respiratory patterns, normal respiration, PB and O II pattern for less than 10 minutes (Table 1).

16 subjects showed clearcut disturbances, PB, CPA, O II pattern for less or more than 10 minutes, PB + abn. BCG and the O III pattern for less than 10 minutes.

Finally 23 subjects, real sleep apneic subjects, showed the whole range of abnormal respiratory or cardio-respiratory patterns including the O III pattern for more than 10 minutes.

Table 1 : Results of the SCSB analysis in 50 subjects with chronic ronchopathy and 7 normal controls.

	NORMAL CONTROLS (7)	SNORERS WITHOUT RESPIRATORY DISTURBANCES (11)	SNORERS WITH RESPIRATORY DISTURBANCES (16)	SLEEP APNEIC SUBJECTS (23)
Normal resp.	7	11	16	15
P.B.	5	7	11	13
C.P.A.	-	-	1	4
O II < 10 min.	1	4	2	6
O II > 10 min.	-	-	10	15
P.B.+abn.B.C.G.	-	-	11	19
O III < 10 min.	-	-	7	-
O III > 10 min.	-	-	-	23
I.R.R.	-	-	3	6
B.C.G. $\pm$	1	2	9	11

These distinctions are of major interest in the therapeutic decision : postural treatment, limited or extended surgery, continuous positive airway pressure.

REFERENCES

Alihanka, J. (1987) : Basic principles for analysing and scoring Bio-matt (SCSB) recordings. Annales Universitatis Turkuensis.

Alihanka, J., Vaahtoranta, K., Saarikivi, I. (1981) : A new method of long term monitoring of the ballistocardiogram, heart rate and respiration. Am. J. Physiol.,240, 384-392.

Polo, O., Brissaud, L., Sales, B., Senegas, E., Besset, A., Billiard, M. : The validity of the static charge sensitive bed in detecting obstructive sleep apneas (submitted).

Salmi, T., Partinen, M., Hyyppä, M., Kronholm, E. (1986) : Automatic analysis of static charge sensitive bed (SCSB) recordings in the evaluation of sleep related apneas. Acta Neurol. Scand., 74, 360-364.

Sleep apnea syndrome (SAS) and respiration

B. Fleury and J. Ph. Derenne

Service de Pneumologie, Hôpital Saint-Antoine, 184 rue du faubourg Saint-Antoine, 75571 Paris 12, France

MOTS CLEFS

Sleep Apnea Syndrome. Pulmonary hemodynamics. Gas exchanges.
Syndrome d'Apnées du Sommeil. Hemodynamique pulmonaire.
Echanges gazeux.

TEXTE

Physiologists as well as chest physicians are both interested in respiratory disturbances during sleep, particularity sleep apneas
Normal respiration requires that air be displaced from the external environment to the alveolar units to make oxygen available for gas exchanges. Apnea results when this process is completely interrupted. Sleep apnea is defined as cessation of airflow at the nose and mouth during sleep (Bradley and al, 1985). For practical clinical purposes sleep apneas are classified into three types : central, obstructive and mixed, although the mechanisms underlying the three types are closely related (Krieger, 1986). In central apnea drive to respiratory muscles is abolished, whereas in obstructive apnea there is continued activation of the inspiratory muscles, particularly the diaphragm, but interruption of airflow due to a complete upper airway occlusion at the level of the oropharynx. Mixed apneas begin as central apnea and are followed by an obstructive apnea. They are generally considered a variant of obstructive apneas. Obstructive and mixed apneas appear to be the most frequent causes of clinical manifestation. The pathogenesis of obstructive apnea is still controversial. Both genioglossus muscles have been demonstrated to play a crucial role in the maintainance of a patent oropharyngeal lumen, particularly during sleep in the supine position, for these are the muscles that force the tongue forward during

inspiration. Loss of their function results in retro collapse of the tongue into the oropharynx, with suffocation as a possible result.
Normal genioglossus function results in regular bursts of electromyographic activity associated with inspiratory effort during sleep. REMMERS et all postulate that airway occlusion during sleep apnea syndrome occurs when the pharyngeal negative inspiratory pressure exceeds the dilating forces of the upper airways muscles. Thus, the dilating forces of the upper airway must exceed the collapsing pharyngeal closing pressure to maintain airway patency. This pathophysiologic hypothesis would also explain how anatomic abnormalities of the upper airway would create a situation whereby negative pharyngeal pressure generated on inspiration would require substantially more compensatory activity of the dilating muscles of the upper airway to maintain patency. Sleep can magnify defects in ventilatory control when mechanical impediments to ventilation exist. The obstructive component could to be the consequence of a defect in the control of the upper aiway dilator muscles ; the structural abnormalities of the upper airways would increase these functional disorders.

The most serious immediate consequence of upper airways occlusion during sleep is the interruption of ventilation and the development of progressive asphyxia. These acute disturbances lead to a series of secondary physiological derangements that eventually give rise to many of the clinical features of sleep apnea syndromes. Chest physicians are particularly concerned with the pulmonary function of these patients during wakefulness and sleep and with the relationship between S.A.S. and pulmonary disease.

Pulmonary function during wakefulness.

The pulmonary function tests are normal or disclose abnormalities in relationship with the obesity or a bronchopulmonary pathology sometimes associated (Krieger, 1986).

The flow volume loop has previously been recommended as a screening method for detecting sleep apneas patients. Specially the presence of either extrathoracic variable obstruction, or a saw tooth pattern seen in the flow volume loop, was suggested as being common in the obstructive sleep apnea syndrome. The sensitivity of the combination of those two tests is excellent, but due to their poor specificity, their diagnostic interest is nonetheless limited (Krieger and al, 1985).

Arterial blood gases may often be at normal levels, though they sometimes demonstrate hypoxemia and/or hypercapnia, both non specific to sleep apnea syndrome.

The definitive diagnosis of breathing abnormalities during sleep requires an analysis of nocturnal polygraphic recording.

Gas exchanges during sleep apnea.

A slight degree of alveolar hypoventilation occurs during sleep in normal subjects. The changes in blood gases during apnea are much more severe (Tilkan and al, 1976). During apnea, in the absence of ventilation, the oxygen required to sustain metabolic activity is progressively withdrawn from the body's endogenous stores of oxygen, while the carbon dioxide produced equilibrates with the body's carbon dioxide stores. Because the body's mobilisable oxygen store is almost two orders of magnitude lower than that of carbon dioxide, during apnea the partial pressure of oxygen in blood falls rapidly in comparison to the slow rise in the partial pressure of carbon dioxide. Arterial hemoglobin oxygen saturation (SaO_2) can be measured continuously diuring sleep by percutaneous oxymetry ; hence considerably more is known about SaO_2 in sleep apnea syndrome than about arterial PO_2 and PCO_2, which at best can be measured only by intermittent sampling of arterial blood. The magnitude and rate of fall of SaO_2 that develops with apnea are highly variable from one patient to another. This variability involves several physiological variables. The duration of apnea is one of the most important. The more prolonged the apnea, the more important the drop in SaO_2 (Catterall and al, 1983). Equally important is the baseline arterial PO_2 (PaO_2), which determines the position of the patient on the oxyhemoglobin dissociation curve at the begining of the apnea (Strohl and al, 1984).

The patients with a high baseline PaO_2 are operating on the flat portion of the dissociation curve, and hence usually desaturate minimally. In contrast, patients, who begin an apnea on the steep portion of the dissociation curve desaturate more rapidly and severely. Factors exerting a major influence on the awake SaO_2, such as chronic airway obstruction, can determine the severity of desaturation during sleep apnea. The lung volume at which apnea begins, functional residual capacity (FRC), can play a role in the case of very small pulmonary volumes with increased potential for airspaces collapse and non homogeneous gas exchanges (Findley and al, 1983). This mechanisms can be present in severely obese patients, and in some patients in whom lung volumes decrease during the course of an obstructive apnea as a result of active expiratory efforts that are able to expel gas through the occluded upper airways. The frequency of disordered breathing events contributes also to the fall of SaO_2 (Sheppard, 1985). Despite the tendency for patients with a high apnea index to have a shorter duration of apnea, these patients demonstrate the more severe oxyhemoglobin desaturation. In addition, oxyhemoglobin desaturation often becomes progressively more severe during chains of repetitive apneas. Inadequate ventilation in the interapneic period, to fully replete oxygen stores in the mixed venous blood, is probably responsible for this phenomenon. Finally, the hypothesis of a different desaturation rate according to the type of apnea is not confirmed by experiments using breath holding during wakefulness as an apnea model (Strohl and al, 1984). The rate and magnitude of fall of SaO_2 is not affected by respiratory efforts and depends primarily on the initial level of SaO_2. The rate of fall of SaO_2 in patients with sleep apnea is similar to that observed during breath holding in wakefulness.

A permanent alveolar hypoventilation does not arise in all sleep apnea syndrome patients. The mechanisms by which the alveolar hypoventilation linked to apnea becomes permanent is not clearly established (Krieger, 1986). It seems independent of the gravity or the long standing character of the apneas. An alteration in ventilatory control has been evoked ; but studies on chemical control of breathing in sleep apnea syndrome show conflicting results. A decrease in ventilatory response to hypoxia and/or hyperoxic hypercapnia is present in some patients, but cannot explain all the cases of permanent hypoventilation. Finally, a role has been recently suggested for a certain degree of bronchial obstruction in association with sleep apnea in the genesis of permanent hypoxia (Bradley and al, 1985).

Pulmonary hemodynamics.

In normal subjects small changes of 2 to 4 mmHg in the pulmonary arterial pressure during sleep have been reported. In contrast to control subjects, patients with sleep apnea syndromes demonstrate substantial elevation in pulmonary arterial pressure (PAP) during sleep (Londsdofer and al, 1972). The PAP rises progressively during the course of apnea and may attain values of 50 to 60 mmHg. Maximal pulmonary arterial pressures are observed in the immediate post apnea period, and coincide with the nadir of oxygen hemoglobin saturation as recorded by percutaneous oxymetry. The severity of the pulmonary hypertension is closely linked with the severity of the nocturnal hypoxemia (Sheppard, 1985). Although the elevations in systolic pressure are greater than the elevations in diastolic pressure, both are similar when expressed as percentage of control. This widening of the pulse pressure suggests that stroke volume may be increased. If stroke volume does increase it would tend to be associatedwith reductions in heart rate. Measurements of cardiac output have been shown to be normal during apnea (Tilkian and al, 1976).

Often the pulmonary artery pressures fail to return to baseline between apnea and rise progressively during chains of repetitive apneas. The pulmonary pressures modifications seem to be related to the increase in pulmonary vasculature resistances consecutive to hypoxia, either directly or by means of its effects upon chemoreceptors.

Although many patients experiencing sleep apnea syndrome have normal hemodynamics during waking hours, a large, poorly defined number do have hemodynamics dysfunction during the day.

The classic description of Pickwickian syndrome includes cor pulmonale and right ventricular failure. Recents findings suggest that permanent pulmonary arterial pressure is frequent when sleep apnea syndrome is severe (64 % of patients with an apnea index greater than 50) (Padszus and al, 1985). The mechanism by which permanent hypertension takes hold is controversial. Permanent pulmonary hypertension is responsible for the right heart failure observed in the more severe patients. Pulmonary hemodynamics changes and right heart failure are reversible with the suppresion of apnea by tracheostomy (Tilkian and al, 1976) or continue positive airway pressure through the nares (Sullivan and al, 1984).

Sleep apnea syndrome and chronic obstructive pulmonary disease (COPD).

On the basis of studies of patients selected because of the existence of daytime hypersomnolence, a large frequency of sleep apnea syndrome in COPD patients has been reported (Guilleminault and al, 1980). This frequency has not been confirmed by study of less biased subjects (Catterall and al, 1983).

Epidemiologic data on the prevalence of the association between COPD and SAS are not available, and further investigations are necessary. Obviously chronic obstructive lung disease can coexist with sleep apnea syndrome, and it is becoming apparent that this combination presents distinct features both clinically and in pattern of hypoxemia and breathing movements during sleep. The combination results in profound hypoxemia particularly during REM sleep and also the characteristic swinging pattern of nocturnal saturation even outside REM sleep.

REFERENCES BIBLIOGRAPHIQUES

Bradley T.D., Rutherford R., Grossman R.F., Lue F., Zamel N., Moldofsky Phillipson E.A (1985) : Role of daytime hypoxemia in the pathogenesis of right heart failure in the obstructive sleep apnea syndrome. Am. Rev. Respir. Dis., 131, 835-839

Catterall J.R., Douglas N.J., Calverley P.M.A., Shapiro C.M., Brezinova V., Brash H.M., Flenley D.C. (1983) : Transient hypoxemia during sleep in chronic obstructive pulmonary disease is not a sleep apnea syndrome. Am. Rev. Respir. Dis., 128, 24-29

Findley L.J., Ries A.L., Tisi G.M., Wagner P.D. (1983) : Hypoxemia during apnea in normal subject : mechanisms and impact of lung volume. J. Appl. Physiol., 55, 1777-1783

Guilleminault C., Cumminskey J., Motta J. (1980) : Chronic obstructive airflow disease and sleep studies. Am. Rev. Respir. Dis., 122, 397-406

Guilleminault C., Tilkian A., Dement W.C. (1976) : The sleep apnea syndromes. Ann. Rev. Med., 27, 465-484

Krieger J. (1986) : Sleep apnea syndromes in adults. Bull. Eur.

Physiopathol. Respir., 22, 147-189
Krieger J. Weitzenblum E., Van devenne A., Stierle J.L., Kurtz D. (1985) : Flow-volume curve abnormalities and obstructive sleep apnea syndrome. Chest, 87, 163-167
Lonsdofer J., Meunier-Carus J., Lampert-Benignus E., Kurtz D., Bapst-Reiter J., Fletto R., Micheletti G. (1972) : Aspects hémodynamiques et respiratoires du syndrome pickwickien. Bull. Physiopathol. Respir., 8, 1181-1192
Podszus T., Mayer J., Penzel T., Peter J.H., Von Wichert P. (1985) : Hemodynamics during sleep in patients with sleep apnea. Sleep Res., 14, 189 (Abstract)
ffmmers J.E., De Groot W.H., Saverland E.K, Anch A.M. (1978) : Pathogenesis of upper airway occlusion during sleep. J. Appl. Physiol., 44, 931-938. Shepard J.W. (1985) : Gas exchange and hemodynamics during sleep. Medical Clinics of North America, 69, 1243-1264
Strohl K.P., Altose M.D. (1984) : Oxygen saturation during BreathHolding and during Apneas in Sleep. Chest, 85, 181-186
Sullivan C.E., Issa F.G., Berthon-Jones M., McCauley V.B., Costas L.J.V. (1984) : Home treatment of obstructive sleep apnea with continuous positive airway pressure applied through a nose-mask. Bull. Eur. Physiopathol. Respir., 20, 49-54
Tilkian A.G., Guilleminault C., Shroeder J.S., Lehrman K.L., Blair Simmons F., Dement W.C. (1976) : Hemodynamics in Sleep-induced apnea. Ann. Intern. Med. 85, 714-719

Chronic rhonchopathy. Ed. C.H. Chouard. © 1988, John Libbey Eurotext Ltd. pp.203-207.

Sleep apnea syndrome: ENT features

Y. Dejean and L. Crampette

Service ORL, Hôpital St Charles, 34059 Montpellier Cedex, France

RESUME

Les dossiers de 100 ronfleurs ont été colligés. Un interrogatoire, un examen clinique ORL, un enregistrement au cours du sommeil (matelas électrostatique) et un scanner pharyngé ont été réalisés pour chaque patient. L'enregistrement permet d'individualiser les ronfleurs simples des ronfleurs à risque et des sujets apnéiques. Le scanner permet de mesurer la surface de la lumière pharyngée à différents niveaux. Les résultats sont analysés, et confrontés. Il apparait que l'interrogatoire est le critère le mieux corrélé à la gravité du ronflement. L'examen clinique et le scanner, par contre, ne montrent pas de différence significative entre les 3 groupes de ronfleurs. Ainsi, sur un plan pratique, l'interrogatoire est l'élément principal pour apprécier l'indication d'un enregistrement du sommeil, alors que les conclusions de l'examen ORL, complété par le scanner ($\pm$ céphalométrie) trouvent leur application principale dans la conduite thérapeutique.

MOTS CLEFS - KEY WORDS

Sleep Apnea Syndrome - ORL evaluation - Sleep Recording - Pharyngeal CT scan.

INTRODUCTION

ORL examination can be undertaken in two main cases :

- for snoring ; this eventuality is the more frequent one. The otolaryngologist has to diagnosticate a sleep apnea syndrome, whose major complaint may be snoring.

- for exploration of apneic patients, previously demonstrated by sleep recording ; in this case, the purpose of ORL evaluation is, above all, to determine potential sites of obstruction.

METHODS

Authors performed investigations in 100 snorers, including clinical symptom study, morphologic evaluation, sleep recording (Static Charge Sensitive Bed - Alihanka, 1987) and pharyngeal CT scan (Haponik et all, 1983 ; Surrat et all., 1983).

Clinical symptom study inquires about hypothesis of sleep apneic events (periodic silences ending by loud snorting, abnormal movements, morning headache or complaint of restless sleep) and excessive daytime sleepiness.

Morphologic evaluation is a standard ORL evaluation of upper airways : nasal status, velopharyngeal features (soft palate characteristics, diameter between posterior pillars, size of tonsils), analysis of posterior tongue pharynx (tongue volume, easiness to see glottic level), and supraglottic larynx. We use fibroscopic method when clinical examination is difficult and when more precision is required in evaluation of an obvious major pharyngeal narrowing.

Sleep recording allows distinction of 3 groups :

- Low Risk Snorers (LRS), with no respiratory abnormalities associated with snoring.

- High Risk Snorers (HRS), with no apneic events, but abnormal respiratory pattern (periodic breathing, increased respiratory resistances, changes in oxygen saturation level) and/or abnormal cardiologic function (improved ballistocardiogram, arrythmia).

- Sleep Apnea Syndrome (SAS) subjects.

CT scan allows measurement of pharyngeal luminal section, especially at velopharyngeal (VP) level and at posterior tongue space (PTS) one.

RESULTS

Sleep recording divides our population in 40 LRS, 40 SAS and 20 HRS.

Clinical symptom study is rather well correlated with the severity of snoring (table I)

	Hypothesis of apneic events	No Hypothesis of apneic events	?
LRS	4	26	10
SAS	31	2	7
HRS	8	4	8

Table I : data of complaint study (? = doubt about apneic events)

However this report discloses that accuracy of complaint study is poor in 25 subjects. Moreover, there is no specific complaint of High Risk Snoring, and 2 SAS subjects were considered, before sleep recording, as LRS.

Clinical examination is not significantly different in the 3 groups.

	LRS	SAS	HRS
Narrowed VP	23	23	12
Narrowed PTS	1	0	0
Narrowed Nasal Airway and VP	7	10	4
Narrowed VP and PTS	2	5	3
Narrowed Nasal Airway, VP and PTS	0	1	0
Normal clinical examination	5	1	1

Table II : Morphologic Status

We do not observe nasal dyspermeability without any pharyngeal site of obstruction associated. The 5 LRS, whose ORL examination is normal are subjects with excessive alcohol intake, or using sedative drugs.

<u>CT scan study</u> brings three main results :

- frequency of upper airway narrowing is not different in the 3 groups (table III)

	LRS	SAS	HRS
Minimal VP surface < 1,50 cm2	13	19	9
Minimal VP surface < 1,50 cm2 and Minimal PTS surface < 2,00 cm2	19	19	9
Other	1	1	2

Table III : results of CT scan measurements

- in SAS patients, pharyngeal narrowing may be more important : virtual luminal section is observed at VP level in 11 SAS subjets, and only in 4 HRS and 3 LRS. PTS surface inferior than 1 cm2 is found in 8 SAS, and only in 4 LRS and 2 HRS.

- in all groups, dyspermeability at the PTS level is demonstrated more often by CT scan than clinically (table IV)

	LRS	SAS	HRS
Clinically demonstrated PTS narrowing	3	6	3
CT scan demonstrated PTS narrowing	16	15	16

Table IV : results of CT scan compared with clinical findings

DISCUSSION

We do not discuss the interest of Static Charge Sensitive Bed sleep recording technique. As otolaryngologists, we only notice that this recording method allows the individualisation of a third category of snorers, the HRS one. The two remaining questions are : how do we consider this group ? and how do we manage HRS ?

Clinical features of snorers are now well-known (Wilms et all, 1982). Our findings are close to those of the literature. However we do not find any supraglottic laryngeal narrowing (even with CT scan contribution), which is generally considered as an uncommon ORL feature in snoring. Nasal dyspermeability is never observed, in our subjects, without associated pharyngeal narrowing. This emphisizes the poor responsability of nasal narrowing in snoring, in accordance with many authors findings. About PTS narrowing, we have to notice that CT scan is more accurate than clinical evaluation. Moreover, this technique allows qualitative examination of PTS narrowing. In 50 % very large inferior tonsillar poles, easily shown by CT scan, determine PTS dyspermeability, without associated retroposition of the tongue basis. This is of interest because of therapeutic consequences ; in these cases, a Uvulo-Palato-Pharyngoplasty including tonsils is adequate, whereas, in other cases, a mandibular or a hyoïd surgery may be provided, taking in to account data of cephalometry (We do not discuss cephalometry in this article about "ORL features", because we consider it as a pre-therapeutic technique and not as a diagnostic one).

The major result of this study seems to be the comparison between ORL features and sleep recording findings : there is no correlation in our population. Thus, it seems wrong to estimate severity of snoring by means of morphologic evaluation, even with CT scan measurements.

CONCLUSION

In a pragmatic point of view, only clinical symptom study brings a (relative) accuracy to estimate snoring consequences, and sleep recording's necessity, whereas morphologic evaluation is not helpfull for these appreciations. However, ORL evaluation, associated with CT scan (and cephalometry in some cases) is very important for therapeutic management : choice (or not) of surgical procedure, and its nature.

REFERENCES

Alihanka, J. (1987) : Basic Principles for Analysing and Scoring Bio-Matt (SCSB) Recordings. <u>Annales Universitades Turkuensis</u>.

Haponik, E.F., Smith, P.L., Bohlman, M.E., et all. (1983) : computerized tomography in obstructive sleep apnea. Am. Rev. Respir. Dis., 127, 221-226

Surrat, P.M., Dee, P., Atkinson, R.L., et all. (1983) : Fluoroscopic and computed tomographic features of the pharyngeal airway in obstructive sleep apnea. Am. Rev. Respir. Dis., 127, 487-492.

Wilms, D., Popovich, J., Conway, W., et all. (1982) : Anatomic Abnormalities in Obstructive Sleep Apnea. Ann. Otol. Rhinol. Laryngol., 91, 595-596.

SUMMARY

SLEEP APNEA SYNDROME (SAS) : ENT FEATURES

Authors performed investigations in 100 snorers, including clinical symptom study, morpohlogic evaluation, sleep recording (Static Charge Sensitive Bed) and pharyngeal CT scan. Sleep recording divides snorers in three groups : Low Risk Snorers (LRS), High Risk Snorers (HRS) and Sleep Apnea Syndrome (SAS) patients. There are 40 LRS, 40 SAS and 20 HRS in our population. Complaint study is well correlated with the severity of snoring. However this report discloses its accuracy is poor in 25 %. Clinical examination is not significantly different in the 3 groups. Measurement by CT scan brings 3 main results : frequency of upper airway narrowing is not different in the 3 groups ;in SAS patients, pharyngeal narrowing may be more important ; in all groups, dyspermeability at the posterior tongue space level is demonstrated by CT scan more often than clinically.

In a pragmatic point of view, only clinical symptom study brings a (relative) accuracy to estimate snoring consequences and sleep recording's necessity, whereas morphologic evaluation is not helpfull to attain these aims. However, ORL evaluation, associated with CT scan ($\pm$ cephalometry) is very important for therapeutic management : choice -or not- of surgical procedure, and its nature.

VII CHRONIC RHONCHOPATHY IN CHILDREN
Chairman: A. Grimfield

Gradual childhood development of obstructive sleep apnea and behavioral sequelae treated with adenoidectomy

L. Scrima, S. Skakich-Scrima and N. Snyderman

Sleep Disorders Center – 594, Department of Medicine & Otolaryngology, University of Arkansas for Medical Sciences, Little Rock, Arkansas 72205, USA

Heavy snoring and/or obstructive sleep apnea (OSA) has been documented in non-obese children and successfully treated with tonsillectomy and/or adenoidectomy. One report on 25 children age 2-14 without OSA or oxygen desaturation, but with heavy nocturnal snoring and restless sleep, indicated that behavioral sequelae were as prominent as the primary presenting complaint (1). This case describes the gradual development of polysomnogram (PSG) documented OSA in a non-obese child, who was referred for mouth-breathing and snoring, and presented a constellation of behavioral symptoms similar to the children of another report (1) who did not have OSA.

At the time of the patient's first PSG, he was a healthy, non-obese, 5.4 year old Caucasian male with a slightly recessed chin, who had been a loud snorer since the age of 3. He was described by his parents as a healthy, very active infant. Between 1.5-2.5 years of age, he was sleeping 9-11 hrs/24 hrs. During his second year, he began to snore softly and was noted to have an elongated uvula. At age 3, prominent snoring began following a severe upper respiratory infection. He became a mouth breather with hypersalivation, drooping lower jaw, and increasing mild speech articulation problems, as well as being a loud snorer with gasping, labored breathing and continuous thumb sucking during sleep. His parents also noted that his total sleep time increased by 1-2 hrs. His sleep was very restless and he became difficult to awaken in the mornings. Behaviorally, he became clumsy, quarrelsome, easily frustrated, impulsive, and had a short attention span for active sequential tasks (e.g., drawing, puzzles). His passive attention span (e.g., for stories being read) remained very good.

A PSG confirmed that the patient had mild OSA (16 apneas/hr of sleep, each lasting 10-30 sec), almost exclusively during REM sleep, and snored in stages 1 and 2 sleep. He also had a 0 min latency to his first REM sleep period. An otolaryngology evaluation found moderately prominent tonsils, a high arched hard palate (believed by some orthodontists to be caused by prominent tonsils forcing the tongue forward and upward) and a slight overbite. A lateral head-neck X-ray also revealed enlarged adenoids. Due to parental preference not to remove the tonsils, only an adenoidectomy was done. A very large obstructive adenoid tuft in the midline was removed, along with the remainder of the excess nasopharyngeal tissue. Pathology report noted hyperplasia of the adenoid tissue with acute chronic inflammation. About 5 weeks after surgery, another PSG was done and documented no apneas nor obstructed breathing; REM sleep occurred in nearly the same amount and percentage as was recorded in the first PSG. The latency to the first REM sleep period returned to within normal expectations (79 min).

This case is suggestive of a number of factors that might have interacted to contribute to the development of OSA in a non-obese child. Chronic nasal congestion secondary to lingering colds or allergies may cause inflammation and enlargement of adenoid and tonsillar tissues. This promotes chronic mouth-breathing and snoring, which may further irritate these tissues. Another feature worth pointing out is the REM onset sleep during the first PSG. It is possible that, since the patient's OSAs occurred almost exclusively during REM sleep, he may have been REM sleep deprived, which can cause REM sleep onset. Clinically, it was reported by the child's parents that mouth-breathing, snoring and restless sleep were no longer present and that he now sleeps an average of 1-2 hrs less per 24 hrs. The behavioral characteristics remain the same but are less extreme. He is more cheerful and is able to focus attention on tasks for longer periods. The gradual onset of loud snoring in this case may be representative of other children with OSA and therefore could be of etiological significance.

1. GUILLEMINAULT C. et al., Eur J Pediatr 1982, 139: 165-171.

Noisy snoring during sleep in infants with pulmonary disease. Isn't pathologic?

E.N. Garabedian, M. Boule, M. Eisenfiz and A. Grimfield

Laboratoire de Physiologie et départements de Pédiatrie et d'oto-rhino-laryngologie, Hôpital Trousseau, 26 avenue Dr Arnold Netter, 75571 Paris, France

ABSTRACT

Pulmonary function was studied in 43 infants suffering from pulmonary disease of various etiology. The age of the children (17 ± 8 months) needed measurements on sleeping children in supine position sedated by chloral hydrate with a dose lower than 50 mg.kg^{-1}. Study of pulmonary function included measurement of lung mechanics (lung resistance and dynamic compliance) which were determined by means of oesophageal balloon technique, while children breathed via a face mask. Infants were studied during periods judged on behavioural criteria to be N.Rem sleep. During measurements noisy snoring appears in 11 infants. Therefore the aim of the study was to set up relationships between noisy snoring pulmonary disease and oto-rhino-laryngologic disease ; and to describe characteristics of lung mechanics and breathing pattern infants during noisy snoring.

KEYWORDS

Pulmonary function test, pulmonary disease, oto-rhino-laryngologic disease, noisy snoring, infants.

INTRODUCTION

The studies of NOONAN (1) and MENASHE (2) established that enlarged tonsils including nocturnal snoring, can lead to upper airway obstruction during sleep with chronic hypoventilation and cor pulmonale.

In infants with pulmonary disease, we observed sometimes noisy snoring during pulmonary function study. Indeed pulmonary function study in infants needed measurements on sleeping children, on supine position sedated by chloral hydrate. So the aim of the study was to :
- evaluate the percentage of snorers infants during pulmonary function study,
- set up relationship between noisy snoring, pulmonary disease and oto-rhino-laryngologic pathology,
- describe lung mechanics and breathing pattern during snoring compared with non snorer infants.

SUBJECTS AND METHODS

SUBJECTS
During 1986, pulmonary function was studied in 43 infants less than 3 yrs (17 ± 8 months), suffering from various pulmonary disease : bronchopulmonary dysplasia n = 11 ; recurent bronchitis and bronchiolitis n = 23 ; congenital diaphragmatic hernia n = 3 ; inhaled foreign bodies n = 2 ; severe infectious pulmonary disease n = 2 ; congenital pulmonary malformation n = 2.

METHODS
The following measurements were made in all infants while they slept, on supine position, sedated by chloral hydrate (dose 50 mg/kg), during periods judged on behavioural criteria to be N Rem sleep

- Lung mechanics : lung resistance (R_L) and dynamic lung compliance (ClDyn) by the oesophageal balloon technique (GAULTIER et al 1974 : infants breathed via a face mask).

- Breathing pattern components : calculated from breathing volume curves, they were tidal volume normalized for body weight (VT_{Bw}) ; respiratory rate (R) ; inspiratory (TI) and expiratory (TE) times ; the fraction of inspiratory time compared with total respiratory cycle duration i.e duty cycle (TI/T_{TOT}) ; and the mean inspiratory flow normalized for body weight (VT_{Bw}/TI) (GAULTIER et al 1983).

In 13 infants, oxygen tension was measured by cutaneous measurement (Radiometer TcPO2 electrode heated to 44°C). Variation in TcPO2 was studied between sleep and awake.

In all, blood gases were measured while they were awake, with arterialized blood sample (GAULTIER et al 1978).

RESULTS

Noisy snoring appears in 11 infants i.e 26% (obstructive apnea was observed in 1 children). So children were separated into two groups :
- group I : snorer infants (S)
- group II : non snorer infants (NS)

and in these two groups we compared pulmonary disease, oto-rhino-laryngologic disease, lung mechanics breathing pattern components and variation in TcPO2 between sleep and awake.

1) Pulmonary disease
The pulmonary disease observed in the S were as following : pulmonary bronchodysplasia n = 2 ; recurent bronchitis and bronchiolitis n=5 ; severe infectious pulmonary disease n = 1 ; congenital pulmonary malformation n = 1.

2) Oto-rhino-laryngologic disease

ORL testings were done in 35 infants (snorer infants n = 8).
The different abnormalities are displayed on the following table.

	ORL Recurent disease	Trachéo-laryngo-abnormalities	Enlarged adenoïds	Enlarged tonsils
S n = 8	3 (37%)	2 (25%)	2 (25%)	4 (50%)
NS n = 27	3 (9%)	5 (15%)	6 (19%)	3 (9%)

It was difficult to evaluate the degree of abnormalities but it seems that ORL abnormalities were mild in the two populations. Indeed the percentage was different : ORL abnormalities in our study are more frequent in snorer infants.

3) Lung mechanics
In S R_L measured during snoring was significantly more increased
(mean ± SD : 570 ± 270%) than in NS group
(mean ± SD : 239 ± 70%) p 0,001.

No significant difference was observed in ClDyn.
S : mean ± SD = 54 + 30 ; NS : mean + SD 67 + 19.

4) Breathing pattern
There was no significant difference between values obtained for the S and NS group in R, TI, TE, TI/T_{TOT}.
VT_{Bw} was significantly lower in S.

5) Variation in TcPO2
In S we measured variation in TcPO2 between sleep and awake in 5 infants.
The mean variation was 23 mmHg ± 7.

In NS we measured variation in TcPO2 in 8 infants. The mean variation was
15 mmHg ± 9.

6) Blood gases
The mean PaO2 for S group was 78 ± 11 and the mean PaCO2 was 39 ± 4.

In the NS group the mean PaO2 was 81 ± 11 and the mean PaCO2 37 ± 4.

DISCUSSION

In S we observed a very hight R_L during sleep and significantly higher than in NS.
On a clinical point of view S infants were not among the most severe pulmonary
disease (for example pulmonary bronchodysplasia).
On a functional point of view, blood gases measured while infants were awake were
not different in the two groups and decrease in ClDyn which reflect distal
obstruction was similar in the two groups. Higher increase in R_L in S can be
supposed to be in relation with pharyngeal resistance created by loss of
pharyngeal tone (REMMERS et Al. 1978). The oto-rhino-laryngologic pathology in S
was mild and did'nt seem explain the noisy snoring and the severe airway
obstruction (PRAUD et Al. 1984). Indeed all infant were not examined by ORL
physician and ORL testing was not performed at the same time than pulmonary
function study. The effect of chloral hydrate can not be excluded. Since in ani-
mals the activity of the genioglossus has been reported to decrease after administration of a hypnotic dose (BROUILLETTE et Al. 1981). Indeed, in studies
comparing natural sleep with sleep facilitated by chloral hydrate administration
at dosages similar to those we used, airway mechanics (STOCKS et Al. 1977),
breathing pattern and alveolar ventilation (LESS et Al. 1982) were
similar.
the large mean decrease in TcPO2 could indicated alveolar hypoventilation secondary to airway obstruction, that agree with lower VT_{Bw} in S.

CONCLUSION

This open study set up a large airway obstruction during some parts of sleep in
snorer infants. The airway obstruction is associated with a important alveolar
hypoventilation. Pulmonary and oto-rhino-laryngologic pathology cannot
explain at present the cause of the snoring and the high airway obstruction.
These preliminary results suggest to study more completely sleep in snorer infants
with a precise ORL examination in order to detect a local cause to the snoring.

REFERENCES BIBLIOGRAPHIQUES

Brouillette, R.T. (1981) : Chloral hydrate depresses genioglossus but not diaphragmatic activity. Fed. Proc. 40, 1379.
Gaultier, C. (1974) : Résistance pulmonaire totale et compliance pulmonaire dynamique (chez l'enfant de 3 à 15 ans). Principe discussion des valeurs normales intérêt de la mesure. Ann. Pediatr. (Paris). 21, 291-298.
Gaultier, C. (1979) : Détermination of capillary oxygen tension in infants and children. Bull. Europ.Physiopathol. Resp. 14, 287-297.
Guilleminault, C. (1982) : Children and nocturnal snoring ; evaluation of the effect of sleep related respiratory resistive load and day time functioning. Eur. J. Pediatr. 139, 165-171.
Gaultier, C. (1983) : Adaptation of the pattern of breathing during lung growth. Am. Rev. Resp. Dis. 127, 234.
Lees, M.H. (1982) : Chloral hydrate and the carbon dioxide chemoreceptor response. A study of puppies and infants. Pediatrics. 70, 447-450.
Menashe, V.D. (1965) : Hypoventilation and cor pulmonale due to chronic upper airway obstruction. J. Pediatr. 67, 198-203.
Noonan, J.A. (1965) : Reversible cor pulmonale due to hypertrophycal tonsils and adenoids : studies in two cases. Circulation. 32, 164.
Praud, J.P. (1984) : Lung mechanics and breathing pattern during wakefulness and sleep in children with enlarged tonsil. Sleep. 7 (4), 304-312.
Remmers, J.E. (1978) : Pathogenesis of upper airway occlusion during sleep. J. Appl. Physiol. 44, 931-938.
Stocks, J. (1977) : Spécific airway conductance in relation to post conceptional age during infancy. J. Appl. Physiol. 43, 144-154.

RESUME

La fonction respiratoire a été étudiée chez 43 nourrissons atteints de pathologie respiratoire diverse. L'âge des enfants (17 $\pm$ 8 mois) a necessité une exploration chez des enfants endormis, prémédiqués avec du sirop de chloral (dose inférieure à 50 mcg.kg) en position décubitus dorsal. L'étude a compris la mesure des paramètres mécaniques (résistance pulmonaire et compliance pulmonaire dynamique) par la technique du cathéter oesophagien. L'enregistrement est réalisé par l'intermédiaire d'un masque facial. Durant ces mesures, réalisées selon des critères de comportements pendant des périodes de sommeil calme, des ronflements sont apparus chez 11 enfants. Le but de l'étude a été de rechercher des relations entre le ronflement, la maladie respiratoire, et/ou la maladie ORL, et de décrire les caractéristiques des paramètres mécaniques et du régime ventilatoire pendant la période de ronflement.

Heavy snorers disease in children

M. Zucconi, F. Cirignotta, E. Sforza, S. Mondini, A. Rinaldi Ceroni*, F. Tartari* and E. Lugaresi

Institute of Neurology and Otolaringology, University of Bologna, Bologna, Italy*

SUMMARY

We studied 10 children with heavy snorers disease using polysomnography. Obstructive apneas or hypopneas were present in 8 out of 10 children with a mean of 35 apneas or hypopneas per hour of sleep. All patients had marked snoring during sleep with " pathological snoring"(associated with a decrease in SaO_2) in some of them. All patients had important adeno-tonsillar hyperplasia and 4 of them underwent adenotonsillectomy with complete disappearance of apneas and snoring. We believe that snoring with O_2 desaturation may also play an important role in the symptoms and consequences of heavy snorers disease.

INTRODUCTION

In adults Heavy Snorers Disease(HSD) is a clinical entity characterized by a continuum from trivial heavy snoring to Obstructive Sleep Apnea Syndrome(OSAS) with a gradual progression from snoring with sporadic apneas to complicated cases with persistent apneas during sleep and alveolar hypoventilation during wakefulness(Lugaresi 1983).

In children too, snoring reflects breathing abnormalities during sleep due to anatomical or functional upper airway stenosis.

Recently Guilleminault(1987) showed that children with heavy snoring throughout the night, without apneas, have the same clinical symptoms as children with clear OSAS. In these children the clinical consequences(somnolence, cardiocirculatory impairment, slow development) may be as severe as in the OSAS group.

In order to evaluate this clinical entity we studied a group of children referred to us for loud heavy snoring that alarmed their parents.

MATERIAL AND METHOD

The group included 10 children(7M,3F) with a mean age of 4.2 ± 1.9 yrs (range 1.5-8 yrs) .Each child underwent an analytic sleep history and clinical examination.

A nocturnal polysomnographic examination including EEG,EOG,EMG of submental and intercostal muscles, microphone, EKG, oro-nasal, thoracic and abdominal respirogram by means of strain-gauge, ear oxymetry (BIOX III BTI,Coulder,Colorado) was performed after clinical evaluation.

Snoring noise and O_2 saturation were also recorded at a low paper speed strip(Linseis 400 B7-SELB-West Germany).

4 children also underwent a second nocturnal polysomnography after adenotonsillectomy.The following were evaluated for each child: the most important clinical symptoms and some details of physical examination, sleep parameters including total sleep time(TST), sleep efficiency(total sleep time and total time in bed ratio)(SE),wakefulness after sleep onset(WASO), percentage of single sleep stages considering St.3 and St. 4 a single sleep phase. Moreover we considered respiratory parameters: apnea plus hypopnea index(A+H)I for total,NREM and REM sleep,mean low O_2 saturation (mean of the dips after each apnea or hypopnea) for total, NREM and REM sleep, the lowest O_2 saturation.

We also measured snoring time(considering an epoch of snoring when most of the epoch was occupied by snoring noise excluding apnea or hypopnea and the snorts at the end of the events), snoring percentage (respect to TST), mean O_2 saturation during snoring and considered "pathological snoring" the percentage of snoring time with O_2 saturation below 90% or below 4% of the level during normal breathing or wakefulness.Mean SaO_2 and lowest SaO_2 were calculated in the same way. Finally we considered(A+H)I, mean low SaO_2 during apnea or hypopnea, snoring percent and mean SaO_2 during snoring after surgery in 4 children.

RESULTS

The most important complaints and some objective data of the 10 children are reported into Table 1.

All children complained of snoring and apnea during sleep; 7 out of 10 had problems in physical development and 3 of them had a typical "pectus excavatum" reflecting their strenous efforts to breathe during the night.

Familiarity for snoring or apneas was clearly found in 7 children. Furthermore 3 children(nos 1,2 and 5) had clinical and radiological findings of pulmonary hypertension. Two of them had been initially admitted to cardiology departments for non invasive and invasive examination of systemic and pulmonary arterial pressures that showed an important(no.1) and slight(no.2) pulmonary hypertension.
Sleep parameters(Table 2) showed a mean TST of 428 min, with a mean SE of 0.86 .There was about 10% of stage 1 NREM with a lot of mini or macro arousals, as an index of disrupted sleep. The other sleep stages were normal.
Respiratory parameters(Table 3) showed a pathological (A+H)I in 8 patients(mean 35.8 ± 8.6) predominating in REM sleep. The mean low O_2 saturation was 79.4% with a severe degree of hypoxia and the most desaturated events in REM sleep in some children(nos 1,2,5).

Lowest O_2 saturation was below 80% in half the children.

Three out of 10 had more than 40% TST with snoring(excluding apnea or hypopnea) and in these patients almost all snoring time was "patholo gical snoring" with mean SaO_2 below 90% and a lowest SaO_2 varying between 82 and 40%(Table 4).

All children at the ENT examination showed an important adenotonsillar hypertrophy . 4 children(nos.1,2,3,4) underwent adenotonsillectomy with almost complete relief of apnea or hypopnea,snoring(mean(A+H) I:3.3;mean % of snoring:3.4) and clinical symptoms.

DISCUSSION

Almost all our children with a clear symptomatology of HSD showed a pathological(A+H)I.Furthermore all but one also had a prolonged snoring time taht in 3 patients was accompanied by a severe O_2 desaturation. These 3 patients were children with objective and subjective signs of pulmonary hypertension.

The "pathological snoring" was characterized by an increase in EMG amplitude of intercostal muscle during NREM sleep, an irregular snoring with some fluctuations in noise and intensity,sometimes a single obstructive breath followed by increased respiratory effort.

We did not analyse respiratory frequency during pathological snoring but the impression was that breathing was more irregular with waxing and waning of frequency, and not always accelerated.

In our opinion, confirmed by our cases, a complete obstruction of the upper airways is not necessary to lead symptoms and cardio-circulatory consequences of HSD. Snoring is an important fact especially if it

TABLE: 1 CLINICAL FINDINGS

PATIENT	SNORING	APNEA	NOCTURNAL MOTOR AGITATION	ENURESIS	DECREASED PERFORMANCE	BIZZARRE BEHAVIOR, IRRITABILITY	EXCESSIVE SOMNOLENCE	DECREASED DEVELOPMENT	PECTUS EXCAVATUM	PULMONARY HYPERTENSION	FAMILIARITY
1	+	+	+	−	+	+	+	+	+	+	+
2	+	+	−	+	+	+	+	+	−	+	+
3	+	+	−	−	−	−	±	−	−	−	−
4	+	+	−	−	−	−	−	±	−	−	+
5	+	+	+	−	−	−	+	+	+	+	+
6	+	+	−	−	+	+	+	+	+	−	+
7	+	+	−	−	−	−	+	+	−	−	−
8	+	+	+	−	−	−	−	+	−	−	+
9	+	+	−	−	−	+	−	+	−	−	+
10	+	+	−	−	−	−	−	−	+	−	+
TOT.	10/10	10/10	3/9	1/10	3/10	4/10	5/10	7/10	4/10	3/10	7/10

TABLE: 2 SLEEP PARAMETERS

PATIENT	TST (MIN.)	SLEEP EFFICIENCY	WASO (MIN.)	STAGE 1 (%)	STAGE 2 (%)	STAGE 3-4 (%)	STAGE REM(%)
1	387	0.85	0	9.1	39.9	22.5	28.5
2	462	0.92	16	14.1	42.1	15.4	28.4
3	463	0.91	34	14.7	52.7	18.4	14.2
4	395	0.85	10	12.2	43.0	27.3	17.3
5	470	0.95	15	8.7	73.6	11.9	5.7
6	479	0.87	8	4.8	51.6	19.2	24.4
7	429	0.90	0	3.5	51.8	20.0	24.6
8	404	0.78	60	9.2	54.0	22.8	13.9
9	421	0.79	56	5.5	49.2	23.0	22.2
10	377	0.78	92	10.1	51.6	21.7	16.5
M:	428.7	0.86	29.1	9.19	50.9	20.2	19.6
SD:	37.6	0.06	30.79	3.79	9.39	4.33	7.31

TABLE: 3 RESPIRATORY PARAMETERS

PATIENT N°	(A + H) I TOTAL	(A + H) I N-REM	(A + H) I REM	MEAN LOW Sa O_2 TOTAL (%)	MEAN LOW Sa O_2 N-REM (%)	MEAN LOW Sa O_2 REM (%)	LOWEST Sa O_2 (%)	SNORING TIME (MIN.)	MEAN SNORING Sa O_2 (%)
1	38.3	16.30	93.82	61.9	73.3	56.9	40	200	83.7
2	74.9	62.9	105.8	67.9	78.5	52.1	40	112	84.7
3	25.3	17.1	74.5	90.4	91.8	88.5	76	99	94.5
4	22.8	22.3	25.6	89.7	90.1	88.2	85	13	92.7
5	76.8	75.6	97.8	44.9	45.3	41.0	40	84	51.9
6	36.4	40.3	24.6	83.7	84.9	77.9	62	206	90.0
7	62.2	44.7	117.1	82.6	89.6	74.4	40	102	93.2
8	6.8	3.3	27.8	88.2	91.5	85.8	82	181	90.2
9	13.8	6.6	39.3	91.9	93.8	90.8	83	66	94.5
10	0.9	0.4	3.9	93.3	94.0	93.0	92	89	95.0
MEAN (SD)	35.8 (8.6)	28.9 (8.2)	61.0 (13)	79.4 (5.1)	83.3 (4.7)	74.9 (5.8)	64 (7)	115 (19.6)	87.0 (4.1)

TABLE: 4 RESPIRATORY PARAMETERS (SNORING)

PATIENT	SNORING TIME (MIN.)	SNORING %	MEAN SA O$_2$ (%)	PATHOLOGICAL SNORING (%)	MEAN SA O$_2$ (%)	LOWEST SA O$_2$ (%)
1	200	51.68	83.72	91.3	83.6	60
2	112	24.24	84.73	94.3	84.33	72
3	99	21.38	94.49	/	/	/
4	13	9.80	92.70	/	/	/
5	84	17.94	51.90	100	51.90	40
6	206	43.01	89.99	46.8	89.9	75
7	102	23.94	93.20	29.8	91.5	88
8	181	44.92	90.25	31.1	88.9	82
9	66	15.80	94.5	/	/	/
10	89	23.60	95.02	/	/	/

is associated with O_2 desaturation, and "pathological snoring" may play a crucial role alongside obstructive apneas, in determining pulmonary hypertension.

The clinical severity of HSD seems related not only to (A+H)I but to the percentage of pathological snoring, mean O_2 saturation during pathological snoring and mean O_2 saturation during obstructive apneas or hypopneas.

Previous reports, since the Sixties, have documented the development of cor pulmonale in children with enlarged tonsils or upper airway obstruction(Menashe 1965,Noonan 1965,Levy 1967,Kravath 1977) with complete relief of cardiocirculatory problems after tonsillectomy (Lind 1982,Grundfast 1982).Despite these findings there is still some reluctance to perform tonsillectomy when children's breathing is not impaired during wakefulness, even though upper airways stenosis during sleep may have an important effect on breathing work with cardiocirculatory consequences.

In two of our patients with pulmonary hypertension adenotonsillectomy relieved snoring and obstructive apneas or hypopneas almost completely.Only rare central apneas with no important O_2 desaturation may remain after surgical intervention.

Measures of pulmonary arterial pressure by a right atrial catheter showed normal values after tonsillectomy in one(n.1) child and resolution of clinical symptoms and EKG abnormality in case No.2.

The other child with pulmonary hypertension is now planning a tempo rary tracheostomy because of associated maxillo-facial abnormality.

Only follow-up clarify whether the problem is completely resolved in these children or whether further evaluation(ENT,Maxillo-facial) is necessary after puberty.

REFERENCES

Grundfast,K.M.;Wittich D.J.Jr.(1982):Adenotonsillar hypertrophy and upper airway obstruction in evolutionary perspective.Laryngoscope 92 ,650-656
Guilleminault,C.(1987):Obstructive sleep apnea syndrome in children. In:Sleep and its disorder in children .Ed. C.Guilleminault pp.213-224.New York:Raven Press.
Kravath,R.E.;Pollak,C.P.;Borowiecki,B.(1977):Hypoventilation during sleep in children who have lymphoid airway obstruction treated by nasopharyngeal tube and T and A.Pediatrics 59 ,865-871.
Levy ,A.M.;Tabakin,B.S.;Hansson,J.S.(1967):Hypertrophied adenoid causing pulmonary hypertension and severe congestive hearth failure.N.Engl.J.Med.207 ;506-511.

Lind,M.G.;Lundell,B.P.W.(1982):Tonsillar hyperplasia in children. A cause of obstructive sleep apneas,CO_2 retention, and retarded growth.Arch.Otolaryngol.108, 650-654.

Lugaresi E.;Mondini,S.;Zucconi,M.;Montagna,P.;Cirignotta,F.(1983): Staging of heavy snorers'disease.A proposal.Bull.Europ.Physiopath.Resp. 19 ,590-594.

Menashe,V.D.;Farrehi,C.;Miller,H.(1965):Hypoventilation and cor pulmonale due to chronic upper airway obstruction.J.Pediatr.67, 198-203.

Noonan,J(1965): Reversible cor pulmonale due to hypertrophied tonsils and adenoids: studies in two cases.Circulation 2(suppl.), 164.

RESUME

Nous avons étudié 10 enfants, soufrant de la maladie des grands ronfleurs par le enregistrement polysomnographique.Apnées ou hypopnées obstructives étaient present dans 8 enfants avec une moyenne de 35 apnées ou hypopnées/heure de sommeil. Touts ces patients ronflaient longuement pendant le sommeil, mostrant en quelque cas un"ronflement pathologique"(associé avec un decrement de la saturation de l'hémoglobine).

Touts les patients souffraient d'une hypertrophie marquée adeno-amygdaloidienne.L'ablation des amygdales et des végétations adénoidiennes(4 cas) a eu pour consequent la desapparition complète des apnées et de ronflement.

Nous croyons que ce ronflement avec desaturation d'oxygène puissent jouer un rôle important dans l'apparition de la symptomatologie et des consequences de la maladie des grands ronfleurs.

Treatment of sleep apnea in children with adenotonsillar hypertrophy by adenotonsillectomy

V. Wooten, G. Peters and Judy Hubbard

The Children's Hospital of Alabama, Birmingham, Alabama, USA

ABSTRACT

Seventy-five children from age 9 months to 16 years in the U.S. were referred for polysomnographic evaluation prior to tonsillectomy and adenoidectomy. Reasons for referral included loud snoring, chronic mouth breathing, excessive nasal secretions, recurrent upper respiratory infections and recurrent ear infections. A retrospective analysis showed that 46 (61.3 per cent) had obstructive sleep apnea syndrome (OSA). Forty-four patients had a tonsillectomy and adenoidectomy, and of these 42 (95.5 per cent) consented to follow-up polysomnography. Thirty-eight out of 42 (90.5 per cent) had resolution of their OSA. The mean lowest oxygen saturation in this group of 38 improved from 84.5 per cent to 92.3 per cent. The average number of apneas also improved from 18.5 per hour pre-operatively to 1.7 per hour. These findings suggest that OSA frequently occurs in children with symptomatic adenotonsillar hypertrophy and that tonsillectomy and adenoidectomy is a highly effective treatment.

KEY WORDS

Adenotonsillar hypertrophy, adenotonsillectomy, tonsillectomy, sleep apnea.

INTRODUCTION

Adenotonsillar hypertrophy (ATH) has been strongly implicated in the pathogenesis of pulmonary hypertension, cor pulmonale, growth failure, sleep disturbance and other symptoms that have been become known to be caused by obstructive sleep apnea syndrome (OSA) (Lind and Lundell, 1982; Menashe, et al 1965; Noonan, 1965). The parents or other caretakers of children with ATH generally complain of noisy respiration during sleep, restless sleep, mouth-breathing and/or difficulty swallowing. The child with ATH may also have chronic rhinorrhea, frequent middle ear infections and recurrent pharyngitis. Unfortunately, fairly stringent surgical indications were recommended in the U.S.A. (Ruben and Weg, 1975) at a time when there were few facilities available to objectively determine the presence of OSA in patients. In addition, there are few studies reported in the literature that indicate how often OSA exists in association with ATH. In this paper we will present data which indicates that ATH in children frequently results in OSA and that adenotonsillectomy (T&A) is a highly effective treatment.

SUBJECTS AND METHODS

Between April 1985 and October 1986, 75 patients with ATH were referred by otolaryngologists for polysomnographic evaluation prior to T&A. These children were seen in the otolaryngology clinic with complaints that included recurrent otitis media and pharyngitis, chronic mouth-breathing, loud snoring and excessive nasal secretions. All of the children were noted to have enlarged tonsils and adenoids on physical examination. The age of the subjects ranged from 9 months to 16 years. There were 41 boys and 34 girls. The mean age of the subjects was 5.7 years. Thirty-one of the subjects ranged in age from 9 months to 4 years, 34 of the subjects from age 5 to 9 years and 10 of the subjects from 11 to 16 years.

Polygraphic recording was performed on a Nihon Kohden 4212P polysomnograph. There was continuous monitoring of the electroencephalogram, chin electromyogram, electrooculogram, electrocardiogram, nasal and oral airflow and thoracic and abdominal respiratory effort. Anterior tibialis electromyograms were recorded in patients over 5 years of age as a screen for nocturnal myoclonus. There was also continuous video monitoring under infrared lighting for each patient. Blood oxyhemoglobin saturation was measured by either a Biox II, Biox III or Nellcor oximeter. Recording of sleep stages was performed according to the methods of Rechtschaffen and Kales (1968). Apneas were defined as a cessation of airflow at the nose and mouth for 10 seconds or longer in duration with or without respiratory effort. Hypopneas, or partial apneas, were defined as events in which there was a substantial (approximately 50 per cent or more) reduction in airflow in association with desaturations and/or arousals. The clinically significant number of events necessary to warrant a diagnosis of sleep apnea was set at 5 or more apneas and/or hypopneas per hour of sleep (the apnea/hypopnea index, AHI). The studies were performed during the patient's normal bedtime hours and a minimum of 3 hours total sleep time including an episode of rapid eye movement (REM) sleep was necessary in order to consider the studies valid. All studies were scored by a trained polysomnographic technician. Repeat polysomnography was performed at least 6 weeks postoperatively on patients having T&A. Remission was defined as an AHI of less than 5 events per hour and a lowest oxygen desaturation above 90 per cent.

RESULTS

Of the 75 patients studied, 46 (61.2 per cent) were found to have clinically significant OSA. The mean apnea/hypopnea index was 22.1 per hour of sleep and the mean lowest oxygen saturation level was 79.1 per cent. Of the patients with OSA, 44 had T&A. One patient was not returned for treatment and the remaining patient was determined to be inoperable due to an enlarged tongue and soft palate. As only 42 (91.3 per cent) returned for a follow-up study, it is this group of patients on which surgical results are based. Their lowest mean pre-operative oxygen saturation was 80.2 per cent and the lowest mean oxygen saturation after surgery was 90.6 per cent. Follow-up polysomnography revealed that 38 of the 42 (90.5 per cent) consenting to a follow up study had remission of the apnea by clinical criteria. The lowest mean oxygen saturation in the 38 children with resolution of OSA was 84.5 per cent prior to surgery and 92.3 per cent after T&A. Their AHI improved from 18.5 to 1.7. The documented treatment failures included a 2 year old girl with a post-operative AHI of 16.9 and a lowest oxygen saturation of 68 per cent, a 7 year old male with a post-operative AHI of 11.6 and a lowest oxygen saturation of 87 per cent, a 6 year old with a post-operative AHI of 10.7 and a lowest oxygen saturation of 53 per cent and a 16 year old female with a post-operative AHI of 9.9 and a lowest oxygen desaturation of 87 per cent. The average post-operative AHI among these four failures was 12.3 and the mean lowest oxygen saturation was to 73.8 per cent.

Eighteen of the 46 patients (39.1 per cent) with OSA were age 9 months to
4 years old. In the 5 to 9 year old group there were 24 (52.2 per cent) with
OSA. Only 8.7 per cent (3) of the children with OSA were in the 10 to 16
year old age range. Of the 18 children with OSA in the 9 month to 4 year
old age group, 16 had T&A. Fifteen (93.8 per cent) had resolution of their
OSA. Twenty-one of the 23 (91.3 per cent) children with OSA in the 5 to 9
year old age range, and 2 out of 3 (66.7 per cent) in the 10 year-and-older
age range also achieved remission of OSA after T&A (see table).

TABLE

	9 mo-4 yrs	5-9 yrs	10+ yrs	Total
No referred	31	34	10	75
+ OSA	18	24	4	46
T&A	16	24	4	44
Post-Operative Polysomnography	16	23	3	42
OSA resolved	15	21	2	38
% Remission	(15/16)93.8%	(21/23)91.3%	(2/3)66.7%	(38/42)90.5%

DISCUSSION

The results of our study indicate that OSA is probably more common in children
with symptomatic ATH than realized. Certainly the otolaryngologists referring
to our center were attuned to the symptoms of OSA and the children that were
referred for polysomnographic evaluation were at least suspected of having
OSA. However, our results indicate that perhaps a high index of suspicion
is worthwhile in children with symptomatic ATH.

It was interesting to find that OSA occurred more frequently in children between
the ages of 9 months and 10 years old with the peak occurrence in the 5-9
year age range. Studies of adults (Dement, et al, 1982) have shown that sleep
apnea becomes more common with increasing age. It may be that the nasopharyngeal
lymphoidal tissue is more sensitive to allergins and infections before the
onset of puberty and becomes hypertrophied. With the onset of adolescence,
the natural attrition of the lymphoidal tissue reduces the likelihood of sleep
apnea. Our study shows that in those patients with OSA due to ATH that T&A
is a highly effective treatment, resulting in a 90.5 per cent cure rate.
This rate of remission is much higher than for adults undergoing either T&A
alone or a uvulopalatopharyngoplasty. These findings tend to suggest that
OSA in pre-pubertal children is more likely to be caused by mechanical airway
obstruction due to enlarged tonsils and adenoids, while OSA in adults is probably
caused by other anatomical and/or neurological factors.

Because ATH has been associated with serious cardiovascular disease, developmental
delays, maladaptive behavior and cognitive impairments, objective searches
for OSA should be undertaken in any child with symptomatic ATH. Despite surgery,
however, four of our patients failed to have remission of their OSA after
T&A and indeed continued to have quite significant illness. Although our
findings indicate that there is resolution of OSA following T&A in the majority
of cases, objective polysomnographic monitoring is necessary to confirm that
the surgery is of benefit.

RESUME

Le but de cette étude rétrospective est de déterminer la fréquence d'apnée obstructive du sommeil (OSA) chez les enfants souffrant d'hypertrophie symptomatique des amygdales et des végétations adénoïdes (ATH) et aussi de déterminer le degré d'efficacité tendant à soulager ce trouble qu'il y a dans l'ablation des amygdales et des végétations adénoïdes (T&A). Des otorhinolaryngologistes ont envoyé 75 patients souffrant de ATH en vue d'une évaluation polysomnographique. L'âge des sujets variait de 9 mois à 16 ans et l'âge moyen était de 5, 7 ans. Il y avait 41 garçons et 34 filles. La plupart d'entre eux souffrait de congestion dans les parties respiratoires supérieures, d'otites fréquentes de pharyngites fréquentes et/ou de respiration bruyante. L'enregistrement polygraphique a été accompli sur un polysomnographe Nihon Kohden, 4212P. Il y a eu un contrôle continu d'EEG, d'EMG des muscles du mentom d'EOG, d'ECG, du flux de l'air nasal et oral par des thermistances et de l'effort respiratoire abdominal et thoracique par impedance. On a contrôlé le tibialis anterieur, par des EMG's chez des patients âgés de plus de 5 ans. La saturation d'oxyhémoglobine sanguine a été mesurée soit par un oxymètre Biox II, Biox III ou Nellcor. On a établi les différents stades de sommeil selon les méthodes decrites par Rechtschaffen et Kales. Les apnées ont été defines comme étant un arrêt du flux de l'air au niveau du nez et de la bouche pendant une durée de 10 seconds ou plus avec ou sans effort respiratoire. Les hypopnées ont été definies comme des cas dans lesquels il y avait une réduction substantielle dans le flux de l'air associé a des désaturations et/ou des réveils. Cliniquement, l'apnée significative a été definie comme un évènement survenant 5 fois ou plus par heure de sommeil (indicateur de l'apnée/hypopnée).

On a trouvé 46 patients sur 75 (61,3 per cent) qui souffraient cliniquement d'OSA significative. Le chiffre indicateur moyen de l'apnée'hypopnée était de 22, 1 par heure de sommeil et la plus basse saturation d'oxygène moyenne était de 79.1 per cent. 42 sur 46 patients (91.3 per cent) avaient subi l'ablation des amygdales et des végétations adénoïdes et avaient une polysomnographie refaite. Avant l'operation, la plus basse saturation d'oxygène moyenne était de 80.2 per cent. Une polysomnographie refaite au moins 6 semaines après l'operation a révélé que 38 sur 42 enfants (90.5 per cent) ont eu une rémission de l'apnée selon nos critères cliniques. La moyenne de saturation oxygène la plus basse après l'operation a été de 90.6 per cent. Notre conclusion devant ces données est que l'OSA est commune chez les enfants souffrant d'hypertrophie symptomatique des amygdales et des végétations adénoïdes et que l'ablation des amygdales et des végétations est extrêmement efficace pour soulager l'OSA.

REFERENCES

Dement, W.C., Miles, L.E. and Carskadon, M.A. (1982): "White paper" on sleep and aging. J. Am. Geriatr. Soc. 30:25-50.

Lind, M.G. and Lundell, B.P.W. (1982): Tonsillar hyperplasia in children: A cause of obstructive sleep apnea, CO_2 retention, and retarded growth. Arch. Otolaryngol. 108:650-654.

Menashe, V.D., Farrehi, C. and Miller, M. (1965): Hypoventilation and cor pulmonale due to chronic upper airway obstruction. J. Pediatr. 67:198-203.

Noonan, J.A. (1965): Reversible cor pulmonale due to hypertrophied tonsils and adenoids: Studies in two cases. Circulation 32:164.

Rechtschaffen, A., Kales, A. (Eds.) (1968): *A Manual of Standardized Terminology, Techniques and Scoring System for Sleep Stages of Human Subjects.* Brain Information Service/Brain Research Institute, University of California at Los Angeles, U.S.A.

Ruben, R.J. and Weg, N. (1975): Contraindications to adenoidectomy. *Bull. N.Y. Acad. Med.* 51:817.

*Many thanks to Katherine Cook for her invaluable assistance in preparing the manuscript.

Apnées obstructives du sommeil chez l'enfant: à propos de 28 observations

S. Bobin*, C. le Pajolec*, P. Attal** and C. Gaultier**

*Service ORL Pédiatrique, Hôpital Le Kremlin Bicêtre, France
**Laboratoire d'Explorations fonctionnelles, Hôpital Antoine Béclère, Clamart, France

RESUME

28 children were evaluated for obstructive sleep apnea (O. S. A.).
All children were studied clinically and a standardized questionnaire was filled by the parents to know the usual habits of the child (sleep, and day behaviour). Sleep monitoring was performed by invasive methods evaluating the different stages of sleep (E.E.G., E.O.G., E.M.G.). Additionally oral and nasal airflow, thoracic and abdominal breathing movements, pulmonary gaz exchanges (transcutaneous PO_2 and PCO_2) were recorded.
Daytime nap was studied in 25 patients and night sleep in 2 patients.
The main cause of O.S.A. was hypertrophy of the tonsils. (23 patients). The other causes were uncommon diseases (Pierre Robin syndrome, Willi-Prader disease, laryngomalacia, Arnold-Chiari malformation).
20 children underwent surgical treatment (adeno-tonsillectomy : 21, staphylorraphy : 1, palatopharyngoplasty : 3, epiglottoplasty : 2).
Long-term results were based on clinical study, on standardized questionnaire, and for 8 children on post-operative sleep evaluation.

MOTS CLEFS

Apnée obstructive du sommeil, enregistrement polygraphique du sommeil, ronflement, enfant.

INTRODUCTION

Depuis la publication de Gastaut en 1966 sur les apnées obstructives du sommeil chez l'adulte obèse et celle de Guilleminault en 1976 rapportant dans la littérature pédiatrique la première série d'enfants présentant des apnées obstructives du sommeil, les travaux consacrés à cette pathologie nouvelle se sont multipliés, qu'ils émanent de physiologiste, de pneumologue, de pédiatre ou d'O.R.L. La présente étude rapporte les données cliniques, polygraphiques, thérapeutiques et évolutives de 28 enfants cliniquement suspects d'Apnée Obstructive du Sommeil (A.O.S) pris en charge dans le service d'O.R.L. pédiatrique de Bicêtre en 1985 et 1986.

PATIENTS ET METHODES :

Il s'agit de 28 enfants vus en consultation avec un tableau clinique évoquant des apnées ou des hypopnées obstructives du sommeil.

Pour chaque enfant, un bilan comportant une anamnèse et examen clinique complet a été réalisé.

Dans 20 cas un questionnaire ayant trait aux différents symptomes diurnes et surtout nocturnes a été rempli par les parents sous contrôle médical.
(tableaux I et II). Questionnaire standardisé. Symptomes nocturnes.

                Ronflement
                Difficulté respiratoire
                Pause
                Agitation
                Réveil
                Soif
                Sueurs

                Réponses possibles :

                      - jamais
                      - parfois
                      - souvent
                      - toujours

(tableau II)   Symptomes diurnes

            Somnolence
            Agressivité
            Appétit médiocre
            Difficulté à la déglutition
            Respiration buccale
            Angines

Ce questionnaire a permis l'établissement d'un score propre à chaque enfant selon la formule proposée par Brouillette dès 1984 :

$$S = 0,71 R + 1,42 D + 1,41 A - 3,83$$

où R est le ronflement, D les difficultés respiratoires, A les pauses respiratoires nocturnes. R et D sont affectés des valeurs suivantes : jamais = 0, parfois = 1, souvent = 2, toujours = 3, A est affecté de la valeur 0 pour non et 1 pour oui.

Dans 27 cas un enregistrement polygraphique du sommeil a été pratiqué dans le service d'Explorations Fonctionnelles du Pr. Gaultier à l'hôpital Antoine Béclère. Le sommeil naturel sans déprivation préalable ni prémédication a été enregistré durant une sieste, (25 cas) ou une nuit (2 cas).

Le tableau suivant dresse la liste des paramètres surveillés.

(tableau III)   Stades de sommeil (EEG, EOG, EMG de la houppe du menton)

          Débit aérien (thermistances nasale et buccale)
          Mouvements thoraciques et abdominaux (magnétomètre)
          Echanges gazeux (pression transcutanée en O_2 et en CO_2)
          EMG des muscles respiratoires
          Rythme cardiaque

La durée retenue pour l'apnée pathologique est supérieure ou égale à 5 secondes.

Une échocardiographie a été demandée chez 5 enfants dont le tableau clinique était préoccupant par son intensité ou son ancienneté.

RESULTATS

Notre série porte sur 19 garçons et 9 filles âgés de 1 mois à 10 ans, la moyenne se situant à 3,5 ans.

Le motif de consultation n'est pas toujours le ronflement nocturne (15 cas) mais parfois des infections O.R.L. récidivantes (6 cas), le bilan d'une malformation (2 cas), un retard staturo-pondéral (3 cas) dont l'un avec malaises anoxiques sévères depuis plusieurs mois, un stridor (1 cas) et une banale hypoacousie (1 cas).

Les réponses obtenues aux questionnaires sont détaillées dans les tableaux suivants.

(tableau IV)
>Ronflement : 16 cas
>Difficultés respiratoires : 17 cas
>Pauses respiratoires : 13 cas
>Agitation : 13 cas
>Réveil : 13 cas
>Soif : 13 cas
>Sueurs : 12 cas

(tableau V)
>Somnolence : 4 cas
>Agressivité : 4 cas
>Appétit médiocre : 10 cas
>Difficultés de déglutition : 8 cas
>Respiration buccale : 16 cas
>Angine : 7 cas

Le score calculé d'après la formule de Brouillette se distribue selon le schéma suivant : (schéma 1).
17 scores sont positifs et 3 seulement sont négatifs. 9 sont supérieurs à 3,5 , chiffre au-delà duquel Brouillette considère comme certain le diagnostic d'A.O.S. 3 sont inférieurs à - 1 éliminant le diagnostic d'A.O.S. du moins cliniquement. Enfin, 8 sont compris entre - 1 et 3,5 ne permettant pas de trancher.

Les résultats des enregistrements polygraphiques du sommeil sont les suivants : 14 patients répondent aux critères définissant le syndrome d'A.O.S. en sommeil nocturne (2 cas) ou de sieste (12 cas), l'enregistrement comportant suffisamment de sommeil paradoxal pour permettre une conclusion.

Pour 4 patients l'absence de sommeil paradoxal ne permet pas de conclure.
1 patient présente des signes d'A.O.S. même en sommeil calme.
8 patients ne répondent pas aux critères définissant le syndrome d'A.O.S. Toutefois, il existe une augmentation du travail respiratoire en sommeil paradoxal.

Le tableau suivant décrit les résultats chez 10 de nos patients âgés de 18 à 63 mois présentant une A.O.S. comparés aux résultats obtenus dans une population témoin de même âge (données personnelles Pr. C. Gaultier).
(tableau VI)

L'examen clinique des patients a permis de retrouver chez chacun d'entre eux une cause favorisante à la survenue de ces apnées.
Hypertrophie amygdalienne : 23 cas, laryngomalacie dont l'une âgée de presque 2 ans présentait un tableau clinique incompatible avec le délai d'enregistrement du sommeil et opérée en urgence,* syndrome de Willi-Prader : 1 cas, Malformation d'Arnold Chiari : 1 cas, syndrome de Pierre Robin : 1 cas.

Les 5 échocardiographies demandées sont normales.

TRAITEMENT :

22 enfants ont été opérés, l'indication étant essentiellement portée sur la clinique. Le geste réalisé a consisté en une adéno-amygdalectomie dans 16 cas, une adéno-amygdalectomie avec uvulo-palato-pharyngoplastie dans 3 cas, une épiglottoplastie dans 2 cas et une staphylorraphie dans 1 cas.

Tous les enfants dont l'enregistrement du sommeil était positif ont été opérés sauf 2, l'un car perdu de vue, l'autre car présentant plus de 60 % d'apnée centrales.

Tous les enfants dont le score de Brouillette dépassait 2,5 et pour lesquels l'enregistrement polygraphique ne comportait pas de sommeil paradoxal ou présentait des signes d'augmentation du travail respiratoire n'autorisant pas encore à l'heure actuelle une conclusion formelle ont été également opérés. Les 3 enfants dont le score de Brouillette était inférieur à - 1 n'ont pas été opérés.

RESULTATS POST OPERATOIRES :

16 questionnaires post opératoires ont été remplis correctement. Les réponses obtenus sont les suivantes :
(tableau VII)
(tableau VIII)

La distribution des scores est la suivante : (Schéma 2)

Tous sont inférieurs à - 1 sauf 1. 8 enregistrements polygraphiques du sommeil ont été réalisés en post opératoire. Dans 4 cas l'absence de sommeil paradoxal interdit toute conclusion. Dans 3 autres cas, le syndrome d'A.O.S. a disparu 3 à 6 mois après l'intervention. Toutefois persistent des signes de travail respiratoire accru.
Dans 1 cas les signes d'A.O.S. n'ont disparu qu'au bout de 13 mois.

COMMENTAIRES :

Nous voudrions insister sur les points suivants :
- la valeur prédictive de la clinique :
Si l'on suit la démonstration de Brouillette, les enfants dont le score dépasse 3,5 ont un syndrome d'A.O.S. certain sans qu'il soit nécessaire de recourir à des enregistrements polygraphiques du sommeil.
Parmi les 8 patients de notre série appartenant à ce groupe, l'enregistrement s'est révélé positif dans 6 cas alors qu'il s'est révélé ininterprétable faute de sommeil paradoxal dans 1 cas et négatif dans 1 autre cas.
Les enfants dont le score est inférieur à - 1, toujours selon Brouillette n'ont pas d'A.O.S. 3 enfants de notre série appartenaient à un tel groupe, leurs enregistrements polygraphiques sont tous 3 négatifs.
Enfin un score compris entre - 1 et 3,5 ne permet pas de trancher.
Parmi les 8 enfants de notre série appartenant à ce groupe, 5 présentaient des enregistrements polygraphiques positifs et 3 négatifs.
Il convient donc de souligner l'excellente valeur prédictive du score de Brouillette ainsi que d'un questionnaire dont nous proposons une version simplifiée, le recours aux enregistrements ne s'imposant qu'en cas de score intermédiaire ou par nécessité médicale (terrain atopique par exemple).

- il faut encore souligner, toujours sur le plan clinique, l'absence dans notre série même dans les cas les plus sévères de retentissement cardiaque.

Certes, nous n'avons pas demandé d'échocardiographie dans la totalité de nos cas mais simplement dans les plus sévères cliniquement.

- 2 laryngomalacies figurent parmi les étiologies dans notre série. Or il s'agit d'une cause d'apnée obstructive du sommeil peu rapportée dans la littérature bien que le collapsus laryngé tout comme le collapsus pharyngé puissent entrainer théoriquement une apnée obstructive.

L'amélioration spectaculaire apportée par la résection de la margelle laryngée confirme le bien fondé de cette hypothèse. Toute laryngomalacie sévère nécessite à nos yeux un enregistrement polygraphique du sommeil afin d'éliminer une telle éventualité.

Enfin, il nous faut souligner la valeur diagnostique remarquable de l'enregistrement du sommeil de sieste sans déprivation de sommeil préalable ou prémédication. Il est toutefois essentiel d'obtenir, durant cet enregistrement une durée suffisante de sommeil paradoxal. La signification lors d'enregistrements considérés classiquement comme négatifs de petits signes traduisant une augmentation du travail respiratoire telle qu'une activité phasique du génioglosse, une respiration paradoxale mérite des études ultérieures, leur présence ne permettant pas encore de déduction thérapeutique.

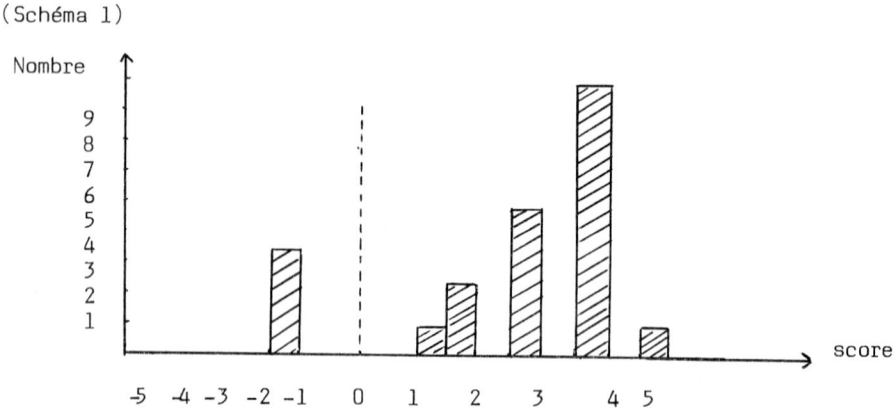

REPARTITION DES ENFANTS SELON LEUR SCORE

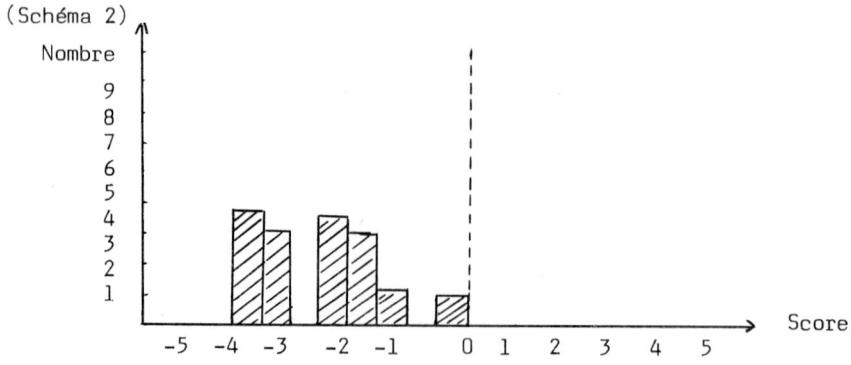

REPARTITION DES ENFANTS SELON LEUR SCORE POST OPERATOIRE

(tableau VI)

	Temoin	Patients	
- TTS MIN	136 (107-186)	112 (53 -157)	
- TSP AS%TTS	14 (6- 20)	15 (7- 30)	
- A/ H > 5 s par heure TTS	4 (0-11)	26 (7- 108)	p 0.01
- AHO %	2 (0-10)	85 (37- 98)	p 0.01
- Delta $PTCO_2$ Maximum	11 (6-15)	22 (9- 37)	p 0.02
- Delta $PTC\ CO_2$ Maximum	7 (4-10)	13 (5-33)	p 0.02

RESULTATS DU SOMMEIL DE SIESTE COMPORTANT DU SOMMEIL PARADOXAL
CHEZ 10 PATIENTS (AGES 18 mois à 63 mois)

TTS : temps total de sommeil
TSP : temps passé en sommeil paradoxal en % TTS
AHO : apnée, hypopnée obstructive

(tableau VII)

Réponses au questionnaire
post opératoire
(16 cas)
Symptomes nocturnes

Ronflement : 2 cas
Difficultés respiratoires : 2 cas
Pauses : 0 cas
Agitation : 5 cas
Réveils : 3 cas
Soif : 4 cas
Sueurs : 3 cas

---

tableau VIII)

Réponses au questionnaire
post opératoire
(16 cas)
Symptomes diurnes

Somnolence : 0 cas
Agressivité : 0 cas
Manque d'appétit : 3 cas
Difficultés à avaler : 0 cas
Respiration buccale : 0 cas

REFERENCES :

Brouillette, R.T., Fernbach, S.K., Hunt, C.E. : Obstructive sleep apnea in infants and children. J. Pediatr., 1982, 100, 31-40.
Brouillette, R.T., Hanson, D., David, R., Klemka, L., Szatkowski, A., Fernbach, S., Hunt, C. : A diagnostic approach to children with suspected obstructive sleep apnea. J. Pediatr, 1984, 105 (1) : 10-4
Gastaut, H., Tassinari, A., Duron, B. : Polygraphic study of the episodic diurnal and nocturnal manifestations of the Pickwick syndrome. Brain. Res. 2 : 167, 1966.
Gaultier, C. : Breathing and sleeping during growth : physiology and pathology. Bull. Eur. Physiopathol. Respir, 1985, 21, 55-112.
Guilleminault, C., Eldridge, F.L., Simmons, B., Dement, W.C. : Sleep apnea in eight children. Pediatrics, 1976, 58, 23-30.
Guilleminault, C., Korobkin, R., Winkler, R. : A review of 50 children with obstructive sleep apnea syndrome. Lung, 1981, 159, 275-287.

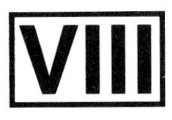 TREATMENTS OF CHRONIC RHONCHOPATHY
Chairman: Y. Dejean

Social problems relating to snoring

Ellis Douek

Guy's Hospital, St Thomas Street, London SE1, UK

It is customary, when looking at an old problem which has recently come to prominence again, to search into the distant past for people's attitude towards it. In this context it is noteworthy that there is no reference to snoring as a problem in the Old Testament, nor does it seem to have received prominence as a medical problem in the Talmudic commentaries on the Bible. This suggests that it was not seen as a disease or as a precursor of disease, such as sneezing but only considered as an aspect of behaviour. Indeed, it is only relatively recently that it has been associated with sleep apnoea and therefore with problems of oxygenation during sleep.

This report is based on twenty-seven patients who presented with snoring as the chief complaint, seventeen patients who had other complaints but where snoring appeared to have a role and a hundred consecutive patients who suffered from nasal obstruction but who also confessed to snoring. One hundred children where snoring was present were also considered. Certain general aspects emerged:

1   Where amusement has a dominant aspect.
2   Where anxiety was the main aspect. This involved not only children but some adults and where a fear of death on the part of the companions dominated.
3   Where social incompetence resulted. Among the patients in this series the following were involved
- The spouse or sleeping companion
- children in school dormitories
- soldiers in Army barracks
- persons in neighbouring rooms or even houses.

Snoring as the main complaint

Of these twenty-seven aged 15-55 patients, two were boarding school boys who suffered from allergic rhinitis. Three were soldiers who could breathe adequately. With all five amusement was the main aspect, with clear cut evidence of social incompetence; in the sense that relationships with their colleagues were damaged as a result.

Of the remaining twenty-two only six were women. None of these had nasal obstruction but all confessed to "catarrh".

The residual sixteen men represented all shapes and sizes from short to tall, thin to fat, long-necked to bull-necked, so that in a general sense the physical appearance did not pick out the snorers.

There was clear evidence of alcohol abuse in five of these men and heavy drinking at night or taking soporifics also had a definite worsening effect.

In those patients there was no question of amusement and the main problem related to the spouse or sleeping companion. Complaints were very serious and a high proportion had to sleep in separate rooms. Even then there were claims that they could be disturbed in other rooms of the house and two patients stated that neighbours had commented. It appeared that the companion was unable to get off to sleep and that in a number of cases they had been woken by the loud noise of snoring. The general understanding of the situation was that in some way the patient was to blame. There was no suggestion that he or she deserved compassion but, on the contrary, merited accusation. This inevitably generated hostility and the patient usually stated that their relationships were at risk. There was no hesitation in submitting to surgery.

Some of the female companions had expressed anxiety that their spouse should die in their sleep though none of the males confessed to such anxiety. Although it was not posible to question in more detail there was some superficial evidence that economic considerations were among the underlying anxieties.

It is of interest that although snoring is common in old people, none of this series was older than 55 years.

Other complaints

This group of patients, seventeen in all aged between 35-65, had a variety of often mixed complaints, and could not easily be further subdivided. They ranged from halitosis; "catarrh" with much hawking and mouth clearing; coated tongue to stomatitis and mouth ulcers.

Eleven were women and only six were men. Snoring was only broached in an oblique manner and was not considered as a separate problem. Here the association between halitosis, coated tongue and snoring appeared to represent a social and perhaps sexual lack of confidence with a conviction that they were a disappointment to their partners or prospective partners. There was a definite tendency to be withdrawn about their relationships and not to be prepared to discuss them in a specific manner. Four of these patients, three women and one man, also complained of awareness of a bad smell or taste although there was no objective evidence of this.

Nasal obstruction

One hundred consecutive patients with nasal obstruction were also considered, 56 were men and 44 were women, aged between 15 and 60. All of them confessed to snoring or at least to some noisy breathing yet attitudes were different. Snoring was readily confessed to but the spouses or companions showed concern rather than anger and hostility. The association with nasal obstruction placed it firmly as a disease of which snoring was only one of the symptoms. No-one suggested that his or her relationship was at risk and when the companion was questioned directly, they all insisted that they were not concerned at all by their own disturbance of sleep, but rather expressed anxiety about their partner's health.

Children

One hundred children aged from birth to 15 years were considered. The cause of the snoring included anatomical abnormalities, enlarged adenoids and nasal allergy.

There was a high rate of anxiety among the mothers and this was in direct and decreasing proportion to age. With babies anxiety was very great but at about the age of four it became a source of amusement. Above the age of 12 or 13 this had turned into a source of annoyance and often seemed associated to other problems of teenagers, with the parents uncertain as to what annoyed them most about their children.

In conclusion

Reactions towards snoring both on the part of those afflicted and on that of their companions followed interesting and often predictable patterns. They quickly became involved with other features of relationships.

The positional treatment of snoring

Jean Michel Pieyre

Spécialiste ORL – FMH Chirurgie Plastique, Hôpital Cantonal de Genève, Genève, Switzerland

SUMMARY

The so-called "positional" method of treating snoring is limited to minor cases, to people who only snore on their backs and have no ENT problems.

Based as it is on conditioning the patient, the method requires the assistance of the spouse, which is indispensable, for the spouse becomes "a sound mirror".

The method is adversely affected by excess weight, over-consumption of alcohol in the evenings, and nervous fatigue. It requires some minimum of intellectual capacity and sufficient motivation.

The method has been tried out personally by the author and gives very satisfactory results. It is certainly one of the neatest ways of putting an end to snoring, but unfortunately there are a number of "ifs"...

THE POSITIONAL TREATMENT OF SNORING

1 - What cases are likely to benefit?

In order to start by outlining the cases likely to benefit from the method, we have prepared the following diagrammatic table.

Stage	0	1	2	3
palato-pharyngeal space	normal	decreased	very decreased	virtual
snoring	0	dorsal sleep position only	all positions	apnea
treatment	0	positional	UPPP	UPPP CPAP tracheotomy

This graphic takes more account of anatomy than physiopathology, but it gives a fairly accurate summary from the practical viewpoint. Only cases of Type 1 can benefit from the so-called conditioning method, because the respiratory area at the palato-pharyngeal level is only slightly reduced.

In the dorsal sleep position, the reduction of palatal muscular tonus leads to subsiding of the uvula and the soft palate. The opening narrows, causing an increase of resistance to breathing and of sound vibration, above all if the patient sleeps in the dorsal position. On the other hand, in the lateral position and flat on the stomach, the tract remains large enough; thus this patient will snore only if he sleeps on his back.

In case No. 2 the tissues are already too loose and the respiratory opening remains insufficient in all sleeping positions: snoring becomes general.

We might ask in passing wether with appropriate palatal exercises to strengthen the musculature of the velum it might not be possible to return from Stage 2 to Stage 1, thus recuperating a number of patients for the method we are discussing.

As to Stage 3, which is that of apnoea and pathological snoring, our method can do nothing. How do we recognize a Stage 1 from the practical point of view? The key question to ask of the snorer, or rather of his spouse, is: <u>Do you snore in all positions</u>? If the patient only snores on his back, the chances are that we are dealing with a favourable Stage 1. If the answer is yes, it is Stage 2. If there is apnoea, it is a Stage 3. This is simplistic, but practice provides a fairly good confirmation of this way of looking at the problem.

Thus two conditions are essential at the outset:

1) The patient should only snore in dorsal decubitus. It will be sufficient to change this position in order to cease snoring; if snoring occurs in all positions, it is pointless to try and condition the patient.

2) The patient should not be suffering from an ENT condition which causes a mayor nasal obstruction, because in such cases, snoring occurs in all positions.

II - <u>Allied but important conditions</u>

1) <u>Obesity</u>: Many patients begin to snore when they put on weight and stop when they regain their normal weight. The role of obesity needs no demonstration in Pickwick syndromes.

2) <u>Over-consumption of alcohol in the evening</u>: there is no need to demonstrate that this is unquestionably a temporary factor in snoring. It temporarily changes a snorer of Type 1 into one of Type 2. Its effect is neurotoxical and nasocongestive.

3) <u>Nervous overstress</u>: is more insidious but can lead to the same consequences.

4) <u>Social status and motivation</u> not to snore any more are deciding factors in a patient's determination to cease snoring.

Let us take two examples:

1) A lorry-driver, relatively obese and hypo-alcoholic, is sent by his wife to see the doctor who cures snoring because she cannot put up with it any longer. For him it is not a problem, but he comes because his wife mede the appointment herself.

2) The intellectual who has just changed wives. He left a 45 year-old for a 25 year-old. She is not sending him, but he is aware that, if she cannot sleep in peace, the balance of their relationship will rapidly deteriorate to his disadvantage. The motivation is not at all the same, nor is the capacity to adapt to the method.

After the consultation, the lorry-driver will go home and find his wife waiting for him on the doorstep; everything that has gone in by one ear has come out by the other. He gives a summary report: all your doctor's good for is telling stories! In any case, I'm not going to have an operation for that!

The intellectual perhaps will not even tell his young companion that he has been to the doctor, but will explain to her in very few words what has to be done. The socio-intellectual level is unquestionably another limitation to this technique of conditioning.

It is thus absolutely essential to take account of these various factors before undertaking any treatment, either holding or surgical, because these adjuvant causes are the main reasons for failure in the two types of treatment, or at least they appear to be from our statistics.

Moreover, they are a perfect symbol of the "resigned" snorer who allows himself become slovenly even when he is sleeping. The psychoanalysts say that snoring or not snoring is in the end a more or less conscious, even affective, form of social behaviour.

III - The method

We have just seen that it is reserved for: snorers who only snore in dorsal decubitus, who have no major ENT condition, who are neither obese nor alcoholic, of a sufficiently high intellectual level, and motivated.

Since these patients only snore on their backs, the method boils down to never sleeping on the back, the only position that is fatal for these cases.

Thus we must:

1) condition the snorer to adopt an anti-snoring position and simply change his position for another anti-snoring one.

2) he is going to make mistakes, above all at the outset, so he must be made aware of them; he needs a "sound mirror". This method originated in the report of the experiments conducted by Josephson and Rosen. Twenty-four participants were divided into three groups of eight, all of them snorers who did not have an ENT condition.

1 conditioned group.
1 sensitized group.
1 control group.

The first group learned not to snore by conditioning: holding up the jaw and seeking an anti-snoring position at all costs; after 15 days it stopped snoring.

The second group, progressively sensitized, had to interrupt a bell which awakened it each time the sound level attained a certain point. After a few nights the snoring was quieter but the alarm-bell kept pace with the snorers' progress and was set off by a weaker and weaker stimulus. Snorers were reduced to either not sleeping or not snoring at all. This group too was cured in approximatively 15 days. The improvement was maintained after one month of interruption of treatment for both groups.

The control group in no way changed its behaviour. This was only a laboratory experiment. However, it can be adapted to everyday life.

Initially the snorer will condition himself by persuasion not to sleep on his back. This seems difficult but it should be recalled that the subconscious never sleeps. From the first night you spend in a new bed, you do not fall out because you know how big it is. If you sleep with someone, you do not knock into them because you instinctively know where they are. Why? Because in principle you change position during the transitions to phase 1, periods of very light sleep, which are the easiest to control. The snorer will fall asleep in a lateral position or flat on his stomach. He does not snore in these positions. The first advantage is that his partner intervenes, reacting like a "sound mirror". The partner sends a signal (a tap on the shoulder or a prod with the finger). This signal must always be the same; this is very important. The snorer is sleeping and is not conscious of what is happening. He must be gradually sensitized to one simple signal which will also be fixed in the snorer's subconscious. Initially, the signal will awaken him, but if he is properly conditioned, he will rapidly understand and will change position. After a few days it all becomes automatic. The signal is given, the position changes and the snore dies away without anyone being the worse or even awakening. After a few weeks, the automatism responses are such that the snorer feels a psychological malaise if he strays into a wrong position and corrects himself unaided. As in Josephson and Rosen's experiments, it takes from 5 to 15 days to achieve sufficient conditioning. This is durable enduring to some extent, but, as the saying goes nothing lasts forever, and constant self-reconditioning is needed; in this way, a snorer can become tolerable. There are two further conditions to be satisfied if the method is to be effective. One is that the patient must not suffer from rheumatism, nor must be undergone surgery on his spinal column, which pratically oblige him to sleep on his back. The other is to have a partner who will participate...

Do not ask me what the percentage of success of the method is. You can give percentage figures for the success of a surgical technique. The positional method involves too many variables to be expressed in figures.

All I can tell you is that for me it has been succesfull and that numerous patients have become bearable thanks to it.

BIBLIOGRAPHY

Josephson SC & Rosen RC, The experimental modification of sonorous breathing. J. Appl. Behav Anal - Summer 13 (2) pp. 373-378.

RESUME

Si on classifie les ronfleurs en 4 groupes, à savoir :
Stade 0 non ronfleur, stade 1 ronfleur en décubitus dorsal <u>seulement</u>, stade 2 ronfleur dans toutes les positions, stade 3 ronfleur pathologique (obstructive sleep apnea syndrome), la méthode de traitement dite positionnelle est réservée au stade 1 uniquement.

Elle se résume en un conditionnement progressif du ronfleur à ne plus jamais dormir sur le dos, moyennant quoi il ne ronflera plus, puisqu'il ne ronfle que dans cette position.

Son partenaire lui sert de miroir sonore, en cas d'échec il l'avertit par un signal, toujours le même, qui renvoie le ronfleur à une position silencieuse. Il est de plus indispensable d'éviter l'alcoolisme vespéral, l'excès de poids et de fatigue nerveuse qui sont des causes aggravantes du ronflement en plus du fait qu'elles perturbent la bonne santé du patient.

Il est enfin indispensable que le ronfleur soit motivé, qu'il ait un quotient intellectuel suffisant pour comprendre la méthode et un minimum de sel-control pour pouvoir l'appliquer.

Prosthetic treatments of chronic rhonchopathy

Bernard Meyer

Hôpital Saint-Antoine, Service ORL, 184 rue du faubourg Saint-Antoine, 75012 Paris, France

SUMMARY :

Snoring is a constant symptom of Chronic Rhonchopathy which can be a severe disease. Prosthetic treatments can try to care the sole snoring by modifying the position of the buccopharyngeal muscles or by stimulating the patient. But in cases of severe Chronic Rhonchopathy with obstructive sleep apnea, and diminution of Sa O2, a tracheotomy canula or a respiratory mechanical method can be necessary. These prosthetic therapies are discussed.

KEYWORDS :

Snoring – Chronic Rhonchopathy – Prosthesis – Stimulator – Tracheotomy canula – Continuous Positive Airway Pressure –

Snoring is a constant symptom of chronic rhonchopathy. It is the first sign to appear, becomes progressively aggravated and finally becomes a familial or even social embarrassment which justifies a request for therapy.

All the other symptoms of the diseases, which constitute more or less severe clinical forms - diurnal somnolence, asthenia, shortness of breath, morning cephalia, sleep disorders, nightmares, repeated awakenings, and even exacerbation of high blood pressure - and which are due to hypopnea, and even to an obstructive sleep apnea and a desorganisation of sleep, are often neglected by the patient, the family and even the general practitioner who do not relate them to the real cause.

When obstructive sleep apnea becomes severe, it begins only then to worry those close to the patient, who request a specific treatment for it.
Nonetheless, regardless of the evident symptoms or those discovered during a check-up, the principle of the treatment is unequivocal, consisting in removing the oropharyngeal obstacle.

This chapter will deal only with prosthetic treatments which, directly or indirectly, can manage to remove this obstacle. Account taken of the physiopathology of chronic rhonchopathy, to which we shall not return, it may be considered that this prosthetic treatment might act :

- by modifying the position of the bucco-pharyngeal muscles
- by increasing muscular tone
- by short-circuiting the upper aerial tracts

The ideal aim of the treatments consists, obviously, in curing the symptoms without disturbing other functions. And yet, it appears that although the medical profession has been concerned for a relatively short time with this disease, nonetheless the good sense or false common ideas have, throughout all time and in all civilisations, tried to fight against the major symptom of rhonchopathy-snoring - most often using suitable procedures, but sometimes using incomprehensible or illogical means which have inspired some imaginative inventors. We shall recall here, quickly, some of these procedures.

1) Some are based on the false notion that a purely nasal respiration should be able to cure snoring. Thus, systems such as chin straps or mouth stoppers, applied to the lips or inserted in the labial vestibule have been conceived.

One can imagine the discomfort, the inefficiency and the risk of aggravating a hypopnea with such a system, which, of course, must be rejected.

2) Others have aimed at imposing a position for the body and the head which might attenuate or eliminate snoring.
In effect, it is well known that ventral decubitus, and sometimes lateral decubitus, can often stop snoring due to the detachment of the soft palate, and in some cases, of the base of the tongue, from the posterior wall of the pharynx.

It is all too frequent for these privileged positions not to be maintained for the entire night. Some procedures may then impose : a tennis ball or a bolster pillow to be sewn into the pajama top are well known examples. Deriving from the same procedure, but more restricting, was a prosthesis made of a splint, covering the entire length of the body, against which the patient straps himself in the desired position.

Outside of the discomfort of such techniques, it is frequent for obesity and/or a rheumatological pathology to prevent the use of these methods.

3) Other prostheses are based on the physical stimulation of the patient. Very frequently, the sole fact of pushing a snorer suffices to make the snoring stop, temporarily. This stimulation, habitually provided by the spouse who is awakened several times a night, in effect provokes a change in muscle tone, a deglutition movement and sometimes a modification in the position of the body and the head, which explain the momentaneous cessation of the snoring.

Prostheses have been designed to automatically bring about a stimulation as soon as the snoring has reached a certain intensity. They are made up of a vibration sensor, sometimes a counter which permits the amount of snoring to be totalled, and of a stimulator which may be visual by virtues of flashes, sonorous or tactile via electrical or pressure stimuli provided by an inflatable bracelet.

A procedure which modifies the position of the mattress as soon as snoring begins.

One of the disadvantages of these methods, at least for those which do not specifically stimulate the patient, is to awaken the spouse sometimes more frequently than the snorer who is not often bothered by his/her own noise.

The other inconvenient is to interfere with the sleeping cycle. In fact, as soon as sleeping becomes deep enough to induce hypotonia and the snoring then involved, the device goes on and changes the sleeping stage or, even, awakes the patient. This effect is especially bad during REM sleep, corresponding to the stage of maximum hypotonia and of highest snoring frequency. In fact, this REM sleep stage, the physiology of which is so important, might get disturbed greatly by these stimulators. Our experience of patients using such devices is low, however all suffered from asthenia, appearing after a few days. Then snoring, even bad enough to involve a diminution of Sa O2 musn't have a therapy altering an other function, already partly compromised by rhonchopathy itself.

Thus, all the procedures described above can be criticized and, in practice, only used in exceptional cases. This is understandable, since they aim at eliminating snoring, a symptom which almost never disturbs the snorer himself, using a procedure which is uncomfortable most of the time, and then, quickly given up.

On the contrary it is the spouse who complains of being awakened several times a night by the snoring. Thus, in practice, the only prosthesis really used, and which is moreover the simplest, is an ear plug, which puts in place an effective silence barrier between the two sleepers. However, these ear plugs must be psychologically accepted and tolerated.

Nonetheless, such a solution is acceptable only if snoring is really an isolated symptom. On the contrary, if rhonchopathy associates to snoring signs of asthenia sleepiness and moreover if obstructive sleep apnea is present, with diminution of Sa O2 it will then be necessary to envisage true therapeutic methods. In the field of prosthetic treatments, two possibilities exist : tracheotomy canula, mechanical respiratory methods.

1 - Tracheotomy canula

Wearing a tracheotomy canula, by short-circuiting the upper respiratory tracts, eliminates all mechanical supra-laryngeal and laryngeal obstacles. This treatment, used in every etiology of acute or chronic respiratory distress, has also been found to be perfectly effective in cases of chronic rhonchopathy.

It eliminates snoring, obstructive sleep apnea and all the symptoms connected with O2 desaturation.

Disadvantages of tracheal canula are numerous and well known. The main disadvantages are as follows :

- physiological : the inhaled air does not undergo hygrometric and thermal transformations or filtration, which are usually the role of the nasal fossa.

- infectious : the wearing of a tracheotomy canula is at the origin of frequent tracheal infections which can become complicated by broncho-pulmonary infections.

- mechanical : tracheal, even sub-glottal stenoses, are not exceptional, being linked with a poor surgical technique and/or a choice, an incorrect adaption and monitoring of the tracheal canula.

- psychological : wearing a tracheotomy canula, even when it is perfectly adapted to the respiratory and vocal tracts, is always felt to be an infirmity.

This is all the more true in cases of chronic rhonchopathy, when the respiratory shunt is used only during sleep.

All these major disadvantages explain why tracheotomy, which, for a very long time, was the elective treatment for severe cases of rhonchopathy accompanied by O2 desaturation, is more and more relinquishing its place to more recent treatments especially surgery and mechanical respiratory methods which have their drawbacks and failures.

2 - <u>Respiratory mechanical methods</u> have been replacing tracheotomy for several years.

A - In 1981, C. E. SULLIVAN (1) was the first to report on the interest of the use of continuous positive pressure during obstructive sleep apnea (CPAP or CPP). This method, envisaged 50 years ago in the treatment of acute pulmonary oedema, consists in providing the upper aerial tracts with a pressure which is slightly higher than atmospheric pressure, while respiration remains spontaneous. SULLIVAN's hypothesis was to create a pneumatic splint to separate the pharyngeal walls, which have a tendency to collapse during nocturnal respiration, due to muscular hypotony during sleep.

In practice, the positive pressure is produced by an electric compressor and sent to the aerial tracts via a nasal mask which keep the mouth free.

The adaptation must be carefully studied in order to be sufficiently tight, at the same time that it remains comfortable. The effective positive pressure is usually less than 15cm of H_2O.

This method has been found to be very efficient, eliminating all of the symptoms of chronic rhonchopathy.

The disadvantages can be linked :

a) to the machine

- If the expiratory resistance encountered by the patient is too high, the machine risks to be poorly tolerated, at least at the beginning. KRIEGER (2) insisted on this point and contributed to the development, in FRANCE, of an apparatus whose expiration circuit resistance did not exceed 3.5 cm $H_2O/1.s^{-1}$.

- If the sonorous level of the motor is too great, it risks to trouble the sleep of the patient and the spouse.

- The device dimension and weight are a handicap for the travelling patient. We have the experience of patients having a profession demanding numerous trips and then asking for an other therapy. However new miniaturized devices will be soon available.

b) to the poor tolerance of the mask when it is poorly adapted or, in exceptional cases, when it provokes a cutaneous irritation. Moreover, the intercurrent attacks of rhinitis may justify the momentaeous discontinuation of the treatment.

c) to the poor psychological tolerance of the patient whose quality of sleep depends on a machine. Nonetheless, if some patients quickly adapt to this sort of daily constraint as long as the improvement in his condition is quick and evident many only adapt themselves progressively. Moreover, after a few months, they accept less well this constraint.

No pulmonary, pleural or gastric complication has been reported, to our knowledge, after months of use, which is easily explained by the low pressure used.

B - In 1983, MAHADEVIA (3) proposed the use of expiratory positive pressure (EPAP or EPP). He noted an improvement in O2 saturation, a decrease in the sleep apnea index and an improvement in the quality of sleep.

Nonetheless, the results reported do not seem as spectacular as those obtained with continous positive pressure.

The interest of these results lies, however, in questioning the mechanisms of action of these various treatments.

- Is it a question of a simple mechanical action ?

The tracheotomy short-circuits only the oropharyngeal obstacle.

The CPP removes the obstacle - The mechanism of the pneumatic splint, a hypothesis put forth by SULLIVAN, was confirmed by D. M. RAPOPORT (4), who revealed, using tomodensitometry, the enlargement of the oropharyngeal canal during sleep. But there could exist other non contradictory hypothesis, by muscular action associated to pneumatic action.

In fact the efficacy of EPP, which has no obvious direct action on the oropharyngeal canal during inspiration, might constitute an argument, on behalf of muscular action. The hypothesis of an imbalance between the depression engendered by the inspiratory muscles and oropharyngeal muscular activity, at the origin of an obstructive syndrome, is usually postulated.

- on the one hand, then the shortening of inspiratory muscles, induced by EPP, decreases their tension. This modification of the physical conditions of the inspiratory muscles might reestablish the broken imbalance with the oropharyngeal muscles.

- on the other hand, then, the EPP might act on the oropharyngeal muscular receptors, at the origin of an increase in their activity. During the use of the CPP, RAPOPORT (4) confirmed an increase in such an activity by means of electromyography of the genioglossis muscles, whose dilating action on the oropharyngeal canal is known.

- In addition, does a central effect exist which one may imagine to act on the one hand on the oropharyngeal dilating muscles and muscle tone notably the velar muscles and, on the other, on respiratory command ?

This central effect would originate in the improvement of the hematosis induced by the preceding mechanisms of action.

CONCLUSION

Prosthetic treatments of chronic rhonchopathy constitute only one of the therapeutic aspects of this disease.

Among the prostheses, one finds the procedures which attempt to act only on snoring, but the efficacy of which is doubtful, and those which are much more serious and effective and fight against the obstructive sleep syndrome ; the latter appear to be too constraining in the benign forms of the disease.

This is the reason for which they are currently competing with surgical procedures, inaugurated by IKEMATSU (5) in 1952 ; this involves a method for treating all phases of the diseases and permits, after all, and in the case of failure, recourse to prosthetic methods.

REFERENCES

1) SULLIVAN C.E., ISSA F.G., BERTHON-JONES M., EVES L.
Reversal of obstructive sleep apnea by continuous positive airway pressure applied through the nares.
The Lancet, 19871 ; April 18 : 862-865

2) KRIEGER J., SAUTEGEAU A., SAUDER P., WEITZENBLUM E., KURTZ D.
Syndromes d'apnées du sommeil. Traitement par la pression positive par voie nasale.
Presse Méd. 19874 ; 13 : 2559-2562

3) RAPOPORT D.M., GARAY S.M., GOLDRING R.M.
Nasal CPAP in obstructive sleep apnea = mechanisms of action.
Bull. Europ. Physiopath. Resp. 1983 ; 10 : 616-620

4) MAHADEVIA A.K., ONAL E., LOPATA M.
Effects of expiratory positive airway pressure on sleep-induced respiratory abnormalities in patients with hypersomnia sleep apnea syndrome.
Am. Rev. Respir. Dis. 1983 ; 128 : 708-711

5) IKEMATSU T.
Study of snoring fourth report : therapy
J. Jpn Otolaryngol. 1964 ; 64 : 434-435

IX TREATMENTS OF CHRONIC RHONCHOPATHY
Chairman: E. Douek

Chronic rhonchopathy. Ed. C.H. Chouard. © 1988, John Libbey Eurotext Ltd. pp.263-272.

Did Napoleon suffer from sleep apneas syndrome?

C.H. Chouard, B. Meyer and F. Chabolle

Service ORL, Hôpital Saint-Antoine, 184 rue du faubourg, Saint-Antoine, 75012 Paris, France

SUMMARY

NAPOLEON would sleep very little. He frequently woke up during night and worked. Brief sleeping time in day repared his fatigue. He had also a short and thick neck. In the last fourth of his life he progressively suffered from obesity, daily unvoluntary sleepiness and his intellectual capabilities undoubtly decreased. Our experience of 48 cases of sleep apneas syndrome diagnosed by mean of polysomonography allow no to think that NAPOLEON suffered from this disease. Historical consequences of this pathology is discussed.

KEYWORDS :

Sleep Apneas Syndrome - History -

NAPOLEON had a reputation for sleeping little, and of awakening refreshed for work. However, in the last quarter of his life, he also suffered from diurnal somnolence. Moreover, as of 1812, he no longer had the illuminations of genius in leading armies which had until then won him victories. In addition, artists have left us a profile of an emperor who might be a patient suffering from Sleep Apneas Syndrome (SAS).

Did NAPOLEON snore ? No one knows. None of his contemporaries has spoken of this detail. Yet, today, snoring is no longer considered as a vulgar fault which should be hidden. We have shown (1) that this sign is the majour symptom of an autonomous disease, "Chronic Rhonchopathy", whose syndrome of sleep apnea is only a clinical form. The aim of this investigation is to demonstrate that NAPOLEON perhaps suffered from it.

MATERIAL AND METHODS

Our experience consists in two parts. In one hand we observed the results of the préoperative clinical examination and polysomnographic registration of 48 patients suffering from SAS (more than 5 apneas per four, each of them more than 10 seconds duration). In the other hand we searched in the large bibliography about NAPOLEON for symptoms able to be reported to a SAS. We have also searched in NAPOLEON's painting and sculpture of this epoch the clinical anatomical features of this disease.

RESULTS

1 - CLINICAL EXAMINATION OF OUR PATIENTS

We only report signs which could have been observed by the NAPOLEON's contemporaries, and which to-day could be retrospectively attached to their real origin.

A-<u>Apneas</u>, more than 10 seconds, disturb the sleep cycles. None except 3 of 48 patients, reach stages III and IV. All pass directly from stage II to Rapid Eye Movement stage. These apneas are responsible for multiple awakes or awakes in more than 70% of cases.

B-<u>Diurnal somnolence</u> is constant. These "absences" or brief naps, which are often invincible, occur during the least physical inactivity. They are short sleeping periods, of only a few seconds (10 to 20 minutes), followed by abrupt awakenings, and the impression that one had slept for very little time. They take place in an arm-chair, in the office, in front of the television, and especially when driving a vehicle. They may be accompanied by the true equivalent of distractions of a few seconds' duration. This somnolence is often overcome with stimulants, or volontary hyperactivity.

C-<u>Asthenia</u> is constant, physical, psychical and intellectual.

D-<u>Snoring</u>, even if its intensity varies during the night, is constantly found in numerous phases of nocturnal sleep. It often appears, very quickly at the onset of diurnal somnolence. It is occasionally minimised by the patient. Exceptionally, it may be difficult to reveal, either for reasons of modesty – as this sign still has a strong pejorative connotation – or by the absence of a husband or wife capable of talking about it. In most of the cases, this is the first sign of the disease, preceding by 1 to 15 years the onset of somnolence.

E-<u>Anatomical particularities</u> (tongue hypertrophy, neck shortness, retrognathia, obesity, nasal obstruction) (Table I) are one or the other nearly constantly found, each explaining the mechanism of snoring, of nocturnal hypoxie chronique, and respiratory efforts developed to combat it. These are real risk factors. The severity of SAS is all the greater in that these risk factors are more numerous in the same patient.

TABLE I
Risk factors repartition
in 48 cases of SAS

	absent	présent
tongue hypertrophia	16	32
neck shortness	12	36
obesity	16	32
nasal pathologia	36	12
rétrognathia	32	16

2 - CLINICAL EXAMINATION OF NAPOLEON

We only report symptoms in favor of SAS in the litterature. Most of them are gathered in two recent books, one from J. TULARD (2), the other from L. CHARDIGNY (3).

A - Functionals signs

NAPOLEON very early revealed sleep disorientation, then, in the last quarter of his life, in a progressively increasing manner, diurnal somnolence and fatigue, with decrease of intellectual faculties.

a) <u>Disorganisation of sleep</u> : NAPOLEON managed to master his sleep pattern, which contributed to his reputation as a super-man, having, in particular, the talent of repairing his fatigue very quickly by sleeping during the day, frequently and anywhere at all, waking a few minutes later, completely relaxed. In fact, he slept little but in a fractioned manner : "in bed at midnight, he woke up at three o'clock to think about the most sensitive affairs, take a warm bath and return to bed at five", TULARD recounts. Although he took advantage of it, he suffered from multiple awakenings : "often awakened several times during the night, nonetheless not affecting the clarity of his ideas, to the contrary, he appreciated a keener presence of mind after midnight", wrote CHARDIGNY. NAPOLEON also had a habit of sleeping almost every day for a few moments during the day. This habit of napping must be compared to those brief restoring periods of sleep which are found in many anecdotes during the Napoleonic epoch. Overcome with fatigue, he dozed off at the State Council, and when he woke up he took up the deliberation at the point when CAMBACERES, continuing the debate in a soft tone, led him. In ELCHINGEN, in 1805, he fell asleep in a chair in front of his standing generals. In LEIPZIG, in 1813, it was the explosion of a bridge which woke him in his chair.

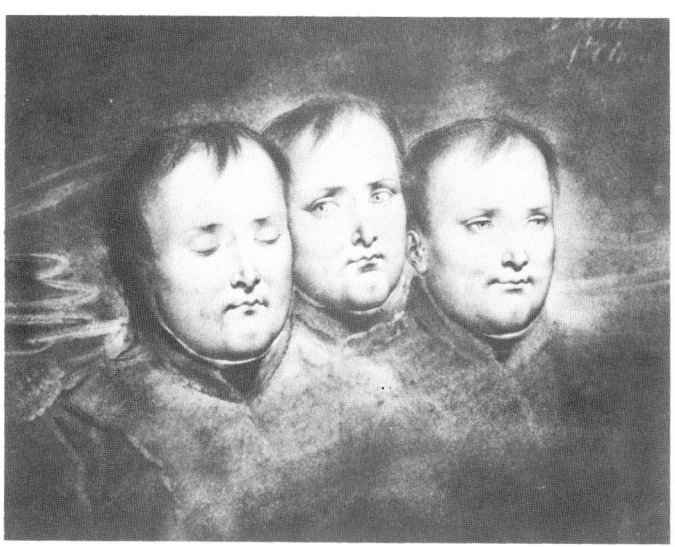

Fig. 1 NAPOLEON sleeping (left) during the representation of the opera from MONVEL "l'amant bourru" at St-Cloud Theatre, then suddenly awaken (middle), and finally smiling when he saw he was oserved (right).
Three sketchs directly drawn by GIRODET who was attending the opera near the Emperor. (Reference in text)

b) <u>Diurnal somnolence</u> : The appearance of veritable somnolence, which is pathological since invincible, is related by all those close to the Emperor beginning in 1812. In April of that year, GIRODET (4) sketched him asleep at the theatre of Saint-Cloud (Fig 1). CHAPTAL(5) noted that the sleep "which he had until then mastered, mastered him in due course". In BANTZEN, in 1813, while NEY was preparing for victory, he slept for two hours on the ground on a coat. This somnolence occurred notably more and more in a coach, when, during the One Hundred Days, he had a sleeping car delivered, a car in which he had had a real bed set up and in which he slept, fully clothed. In a painting, CHARLET (6) shows us the emperor in a thatched cottage, on the eve of Montmirail in 1814, near the fireplace, asleep in a chair. Two days before Waterloo, General REILLE saw him exhausted, languid, scarcely hearing what was said to him. On Saint-Helen's (7), he was constantly given, at all times, to irrestible nodding off. This somnolence was often limited to distractions, strange attitudes, a sort of absence, a real sleeping while awake of a few seconds' duration, which alarmed those close to him as of 1812 and even led to whispers of epilepsy.

c) <u>Fatigue</u> was alluded to by NAPOLEON as of 1808. In a letter to Josephine he wrote : "I attended the Weimar ball. The emperor Alexander danced ; but I didn't ; 40 years are 40 years." He himself was aware of a decrease in strength as of 1812 : "instead of a glass of lemonade, now it's a glass of coffee ... the need of which I feel." This asthenia became more and more marked beginning in 1814, and in his letters to the young empress the word "fatigue" was very frequently mentioned.

d) <u>The decrease in his intellectual activity</u>, intermittent at the onset, then evident at Saint-Helen's (8), was noted as of the Russian campaign in words more or less covered by many of his companions. "War, he said, is an art full of movement". Yet, as CHARDIGNY noted, in Russia he plodded along. He plodded in Vilna, in Vitebsk. He sunk in Moscow. And in Moskova, against the principles which had made his reputation, he undertook an attack from the front. As of his return from Elba he disappointed his partisans : his former Police Prefect, PASQUIER, saw then in him signs fo a "profond decadence". The Emperor's neglected appearance on Saint-Helen's, described by his companions, is seen in the painting by Van STEUBEN (9), representing NAPOLEON dictating his memoirs to General GOURGAUD.

B- <u>Physical signs</u>
The physical examination of the Emperor revealed a short neck, a definite retrognathia, increasing obesity and an intermittent nasal obstruction.

a) <u>The short and thick neck</u> was pointed out by all the contemporaries who approached NAPOLEON. In all the paintings and busts of the period, this shortness, which became more and more accentuated with age and increasing weight, can be seen. The short and stiff collar of the uniform, in the portraits by GROS (10), brushed against the horizontal branch of General BONAPARTE'S lower jaw, or marks the full cheeks of the ageing emperor painted by DAVID (11).

b) <u>Retrognathia</u> is variable depending on age. Quite observable on the busts, it seems to be absent on the CORBET (12) marble, mild in the work by HOUDON (13), more marked on the BARTOLINI Emperor wearing his laurels (14). On the latter work, which reveals the neck, the thyroid cartilage is very visible, but the limits of the mandible level are already bloated. In hte portraits, only the profiles or 3/4 poses permit the retrognathia to be assessed.

They are rare in the imperial epoch. It is absent in the Gros Bonaparte, and that of INGRES (15). However, it is suggested in the already bloated features of NAPOLEON on the imperial throne (16).

Conversely, in all representations of NAPOLEON, a broad jaw with a marked mandible angle is noted, leading to a suspicion of lingual hypertrophy.
In addition, at all ages the protrusion of the anterior apophyses of the symphysis menti is well represented. This hypertrophy, by lengthening the inferior maxilla, hollows out the cleft in the chin, which is particularly clear on the BARTOLINI marble, and in the emperor's nephews at Saint-Cloud, in the painting by DUCIS (17). It is also found in the Saint-Helen's death mask. Finally, it is often noted in many of Napoleon's descendants.

c) <u>Obesity</u> appeared as of 1812. Already at this period the Emperor was saying to himself : "I have become too fat". Most of the comentators mention it. It is seen in many paintings recalling the final years of his reign. It is marked on the sleeping Napoleon by CHARLET. It was obvious for the companions on Saint-Helen's.

d) <u>Nasal obstruction</u> must be suspected, intermittent though certain that it was, at the time of the exacerbations of rhinitis which were more and more frequent as of 1812, and which were doubtless complicated by sinusitis, given the overall reverberations which often accompanied the latter. On the evening of the battle of Moskova, NAPOLEON was suffering from a bad cold, with fever.

Then, before Moscow, it was necessary to stop for three days, as he was aphonic and completely exhausted. The same was true at Dresden, in 1813, where the victory was had under driving rain. Indeed, the empress, Marie-Louise, in her letters often expressed the fear that he would take cold.

Moreover nose fracture and septum deviation are evident on Saint-Helen's death mask

DISCUSSION

Among the clinical signs which allow, in NAPOLEON, the suspicion of SAS, retrognathia is the most debatable, since it seems to vary from one artistic representation to another. Nonetheless, it is necessary to emphasise the risk of error which might result from a superficial observation of the imperial profile if it ignored the markedness of this protrusion of the symphysis menti. In effect, the latter lengthens the appearance of the jaw and might mask a shortness of mandible to an artist, moreover one who was concerned with accentuating the exemplary character of his illustrious model. It is permitted to think that this, and the increasing weight gain of the emperor, erased the bone delimitations, explaining this apparent morphological discordance between the young years and middle age. Moreover, with ZIESENISS (18), who pointed out to INGRES the anatomical variations found from one portrait to another, it is necessary to recall the difficulty the artists had in getting their illustrious model to pose for them ; indeed, GROS complained of this with regard to General BONAPARTE, as DELESTRE (19) reported.

The shortness of the neck might be discussed, since no portrait revealing the sub-clavicular hollows, always hidden by the clothing, exists. The BARTOLINI marble, which has been reproduced in several paintings, notably the portrait of Elisa by LETHIERE (20), is the only exception ; however, this representation of a Roman-style Emperor confirms the existence of a thinck neck.

The morphology and sleep disorders of NAPOLEON thus very strongly lead to a suspicion of SAS. He did not suffer from it while he was young, but, on the contrary, took advantage of his multiple awakenings, doubtlessly connected to apnea occurring during his paradoxical sleep, to deal with the preoccupations of the moment.

With age, the Chronic Rhonchonpathy of the Emperor began to make itself felt, and although his robust temperment was able to struggle against asthenia for some time, which must of course have affected him, he required more and more sleep, of a few minutes' duration, during the day in order to compensate for the chronic asphyxia of his sleep and his constant efforts to fight it.

This thus explains the Emperor's sudden falling into a highly restoring sleep, of short duration, followed by quick and perfectly lucid awakening. This is found to have been exactly described in the same manner by many of our patients, be they intellectuals or manual labourers.

These short and repairing cases of somnolence, long exalted as one of Napoleon's virtues, were not considered to be pathological until they became almost daily occurrences.

Snoring always accompanies the nights of patients suffering from SAS. Yet, no trace of this disorders is found in writings on Napoleon. One may wonder why this sign, a key symptom of the disease of chronic rhonchonpathy, is not found in that illustrious patient. One explanation is possible. The Emperor, deeming it indispensable to his prestige as a demi-god, to make all believe, with the complicity of those who surrounded him, that he was exemplary. It was not modesty which suppressed word of such nocturnal noise. In fact, NAPOLEON never tried to hide the fact that he suffered from hemorrhoids or constipation. As we have shown (21) it was because of common decency that this detail was hidden, because at the time the pathological nature of snoring, of which only the trivial side was perceived, was not known.

Finally, it should be pointed out that no other sleep disorders experienced by Napoleon exist which would allow account to be taken of the pathological signs observed, and notably of their association to a legendary intelligence and hyperactivity, which decreased progressively only during the last ten years of his life.

CONCLUSION

What would have happened if NAPOLEON had had the benefit of modern treatment for SAS, surgery of the velum or continuous positive airway pressure ? Tactical errors would surely have been avoided, the retreat from Russia would not have taken place, and Waterloo, as POINSOT (22) imagined, would have been a victory for France. NAPOLEON admired England. As a liberator of people, he desired, as TULARD noted, "the agglomeration and conferation of great peoples". Europe would then have doubtless been born with him, and the world would not have known the last two World Wars.

BIBLIOGRAPHIE

1 - **CHOUARD C.H., YALTY J., MEYER B, CHABOLLE F, FLEURY B., YERICEL R., LACCOURREYE O. & JOSSET** La Rhonchopathie chronique ou ronflement - Aspects cliniques et indications thérapeutiques .Ann. O.L. Paris, 1986,103,319-327
2 - **TULARD J.** NAPOLEON ou le Mythe du Sauveur. FAYARD Edit. - PARIS, 1977
3 - **CHARDIGNY L.** L'homme NAPOLEON .PERRIN Edit.- Paris, 1987
4 - **GIRODET A.L.** 3 portraits de NAPOLEON au théâtre de saint-Cloud - Dessin du 13 Avril 1812 Coll Comte de Dreux-Bréze, in Napoléon tel qu'en lui-même, Archives Nationales de l'Hôtel de Rohan Juin-Déc.1969, n° 327.
5 - **CHAPTAL J.** Mes souvenirs sur NAPOLEON 1883. (cité in CHARDIGNY)
6 - **CHARLET T.N.** Napoléon le soir de Champaubert (10 Février 1814) à la veille de la victoire de Montmirail-Musée de la Légion d'Honneur
7 - **TULARD J.** NAPOLEON à Sainte-Hélène - Robert Laffont Edit. - PARIS, 1981
8 - **LAS CASES E.A.** Mémorial de Sainte-Hélène; DUNAN Edit. - PARIS, 1951
9 - **VAN STEUBEN** Napoléon à Sainte-Hélène dictant ses mémoires au Général GOURGAUD-Huile - Coll. Partic., in Napoléon tel qu'en lui-même, Archives Nationales de l'Hôtel de Rohan Juin-Déc.1969, n° 662.
10 - **GROS A.** Napoléon Bonaparte au pont d'Arcole - Musée du Louvre
11 - **DAYID JL** Le sacre de Napoléon - Musée du Louvre
12 - **CORBET** : Buste de BONAPARTE - Musée de Yersailles
13 - **HOUDON J.A.** : Buste de BONAPARTE - Musée de Yersailles
14 - **BARTOLINI** : Buste de NAPOLEON en Empereur romain - Musée de Yersailles
15 - **INGRES J.** Bonaparte 1° Consul - Musée de Liège
16 - **INGRES J.** Napoléon sur le Trône impérial - Musée des Armées
17 - **DUCIS L.** NAPOLEON et ses neveux et nièces au Château de Saint-Cloud. Musée de Yersailles.
18 - **ZIESENISS C. O.** A propos de l'Exposition Ingres au Petit Palais. Rev. Institut NAPOLEON 106 - Jan 68, pp. 21-26.
19 - **DELESTRE J.B.** Gros, sa vie et ses ouvrages. Jules Renouard Edit., Paris 1867
20 - **LETHIERE** Portrait d'Elisa - Musée de Yersailles.
21 - **CHOUARD C. H** Vaincre le Ronflement et retrouver la forme. RAMSAY Edit. - PARIS 1986
22 - **POINSOT J.** Comment NAPOLEON guéri aurait gagné à Waterloo ? (1978)

Objective monitoring of therapeutical success in heavy snorers: a new technique

T. Penzel, G. Amend, J.H. Peter, T. Podszus, P. von Wichert and M. Zahorka

Medizinische Poliklinik, Philipps-Universität, Baldingerstrasse, 3550 Marburg, FRG

ABSTRACT

Heavy snorers have been found to suffer from a variety of diseases, especially cardiovascular complications. We therefore developed a new technique of quantified snoring analysis which can be used for ambulatory screening, therapeutical monitoring, or in combination with recordings of other relevant parameters. Snoring was recorded in a silent chamber equipped with polysomnographic facilities, using dB(A)-meter, bedside microphone, 2 laryngeal microphones for validation, and another one connected to a low-frequency (50-800 cps) filter. The filter permitted the distinction of snoring and physiological breathing sounds via the determination of low-frequency power in total power. The analogue signal filter, which permits on-line snoring analysis, was subsequently used in a pilot study, preparatory to a full-scale investigation in the therapeutical efficiency of Sonarex® nasal surfactant. Finally, we succeeded in combining the filter device with a continuous calculation of heart rate in a portable unit for purposes of diagnosis and ambulatory monitoring of therapy.

Polysomnography - sleep apnea - snoring - time series analysis

INTRODUCTION

Snoring has long been underestimated as a risk factor in connection with the clinical pictures of a variety of cardiovascular diseases. Several authors (Koskenvuo et al., 1987; Lugaresi et al., 1980; Mondini et al., 1983) have reported high prevalence rates of hypertension, angina pectoris, and arteriosclerosis among heavy snorers. Loud and irregular snoring is also a leading symptom of obstructive sleep apnea. One of the main obstacles for a systematic use of snoring parameters in Internal Medicine is the fact that snoring is not easy to objectify, which, however, is a prerequisite for the definition of specific snoring patterns as diagnostic criteria, or systematic monitoring of therapeutical success in the medical treatment of snoring. This is especially important as it can help to solve the question if an efficient therapy of snoring will lead to an overall improvement in the clinical pictures of which it is a part. We therefore concentrated on the development of a quantified snoring analysis compatible with time-related recordings of other parameters. Several years of experience in the diagnosis and treatment of sleep apnea convinced us that the high prevalence of this clinical picture demanded the development of a diagnostic unit for ambulatory use.

Requirements

The new technique was required to facilitate the recognition of snoring patterns over the night, but should also permit an assessment of the severity and the clinical relevancy of snoring. A recording of the volume of nocturnal breathing sounds would therefore be incomplete. The analysis of breathing sounds should yield information on the proportion of snoring in the sound recordings, independent of volume, and the coincidence of snoring events and critical changes in other parameters. Further, the method should be easy to use and permit ambulatory screening for, and monitoring of therapeutical success in, clinical pictures going along with heavy snoring.

DESIGN

In search of adequate parameters for the investigation and assessment of snoring we conducted a series of studies in a silent chamber equipped with the usual sleep laboratory facilities. The subjects were patients with an initial result of sleep apnea who underwent full scale polysomnography for differential diagnosis.

In addition to EEG, EOG, and EMG we recorded thoracic and abdominal respiratory activities by means of inductive plethysmography, nasal airflow by thermistor, and oxygen saturation as well as partial arterial oxygen tension transcutaneously. The acoustic recordings included a bedside microphone and dB(A)-meter. Two laryngeal microphones of different gain were used for validation. The recordings were subjected to a variety of computer routines resulting in the parameters described below. On the basis of the results, we developed a frequency filter. After extensive tests with an additional laryngeal electret microphone connected to the filter, the technique was used in a pilot study of therapeutical success in 4 heavy snorers.

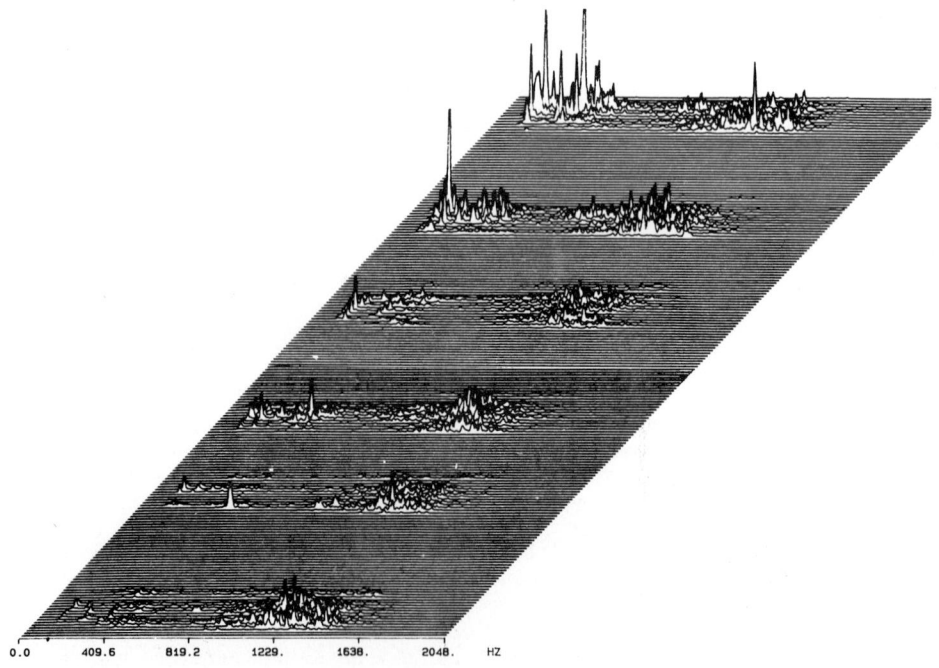

Fig. 1: Fourier power spectra up to 2048 cps in steps of 0.125 s over a period of 25 s. High power in low frequencies is indicative of snoring.

RESULTS

Digitized frequency analysis of breathing sounds
The acoustic signal was subjected to a Fourier transform by means of an Intertechnique signal-analyzing computer. The power spectra were calculated in steps of 0.125 s up to 2048 cps. Figure 1 shows the successive spectra of 25 s. The patient breathes 6 times, and normal respiratory sounds are gradually superseded by snoring. Normal breathing and snoring are characterized by powers in different frequency bands, separated by a clearly visible gap at about 800 cps.

By analyzing the distribution of frequency powers in segments of 0.125 s each, we arrived at a power distribution function which is independent of volume. For each frequency, we calculated the power proportion within 100 per cent of total power recorded in the respective time segment. By successively adding up the proportions assigned to each frequency, we arrived at the frequency-related distribution of power within each segment (Fig. 2). By determining the value of this distribution function at frequency 800 cps, we found a useful parameter. Defining 100 per cent of total power as 1.0, the parameter would assume values between 0.0 and 1.0. If a specific segment is characterized by normal breathing sounds, there

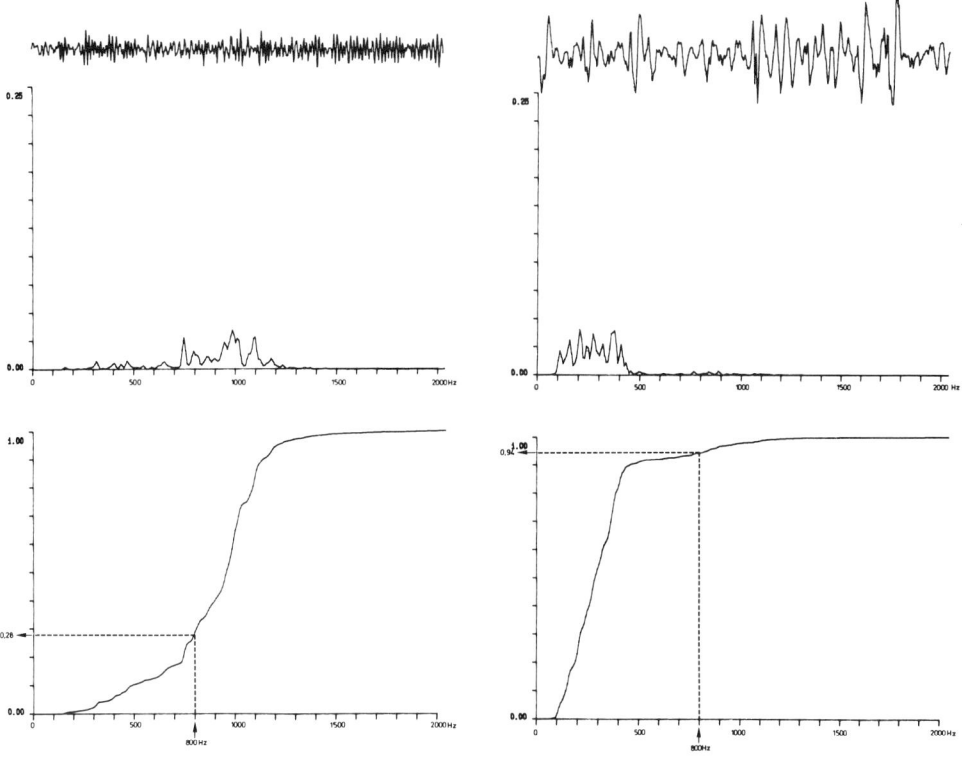

Fig. 2: Example of digitized analysis of breathing sounds for the determination of the criterion 'snoring power'. Laryngeal acoustic signal (top), power spectrum (middle), power distribution (cumulative proportions of powers pertaining to the individual frequencies) within 100 per cent of total power (= 1.0), all in one segment of 0.125 s. Normal respiratory sounds with small proportion of low frequencies (left); heavy snoring with high proportion of low frequencies (right); position of the 800-cps-parameter value indicated.

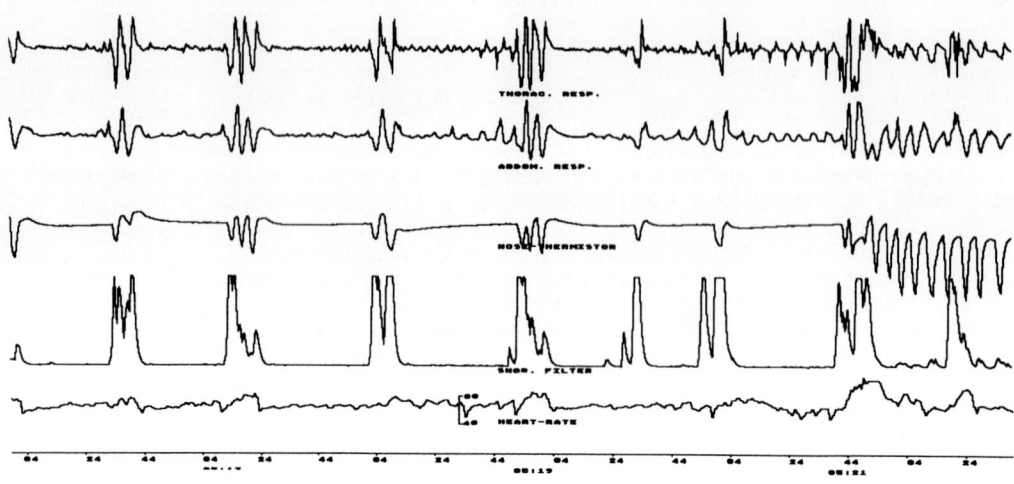

Fig. 3: Excerpts from a multi-parameter recording including snoring power from the analogue filter device. From the top: thoracic respiration; abdominal respiration; nasal airflow; snoring power; beat-to-beat calculation of heart rate. The record illustrates a 6-min-period with successive apneas alternating with compensatory hyperventilation accompanied by heavy snoring and critical increases in heart rate.

is a high proportion of frequencies > 800 cps. Accordingly, the parameter value is below 0.5 (Fig. 2, left). Vice versa, a high proportion of frequencies < 800 cps, indicative of snoring, results in a value above 0.5 (Fig. 2, right). Between inspiration and expiration, the value was found to remain close to 0.5.

Volume of breathing sounds as accessory parameter
As a second parameter we used volume. This parameter permits the distinction between snoring sounds at low volume, which were found to be characteristic of hypoventilation and phases immediately before the termination of obstructive apnea episodes, and very loud snoring, which was found to be indicative of apnea-terminating hyperventilation.

Analogue snoring filter
On the basis of the two parameters absolute volume and snoring power we developed an analogue snoring monitor consisting of automatic gain control and frequency filter, which is susceptible to the relative power of low frequency signals. The device permits continuous on-line analysis of breathing sounds. Parallel recordings of EEG and EOG, evaluated by a different computer program, supply information REM-sleep and ups and downs in vigilance. A long-term ECG shows variations in heart rate, which have a high diagnostic value in sleep-related breathing disorders (Guilleminault et al., 1984; Penzel et al., 1986). Figure 3 shows a synchronized recording of several parameters, illustrating successive apneas terminated by bursts of heart rate, heavy snoring, indicated by high snoring power, and pronounced respiratory efforts.

In a further step we succeeded in miniaturizing the low frequency filter. In collaboration with Madaus Medical Electronics we developed a diagnostic unit composed of the analogue snoring filter and a routine for beat-to-beat calculation of the heart rate. This compact analyzer is a portable device for applications in ambulatory diagnosis and monitoring of therapeutical success. All data are stored in a built-in 64-K-RAM and can be evaluated by means of a Personal Computer.

APPLICATIONS

After the new technique of objective analysis of respiratory sounds had been developed, tested, and continuously perfected in studies of more than 50 patients, we conducted a pilot study with 4 heavy snorers, monitoring therapy with Sonarex® nasal surfactant. The method was found to work well, and the portable recorder will soon be on the market. The therapeutical efficiency of Sonarex® suggested by the pilot study will soon be tested in a program with a larger number of patients. Other applications of the method include long-term monitoring of patients with various sleep-related breathing disorders and screening for sleep apnea and heavy snoring. The main advantage of the technique here discussed is, in this respect, that it can be easily handled and is not limited to hospital use. The on-line calculation of the snoring parameters in comprehensive recordings, on the other hand, permits the recognition of snoring patterns in combination with the evaluation of cardiovascular, respiratory, and EEG-parameters and, thereby, an assessment of the detrimental dimensions of snoring.

REFERENCES

Guilleminault, C., Connoly, S., Winkle, R., Melvin, R. (1984): Cyclical variation of the heart rate in Sleep Apnea Syndrome: Mechanism and usefulness of 24 h electrocardiography as a screening technique. Lancet I, 126-131.
Koskenvuo, M., Kaprio, J., Telakivi, T., Partinen, M., Heikkilä, K., Sarna, S. (1987): Snoring as a risk factor for ischaemic heart disease and stroke in men. Brit. Med. J. 294, 16-19.
Lugaresi, E., Cirignotta, F., Coccagna, G., Piana, C. (1980): Some epidemiologic data on snoring and cardiovascular disturbances. Sleep 3, 221-224.
Mondini, S., Zucconi, M., Cirignotta, F., Aguglia, U., Lenzi, P., Zauli, C., Lugaresi, E. (1983): Snoring as a risk factor for cardiac and circulatory problems: An epidemiological study. In Sleep/Wake Disorders, eds C. Guilleminault and E. Lugaresi, pp 99-106.
Penzel, T., Fuchs, E., Hügens, M., Koehler, U., Meinzer, K., Peter, J.H. (1986): Herzfrequenzschwankungen bei Patienten mit Schlafapnoe. Biomed. Technik 31 (Suppl), 142-143.

RESUME

On a observé que les sujets atteints de ronflement important présentaient une pathologie variée, en particulier des complications cardio-vasculaires.
Nous avons donc étudié une nouvelle technique d'analyse quantifiée du ronflement, qui peut être utilisée en screening ambulatoire, ou en monitorage, combiné à l'enregistrement de paramètres associés. Le ronflement a été enregistré dans une pièce insonorisée, par enregistrement polysomnographique, en utilisant la mesure du son en décibels, à l'aide d'un micro placé près du lit, de deux microphones laryngés pour validation, et un autre branché sur un filtre basses fréquences (50-800 cps). Le filtre a permis de faire la distinction entre le ronflement et les bruits physiologiques de la respiration, en établissant un rapport entre les basses-fréquences et la totalité des fréquences. Le même filtre permettant d'identifier le bruit du ronflement a été utilisé pour un essai pilote, en avant-première à un essai clinique plus large afin de tester l'efficacité du Sonarex

qui est un surfactant nasal.

Finalement, nous avons réussi à associer l'utilisation du filtre et l'enregistrement en continu du rythme cardiaque par une unité portable permettant à la fois une observation diagnostique et une action thérapeutique.

Polysomnographic evaluation of the effect of uvulopalatopharyngoplasty (UPPP) on obstructive sleep dyspneas

K. Togawa, S. Miyazaki, K. Yamakawa, Y. Itasaka and M. Okawa*

Department of Otolaryngology and Department of Neuropsychiatry*, Akita University School of Medicine, 1-1-1 Hondo, Akita 010, Japan

ABSTRACT

Based on the polysomnographic data and physical findings of snoring patients, uvulopalatopharyngoplasty(UPPP) with or without intranasal corrective surgery were applied on 34 cases. This time, we report the therapeutic effects and complications of the surgery upon 16 cases who had been followed up for more than one year. The results were satisfactory in most cases except for a few. After surgery, excessive respiratory effort decreased within normal range. Variations in transcutaneous pO_2 and pCO_2 (tc.pO_2, tc.pCO_2) were almost disappeared. Three cases complained of remaining of snoring. The reasons were the failure of weight reduction and re-narrowing of oropharyngeal airway. Patients experienced the improvements of snoring, excessive day-time sleepiness and falling asleep, midnight awakening and dried mouth in the morning. There were a few complications of UPPP. After 6 months postoperatively, they complained of dull taste, sensation of dysphagia and pharyngeal discomfort. UPPP can play a significant role in the treatment of obstructive sleep disturbance and snoring, and the complication of which were not serious.

KEYWORDS

Sleep apnea, snoring, polysomnography, uvulopalatopharyngoplasty (UPPP)

INTRODUCTION

Snoring is no doubt a sign indicating the existence of stenosis in the upper airway during sleep. Polysomnography is the best maneuver to evaluate the severity of the respiratory disturbance and its influence upon cardio-respiratory and sleep conditions. UPPP is one of the surgical approaches to obstructive sleep apnea and snoring of the upper airway origin especially due to the ptotic pharyngopalatal arch and tonsillar hypertrophy. For the judgement of applying UPPP, polysomnography was performed on all cases preoperatively. Among the parameters we recorded, the intraesophageal pressure-change(P.es) was very useful to evaluate the respiratory effort exactly. In this text, the effects and complications of UPPP are discussed.

SUBJECTS AND METHODS

Thirty-four patients aged 20 to 73 years who complained of snoring or sleep problems were examined by polysomnography. 23 cases among them showed respiratory disturbance during sleep due to the upper airway narrowing. They were candidates of receiving UPPP. 16 cases underwent the surgery, but 7 cases refused it. Table 1 shows the summary of preoperative condition of these patients; 8 patients were obese (BWI 130-146%). 13 patients had ptotic pharyngopalatine arch and 5 patients had tonsillar hypertrophy. 5 patients complained of sleep disturbances and 7 cases complained of daytime excessive sleepiness. Additionally, nasal allergy(31%), hypertention(13%), polycythemia(13%) and liver function disorders(13%) were found among them.

Table 1. Prepoerative condition of 16 cases who underwent UPPP

PATIENT		AGE/SEX	OBESITY (BWI,%)	LPA/TH	RETRO-GNATHIA	NASAL ALLERGY	DAYTIME SLEEPINESS	SUJ.SLEEP DISTURB.	DRIED MOUTH
1	KM	29/M	146	+ / ++	−	−	++	−	−
2	AK	46/M	140	+ / ++	−	−	+	±	++
3	SS	57/M	140	++ / ±	+	+	±	++	+
4	HK	47/F	138	+ / −	±	−	−	−	+
5	HT	33/M	137	+ / ±	−	−	−	+	−
6	KY	25/F	137	± / +++	−	+	−	++	−
7	IK	73/M	136	+ / −	−	−	−	−	−
8	SM	32/M	135	− / +++	−	−	±	+	+
9	SS	59/F	123	+ / −	−	−	+	±	+
10	MT	53/M	122	+ / −	−	+	+	?	+
11	TK	57/M	119	+ / −	−	−	++	±	+
12	NH	41/F	109	+ / −	−	+	−	+	+
13	TY	21/M	106	+ / −	−	−	+	−	+
14	OT	20/F	101	+ / −	−	−	−	−	−
15	AK	57/F	88	+ / −	±	−	+	−	−
16	FY	27/F	88	− / ++	−	+	−	?	−

Abbreviation: BWI, body weight index; LPA, low position of pharyngopalatine arch; TH, tonsillar hypertrophy; SUJ, subjective.

Parameters recorded by polysomnography were EEG, EOG, EMG, ECG, tidal volume, Pes tc.pO2 & pCO2, expiratory O2 and CO2 contents (FeO2 & FeCO2). These were recorded on a data-recorder and analyzed later. Fig 1 shows a part of the data recorded from SM case preopratively. Periodical breathing pattern with obstructive sleep apneas are clearly demonstrated. Postoperative polysomnography was carried out on 14 cases, however 2 cases did not fall in asleep during the examination.
In addition, we sent out questionnaires to all of 16 patients 1 year later; the items of questionnaires were remaining of snoring, sleep disturbance, daytime excessive sleepiness, body weight reduction, etc.

Figure 1. Preoperative respiratory monitoring of a case with marked-obesity and tonsillar hypertrophy (32y. male)

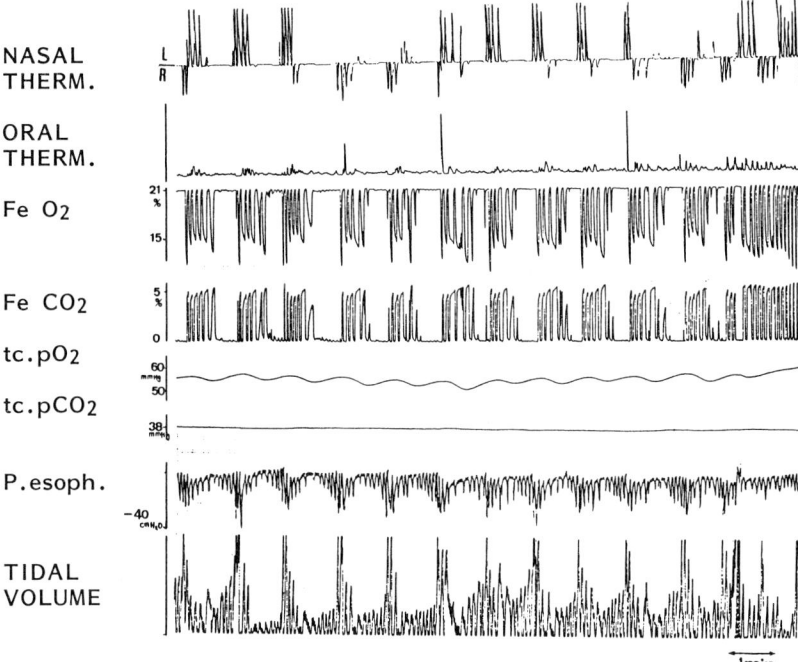

RESULTS

The grade of response to UPPP varied among individual patients. Most of them enjoyed satisfactory improvements (Table 2). Especially obese patients with tonsillar hypertrophy achieved remarkable improvement. Fig. 2 shows a part of the postoperative polysomnography from the same case as Fig. 1. In general, obstructive apnea and hypopnea decreased considerably or almost disappeared. The value of P.es lessened to one-third or one-fifth of the preoperative value. Variations of $tc.pO_2$ and $tc.pCO_2$ also were minimal. They recovered to breathe through the nose, and felt decrease in nasal resistance after surgery. On EEG, the episodes that they showed typical frequent sleep/wake pattern preoperatively were almost disappeared. They got sound sleep with no or occasional slight snoring. One case with moderate obesity and ptotic pharyngopalatine arch obtained sound sleep without snoring until 6 months after surgery. However, 1 year later, he regained his weight and his oropharyngeal airway became narrow again. Two patients complained of remaining of snores after surgery. However, their postoperative polysomnographic data showed moderate improvement as to respiratory effort during sleep. Snoring sound was also much weaker than that before surgery.

Complicatios of UPPP were as follows; soon after the operation, two obese patients suffered from severe respiratory distress due to the pharyngeal wall swelling derived from postoperative edematous reaction. One patient underwent tracheostomy for the instant respiratory management. During the early period of recovery (from 1 to 7 days), the patients complained of the regurgitation of fluid into the nose (18%) and cough (13%). After 6 months postoperatively, they complained of dull taste (13%), sensation of dysphagia (6%) and pharyngeal discomfort (31%). As for dull taste, two female patients felt inconvenient, as they could not taste their cooked food how it had been seasoned.

Table. 2 Results of pre and postoperative polysomnography

PATIENT		WEIGHT CHANGE(Kg)	EP CHANGE (cmH₂O)	tc.pO₂&pCO₂ CHANGE			OBST. APNEA or HYPOPNEA			SURGERY	EFFECT OBJ/SUJ
1	KM	?	50 − 8	++	−	−	++	→	−	UPPP+N**	G / G
2	AK	−4	70 − 12	++	−	−	+++	→	−	UPPP+N	G / G
4	HK	−2	34 − 12	+	−	±	+	→	−	UPPP	G / G
7	IK	0	27 − 15	+	−	−	+++	→	−	UPPP	G / G
8	SM	0	30 − 10	±	−	−	++	→	±	UPPP	G / G
9	SS	−1	28 − 22	+	−	−	+	→	−	UPPP	G / G
10	MT	+2	44 − 34	++	−	+	+++	→	+	UPPP+N	P / P
11	TK	−6	26 − 20	+	−	+	+	→	±	UPPP	G / P
12	NH	+2	20 − 12	+	−	±	++	→	+	UPPP+N	P / G
13	TY	0	40 − 8	+	−	+	++	→	−	UPPP+N	G / G
14	OT	?	30 − *	±	−	±	++	→	−	UPPP	G / G
15	AK	0	28 − 12	+	−	−	+	→	−	UPPP+N	P / G

Abbreviation: *, failed to monitoring; **, nasal corrective surgery; OBJ, objective; SUJ, subjective; G, good; P, poor.

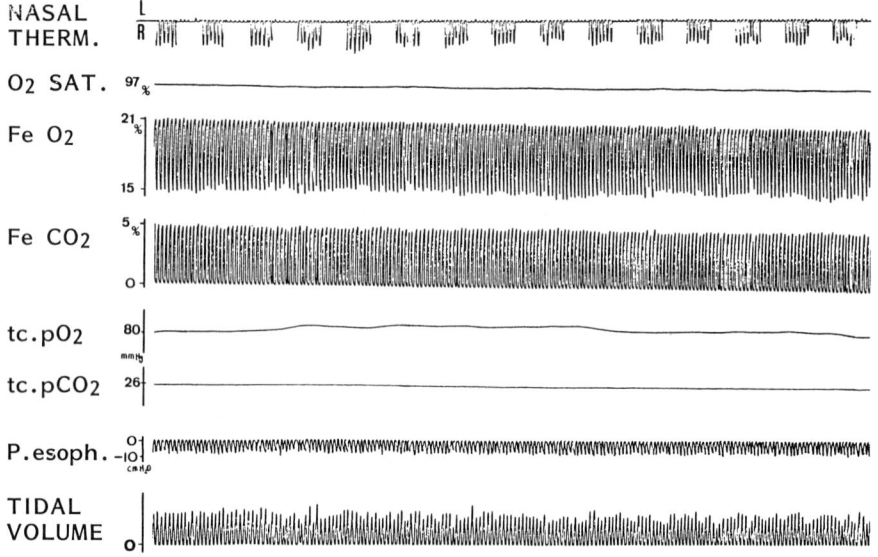

Figure 2. Postoperative respiratory monitoring of the "Fig. 1" case

DISCUSSION AND CONCLUSION

UPPP can play a significant role in the surgical management of obstructive sleep dyspnea. Most patients gained wide oropharyngeal space by the surgery and recovered sound sleep without obstructive sleep apnea or hypopnea. Effects of UPPP were great on the cases of ptotic pharyngopalatine arch with tonsillar hypertrophy. Someone might say "tonsillectomy alone would benefit for the relief of respiratory disturbance". We are against to this idea. Bilateral palatopharyngeal arch should be resected at least its upper part. For the relief of sleep apnea of children due to adeno-tonsillar hypertrophy, adeno-tonsillectomy is a recommendable treatment. In case of moderate obesity with low palatopharyngeal arch, the surgery relieves the respiratory effort during sleep considerably even if slight snoring might be remained. However, in such cases with retrognathia, macroglossia, uncontrollable obesity, effects of surgery would not be satisfactory.

There were a few complications of UPPP. Acute upper airway obstruction due to edematous swelling of the palatopharyngeal mucosa right after the surgery is the most serious one, though it might be quite rare. In such case as marked obese patient with short neck, special care for respiration should be paid. Dull taste and pharyngeal discomfort were perhaps derived from palatopharyngeal arch resection and subsequent scar formation. However, the same discomfort may happen after tonsillectomy alone, and usually disappear within a few years.

Polysomnography is very usuful to diagnose and evaluate the severity of sleep dyspnea. At the same time, both local and general physical-examinations are indispensable for the selection of treatment. UPPP is one of the recomendable treatments. However, we must not overlook the importance of body weight reduction and any latent general disorders.

RESUME

Le ronflement est, sans aucun doute un signe de sténose dans les voies respiratoires supérieures durant le sommeil. La polysomnographie sur ces patients a révélé qu'ils avaient des troubles de la respiration et du sommeil. En se basant sur les données polysomnographiques et les études physiques des ronfleurs, l'uvulo-palatopharyngoplastie (UPPP), avec ou sans intervention chirurgicale intranasale corrective a été appliquée sur 31 cas. Dans cette étude, nous rapportons les effects thérapeutiques et les complications des interventions chirurgicales des 16 cas qui ont été suivis pendant plus d'un an. Les resultats sont satisfaisants dans la plupart des cas, sauf pour quelques cas. Après l'opération l'effort respiratoire représenté par le changement de pression intra-oesophagienne (EP) diminue jusqu'à son niveau normal. Les variations en pO_2 et pCO_2 sous-cutanés représentant les troubles respiratoires ont également disparu. Deux patients se plaignent de continuer a ronfler. Les raisons sont l'échec de la diminution de poids et le rétrécissement des voies respiratoires oropharyngiennes. Les résultats suivants ont été obtenus: guérison du ronflement: 81%, guerison du besoin excessif de sommeil dans la journee: 66%, guérison de l'endormissement: 50 %, guérison des reveils en pleine nuit: 71%, guérison de la bouche seche: 100%. Il y a eu quelques cas de complications à la suite de l'UPPP. Durant une courte période après l'intervention chirurgicale, des patients se sont plaints des régurgitations des fluides dans le nez (18%), toux (13%) et dyspnee (13%). Six mois après l'intervention, des patients se sont plaints de la perte du goût (13%), sensation de dysphagie (6%), malaise pharyngien (31%). La perte du goût et le malaise pharyngien peuvent provenir de la résection du palais et sa cicatrisation. L'UPPP peut jouer un rôle significatif dans le traitement chirurgical des troubles du sommeil dus aux obstructions et du ronflement, et ses complications ne sont pas sérieux.

REFERENCES

Togawa, K. (1974) : Snoring -how to manage-. (Japanese) Otolaryngology (Tokyo) 46, 685-690.
Togawa, K. Konno, A. et al (1982) : Influence of nasal obstruction on sleep. (Japanes) Pract.Otol. (Kyoto) 75, 2505-2515.
Fujita, S. (1984) : UPPP for sleep apnea and snoring. Ear Nose Throat Jour. 63, 227-235.
Togawa, K. Miyazaki, S. (1985) : Polysomnographic study of snore. Myers, E.N. Ed. New Dimension in Otorhinolaryngology -Head and Neck Surgery Vol 2, 1112-1113.

Effect of nasal application of asonor on snoring

Poul Jennum

Department of Clinical Neurophysiology, Sleep Laboratory, Glostrup Hospital, DK-2600 Glostrup, Denmark

SUMMARY

In order to test the effectivity of a new polyglycoside (Asonor) in reducing snoring, 12 representatively selected men, characterized by regular snoring without apneas and hypopneas, nocturnal respiration was determined with and without Asonor.

Snoring was detected by changes in respiratory pattern determined by use of inductive plethysmography, after determination of cross-correlation coefficient.

With Asonor, cross correlation value increased significantly ($p=0.024$). The relative amount of partially changes in the respiratory movement characteristic for snoring was reduced 15% ($p=0.006$).

These preliminary results indicate, that nasal application of Asonor can be used as a treatment in reducing regular snoring.

INTRODUCTION

Snoring is very prevalent in the adult population, and are possibly associated with social problem and might be a risk factor for cardiovascular disease and manifestations (1-3). Therefore there are are major interest in order to reduce snoring.

Tonsillectomia, nasal surgery, and UPPP (uvulopalatopharyngoplastic) (4) are found effective among some snorers, but until now no medical treatment has been found effective in reducing snoring.

Asonor is a compound consisting of natural saline and polyglycoside solution (including solution P, polysorbate, benzalconium, glycerole ect.). Though subjective report indicate, that Asonor reduce snoring, the following study was performed in order to study, 1) whether Asonor reduce snoring, 2) to test the treatment effect.

SUBJECTS AND METHODS

12 men were selected from a representative epidemiological study which are actually ongoing in the Glostrup area, near Copenhagen in Denmark. Mean age was 38 (30-60).

All were selected if they complained of snoring, and showed snoring by night polygraphic measurements by use of inductive plethysmography.

None of the participants had any known sickness excluded by questionaire, a normal clinical examination, and a normal resting blood pressure (<160/95 mmHg). General inspection of the upper airway was found normal with no apparent gross abnormalities None of the participants toke any medication.

The study design was:
1. day no treatment
2. day Asonor
3. day no treatment

Each person were informed, to take 4-5 drops of Asonor in each nostril 5 - 10 minute before bedtime. Respiratory measurements were performed ambulatory, by use of inductive plethysmography (5, 6). The abdominal and thoracic signal were analog digital converted with a 12 bit analog digital converter with a sample rate of 10 Hz (Data Translation 2814). The signal was stored on a 20 mB hard disk on a MS-DOS computer (Olivetti M21).

Cross-correlation (r) product was calculated every second with a sliding window of 3 seconds. Normal respiration give rise to a cross correlation product of 1 or near 1, decreasing cross correlation product indicate increasing paradoxical movements, characteristic for snoring and obstructive apneas.

Normal value for respiration was arbitrary set to $r > 0.80$, and regular snoring: $0.20 < r < 0.80$.

SPSS-PC+ (Statistical Program for the Social Science, Chicago, 1986) was used for statistical analysis.

All values are given as mean +/- SEM (Standard Error of the Mean). 2-tailed Student's t-test for paired comparisons was used. P values below 0.05 were considered significant for all variables.

RESULTS

From the first to the second night there was a slight non-significant increase in the mean cross correlation coefficient (0.758 +/- 0.056 vs. 0.773 +/- 0.056; p = 0.061). From night 2 to night 3 (0.749 +/- 0.052), a significant reduction i the mean cross correlation value was found (p = 0.021) (figure 1).

The relative amount of cross correlation value less than 0.80 decreased significantly (p = 0.024) from night one (0.412 +/- 0.059) to two (treatment night) (0.369 +/- .0.67), and increased significantly to night three (non-treatment night) (0.434 +/- 0.061; p = 0.006).

There was a significant association between changes in cross correlation value and in the area under the curve for r < 0.80, namely for the first night (r = 0.831, p = 0.0008), second night (r = 0.844; p = 0.0006), and third night (r = 0.801; p = 0.0017).

A positive, but non-significant, association between treatment effect and the mean cross correlation value on night 3 was observed (r = 0.263; p = 0.41).

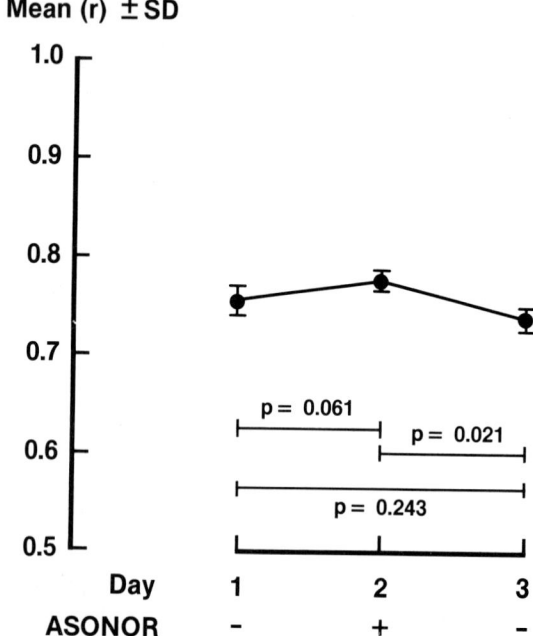

FIGURE

Figure 1

Cross correlation value with and without Asonor.

DISCUSSION

This open study of nasal application of Asonor, show that the specific changes in the respiratory pattern, characteristic for snoring can be significant reduced by using Asonor in some patients, with a treatment effect of approximately of 15% ((0.434-0.369)/0.434). The range of the individual responses were 2-25%.

None of the participants reported any side effect, and no complained of poorer sleep during night 2 compared to the first or third nights.

Though the study desigh was open caution should be made to the results. Therefore further studies should include blind controlled studies.

However, it is interesting, that a non specific polyglycoside solution seems to reduce the abnormal nocturnal respiratory pattern, characteristic for snoring in a general representative selected population. The treatment effect was different, but is in accordance with non-published open observations, that Asonor reduce subjective reported snoring in approximately 60% of the snorers.

Several mechanism are suggested to be involved in the partially upper airway clossure, that are characteristic for snoring, including increased nasal resistance, anatomical factors, neuromuscular tone, inspiration, upper airway activation during inspiration, and gravity among others among others (7, 8). Nasal installation of Asonor might affect several of these, including changes in nasal resistance, a lubricating effect, or changes in the inspiratory activation in the upper airway.

Changes in covariation between thoracic and abdominal signal was used in order to give an simple, quantification of snoring, which are easy to reproduce, and not depended upon other acustical signal in the surroundings (ex. sleeping partner or dog). No validation in order to test the association and snoring sound has been made.

Controlled, blinded clinical trials with objective sound measurements needs to be performed, before we can say whether Asonor reduce snoring, and patophysiological studies should be performed to explain the apparent positive effect of nasal application Asonor has upon regular snoring.

References

1. Koskenvuo M, Karpio J, Partinen M et al. (1985): Snoring as a risk factor for hypertension and angina pectoris. Lancet I, 893-5

2. Jennum P, Schultz-Larsen K, Wildschiødtz G. (1985): Snoring as a medical risk factor. II. Relation to oral glucose tolerance test. Sleep Res 14, 171

3. Partinen M, Palomaki Heikki. (1986): Snoring and cerebral infarction. Lancet II, 1325-6

4. Moran WB, Orr C. (1985): Diagnosis and management of obstructive sleep apnea. Arch Otolaryngol 111, 650-8

5. Staats BA, Bonekat W, Harris CD, Offord KP. (1984): Chest wall motion in sleep apnea. Am Rev Resp Dis 130, 59-83

6. Zimmerman PV, Connellan SJ, Middleton HC, Tabona MV, Goldman MD, Pride N. (1983): Postural changes in rib cage and abdominal volume-motion coefficients and their effect on the calibration of a respiratory inductance plethysmography. Am Rev Resp Dis 127, 209-14

7. Guilleminault C, Lugaresi E (ed.) (1983): Sleep/wake disorders: Natural history, epidemiology and long-term evolution. Raven press. New York

8. Sullivan CE, Issa FG, Berthon-Jones M, Saunders NA. (1985): Pathophysiology of snoring. In Saunders NA, Sullivan NA (ed.). Sleep and Breathing. Lung Biol Health Dis 21, Marcel Dekker, Inc., New York

RESUME

Afin de tester l'efficacité d'un nouveau polyglucoside (ASONOR) ayant pour effet de diminuer le ronflement, 12 sujets représentatifs ont été sélectionnés, caractérisés par un ronflement régulier sans apnée ni hypo-apnée. Leur respiration nocturne a été étudiée avec et sans ASONOR.

Le ronflement était signalé par les changements de mode respiratoire par pléthysmographique inductive après détermination du coefficient de corrélation croisée.

Avec ASONOR, la valeur du coefficient de la corrélation croisée augmente de manière significative (P = 0.024). L'importance du changement partiel des mouvements respiratoires caractéristiques du ronflement, était diminuée de 15 % (P = 0.006).

Ces résultats préliminaires montrent que l'application nasale d'ASONOR peut être considérée comme traitement visant à diminuer le ronflement régulier.

Elimination of snoring by means of nasal continuous positive airway pressure reduces airway resistance and respiratory work in obstructive sleep apnea patients

J. Krieger and D. Kurtz

Service d'Exploration Fonctionnelle du Système Nerveux, CHU, 67091 Strasbourg, France

ABSTRACT

In snorers, upper airway resistance to airflow is increased ; the consequence is the need for higher (more negative) intrathoracic inspiratory pressures to maintain ventilation at a sufficient level, thus leading to increased respiratory work.
To assess the effects of nasal continuous positive airway pressure (CPAP) on these parameters, we measured, in 9 patients with obstructive sleep apnea syndrome (OSAS) : tidal volume (V_T), peak inspiratory airflow ($\dot{V}$ max ; pneumotachography) and peak intrathoracic pressure (Poes ; oesophageal balloon) during 10 consecutive breaths randomly chosen in a stage 2 NREM sleep period when snoring persisted after elimination of apneas, and in a period of the same sleep stage when snoring had disappeared after an increase in the CPAP level
The elimination of snoring required an increase in nasal CPAP from 6.8 ± 1.0 to 8.6 ± 1.1 cm H_2O ($p < 0.01$). It resulted in a decrease in Poes from -11.6 ± 1.7 to -4.2 ± 0.5 cm H_2O ($p < 0.001$) ; $\dot{V}$ max did not increase significantly but tidal volume increased from 397 ± 18 to 466 ± 21 ml ($p < 0.05$) ; the consequence was a lower total airway resistance at peak airflow (from 51.0 ± 5.9 to 33.0 ± 6.3 $cmH_2O.l^{-1}.s$; $p < 0.01$) and lower index of respiratory work (from 6.8 ± 1.1 to 5.1 ± 2.3 cm $H_2O.l$; $p < 0.05$).
Thus, the elimination of snoring by nasal CPAP results in higher ventilatory flows and volumes with lower intrathoracic pressures, consecutive to a reduction in airway resistance, thus leading to decreased respiratory work.

KEYWORDS

Snoring, obstructive sleep apnea syndromes, airway resistance, respiratory work, nasal continuous positive airway pressure.

INTRODUCTION

Nasal continuous positive airway pressure (CPAP) has been proposed by Sullivan et al. (1981) for the treatment of

obstructive sleep apnea syndromes. Its efficacy has been widely confirmed both in the elimination of obstructive apneas, the restoration of polygraphically normal sleep and the elimination of clinical symptoms.
It has been shown that nasal CPAP not only eliminates sleep apneas but snoring as well (Berry and Block, 1984) ; the pressures which eliminate snoring are slightly higher than those which eliminate apneas.
On the other hand, snorers have been shown to have increased airway resistance, requiring higher (more negative) intrathoracic pressures to maintain ventilation at a sufficient level, thus leading to increased respiratory work (Skatrud and Dempsey,1985). In the present work, we evaluated the consequences of the elimination of snoring by means of nasal CPAP on total airway resistance and estimated respiratory work, in patients with obstructive sleep apnea syndromes.

SUBJECTS AND METHODS

Nine consecutive obstructive sleep apnea patients participated in the study. They were aged 44 to 63 years (mean ± sem : 53.9 ± 1.76 years).
Obstructive sleep apnea syndrome (OSAS) was diagnosed by means of standard polysomnography including EEG, EOG, EMG ; a pneumotachograph (Fleisch n° 2 with Godart Statham transducer and electronic integrator) attached to an airtight nasobuccal silicone rubber mask measured ventilatory flows and volumes ; an oesophageal balloon connected to a Validyne pressure transducer measured intrathoracic pressure. All patients had severe obstructive sleep apnea syndromes (OSAS) with apnea indexes ranging from 24 to 131 (68.9 ± 12.0) apneas/hour of sleep.
During a second polygraphically recorded night during which the same parameters were monitored, the effects of nasal CPAP were tested. The pneumotachograph was inserted in the expiratory line of the CPAP tubing : it measured the flow of the CPAP device compressor as modulated by the patient's ventilatory flow. The CPAP level applied by means of a nasal mask was continuously recorded.
The nasal CPAP level was progressively increased by 1 cmH$_2$0 increments ; ten consecutive breaths were randomly chosen during a period of stage 2 sleep when snoring persisted after the elimination of apneas, and were compared with ten consecutive breaths chosen during the first stage 2 sleep period during which snoring had disappeared as a result of an increase in the CPAP level.
These two sets of breaths were characterized by their tidal volume (V_T), peak inspiratory airflow ($\dot{V}$ max) and corresponding oesophageal pressure (Poes). Total airway resistance (R) at peak airflow was computed as the ratio of the difference between nasal mask pressure minus intrathoracic pressure (ΔP) over peak inspiratory flow.
Since a pressure/volume curve was not available, respiratory work was approximated by a respiratory work index (I_{RW}) computed as the product of ΔP by V_T.
The values obtained in the snoring and nonsnoring conditions were compared by means of a Student t test for paired values.

RESULTS

Figure 1 illustrates the effects of the elimination of snoring (indicated by a vibration in the inspiratory part of the flow curve) in a representative patient : an increase in the applied CPAP level dramatically decreased intrathoracic inspiratory pressures (Poes), while the airflows ($\dot{V}$) and volumes (VT) were increased.

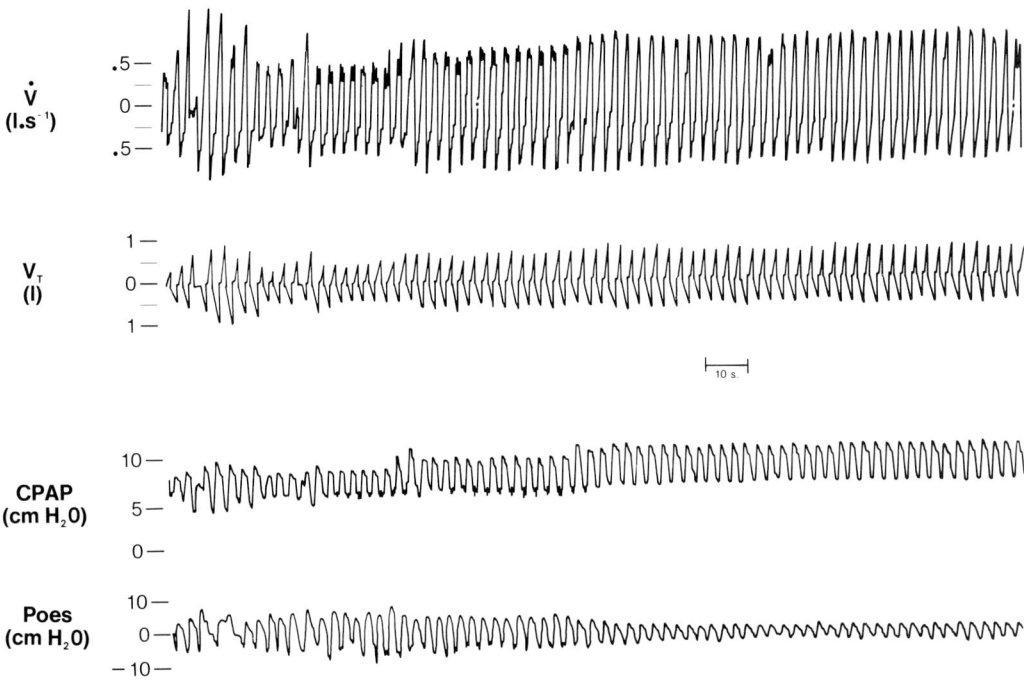

Table 1 summarizes the results obtained in 9 patients ; the mean increase in CPAP necessary to eliminate snoring was about 2 cm H_2O ; it resulted in a decrease in intrathoracic pressure ; ventilatory flows were increased. However, the increase in peak inspiratory flow was not significant, possibly because of the particular shape of the inspiratory flow curve during snoring, which begins with a very sharp peak, followed by a plateau (Krieger and Kurtz,1987 ; see Fig 1) ; because of this particular shape, inspiratory peak airflow is artificially increased during snoring. On the other hand , tidal volume, were significantly increased. Total inspiratory airway resistance at peak flow was dramatically decreased ; the respiratory work index decreased to a lesser extent.

Table 1 - Respiratory parameters (means ± sem) during the snoring and nonsnoring condition in 9 obstructive sleep apnea patients treated with nasal CPAP.

	CPAP level (cm H_2O)	Poes (cm H_2O)	$\dot{V}$ max (ml.s-1)	V_T (ml)	R (cm$H_2O.l^{-1}.s$)	I_{RW} (cm$H_2O.l$)
Snoring	6.8±1.0	-11.6±1.7	344±29	397±18	51.0±5.9	6.8±1.1
Nonsnoring	8.6±1.1	-4.2±0.5	398±47	466±21	33.0±6.3	5.1±2.3
p	< 0.01	< 0.001	ns	< 0.05	< 0.01	< 0.05

CPAP = continuous positive airway pressure, measured at end expiration in the nasal mask
Poes = intrathoracic pressure at peak inspiratory flow
$\dot{V}$max = peak inspiratory airflow
V_T = tidal volume
R = total airway resistance at peak airflow
$\dfrac{(Poes - P\ nasal\ mask)}{\dot{V}\ max}$
I_{RW} = Index of respiratory work
(Poes - P nasal mask) x V_T

DISCUSSION

Previous studies had shown that snorers had higher airway resistances and greater respiratory work during sleep than non-snorers (Skatrud and Dempsey, 1985).
Our results demonstrate that in OSAS patients the elimination of snoring by means of nasal CPAP results in a decrease in airway resistance and suggest a decrease in respiratory work which could only be approximated in our study.
The consequences of the elimination of snoring by nasal CPAP are further suggested by our clinical observations in three patients. These patients were referred for a suspected obstructive sleep apnea syndrome because of heavy snoring associated with chronic tiredness. The polysomnographic recording eliminated the presence of significant obstructive sleep apneas, but demonstrated snoring and markedly elevated intrathoracic pressures. Because of previous observations concerning the effects of CPAP on snoring in OSAS patients we proposed CPAP in these non OSAS snorers. The result was a restitution of the restorative value of sleep after a single night on CPAP. All three patients asked for home treatment with nasal CPAP. After a follow-up period of over 3 month, the beneficial effects on chronic fatigue persisted.
On the basis of our observations, we hypothesize that increased respiratory work could be a factor in chronic tiredness in snorers.

RESUME

Chez les ronfleurs, la résistance des voies aériennes supérieures est augmentée ; il en résulte la nécesité de pressions intra-thoraciques inspiratoires plus élevées (plus négatives) pour maintenir la ventilation à un niveau suffisant et donc un travail ventilatoire augmenté.
Pour évaluer les effets de la pression positive continue sur ces paramètres, nous avons mesuré chez 9 patients atteints de syndromes d'apnées du sommeil à apnées obstructives le volume courant (V_T), le débit inspiratoire maximum ($\dot{V}$ max ; pneumotachographie), la pression intrathoracique correspondante (Poes au moyen d'un ballonnet oesophagien). Dix cycles respiratoires consécutifs ont été choisis au hasard pendant une période de stade 2 où persistait un ronflement après la suppression des apnées et ont été comparés à 10 cycles respiratoires choisis dans le même stade de sommeil après élimination du ronflement par augmentation du niveau de pression positive continue.
L'élimination du ronflement, obtenue pour une augmentation de pression de 6,8 ± 1,0 cm H_2O à 8,6 ± 1,1 cm H_2O ($p < 0,01$) entraîne une diminution des pressions intrathoraciques de -11,6 ± 1,7 à -4,2 ± 0,5 cm H_2O ($p < 0,001$). Simultanément, $\dot{V}$ max n'augmente pas de façon significative, mais V_T augmente de 397 ± 18 à 466 ± 21 ml ($p < 0,05$). La résistance inspiratoire totale des voies aériennes décroît de 51,0 ± 5,9 à 33,0 ± 6,3 cm $H_2O.l^{-1}.s$ ($p < 0,01$) ; un index reflétant le travail ventilatoire (P X V_T) décroît de 6,8 ± 1,1 à 5,1 ± 2,3 cm $H_2O.l$ ($p < 0,05$).
Ainsi la suppression du ronflement par la pression positive continue est suivie de débits et de volumes ventilatoires plus élevés pour des pressions intrathoraciques plus basses, en raison de résistances plus faibles des voies aériennes, entraînant un travail ventilatoire moindre.

REFERENCES

Berry, R.B. and Block, A.J. (1984): Positive nasal airway pressure eliminates snoring as well as obstructive sleep apnea. *Chest* 85, 15-20.
Krieger, J. and Kurtz, D. (1987): Problems in the application of nasal continuous positive airway pressure (CPAP) for the treatment of obstructive sleep apnea. In *Sleep Related Disorders and Internal Diseases*. Springer Verlag, Heidelberg, in press.
Skatrud, J.B. and Dempsey, J.A. (1985): Airway resistance and respiratory muscle function in snorers during NREM sleep. *J. Appl. Physiol.* 59, 328-335.
Sullivan, C.E., Issa, F.Q., Berthon-Jones, M. and Eves, L. (1981): Reversal of obstructive sleep apnoea by continuous positive airvay pressure applied through the nares. *Lancet* i, 862-865.

Efficiency of continue positive airway pressure (CPAP) after uvulopalatopharyngoplasty (UPPP) failure for obstructive sleep apnea syndrome (OSAS)

B. Fleury, F. Laffont, F. Chabolle and J. Ph. Derenne

Hôpital Saint-Antoine, 184 rue du faubourg Saint-Antoine, 75012 Paris, France

Obstructive sleep apnea syndrome (OSAS) is most often characterized clinically by sleep fragmentation, daytime hypersomnolence and snoring. When the patency of upper airway during sleep is definitively restored by tracheostomy a reversal of daytime sleepinesse is obtained (GUILLEMINAULT et al, 1981). However tracheostomy, owing to its particular technical difficulties, its discomfort and its possible complications is not a simple treatment to implement.

When no evident anatomical conditions predisposing to apnea are found in OSAS patients, two therapeutic approaches have been recently described : an alternative surgical approach to the tracheostomy, the uvulopalatopharyngoplasty (UPPP) (FUJITA et al, 1981) and an non surgical approach, the continuous positive airway pressure (CPAP), (SULLIVAN et al, 1981) delivered by a nasal mask.

UPPP is a curative surgical treatment but has some failure rate, probably due to an obstructive process in the oropharynx lower than the soft palate (FUJITA et al, 1983).

MATERIAL - METHODS

4 patients with an OSAS were studied three months after UPPP.
The were 4 men, (mean + SD) 49 + 9,5 years old, with an overweight (184 + 30 % of the ideal body weight).
A the date of the study they had daytime hypersomnolence and a snoring evocating the persistence of an OSAS. New polysomnography was performed. This included EEG, EOG, chin EMG for sleep staging, oral thermistor for air movement, inductance plethysmography for respiratory effort and oxygen saturation (OH MEDA 3700 pulsatile oxymeter). Apneas were defined as a cessation of air movement at the nose and mouth for greater than 10 s.

The polysomnography had confirmed the persistance of chains of obstructive apneas in the four patients (Table I).

PATIENT	Apnea Index/Hour	
	NREM Sleep	REM Sleep
1	37	16
2	70	80
3	40	70
4	48	44

Table 1

NASAL CPAP

Each patient underwent a trial of nasal CPAP after given informed consent. Positive airway pressure was applied through a nose mask (P + SEFAM, France).
Pressure were gradually increased until suppression or significant reduction of the number of apneas was obtained.
To test the efficiency of CPAP after failure of UPPP in OSAS patients was the purpose of the study.

RESULTS

Two patients were able to tolerate the mask for the entire night (8 hours) and two had tolerated it only for two hours.
The evolution of the apnea index during NREM and REM sleep is shown in figures 1 and 2.

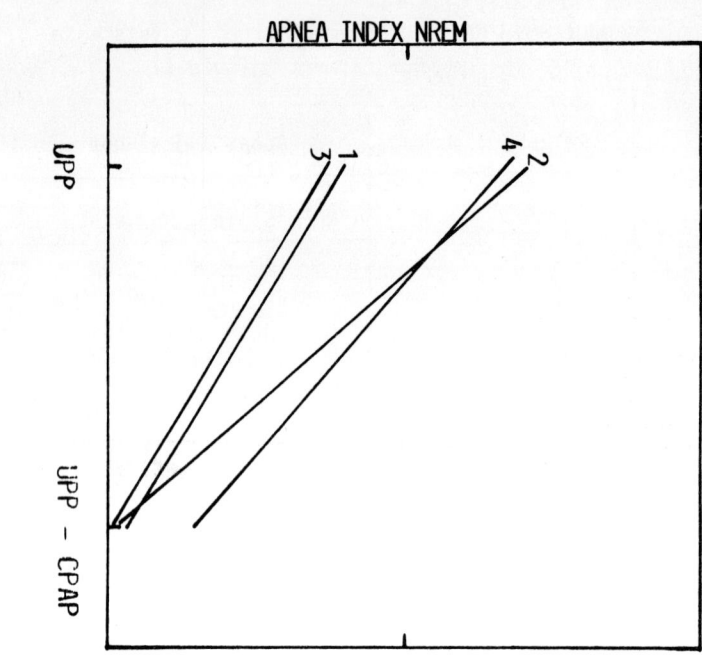

Fig I

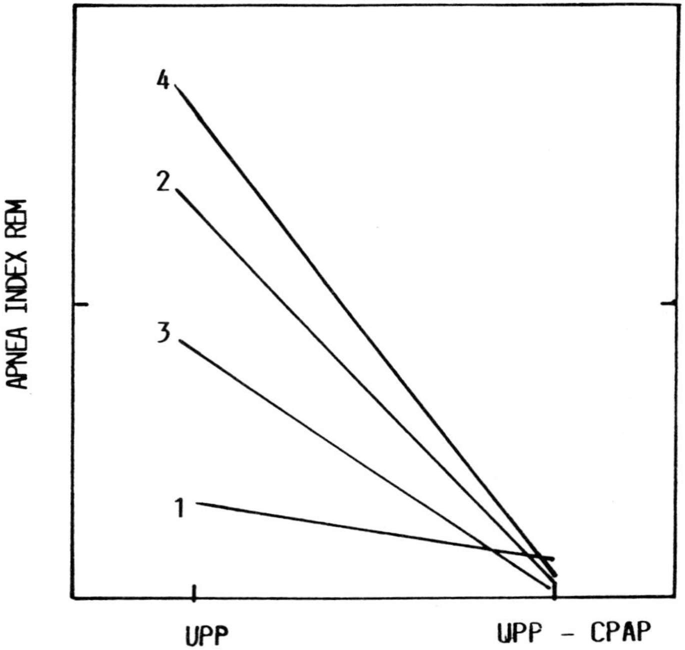

Fig II

Evolution of the apnea index after UPP with and without CPAP

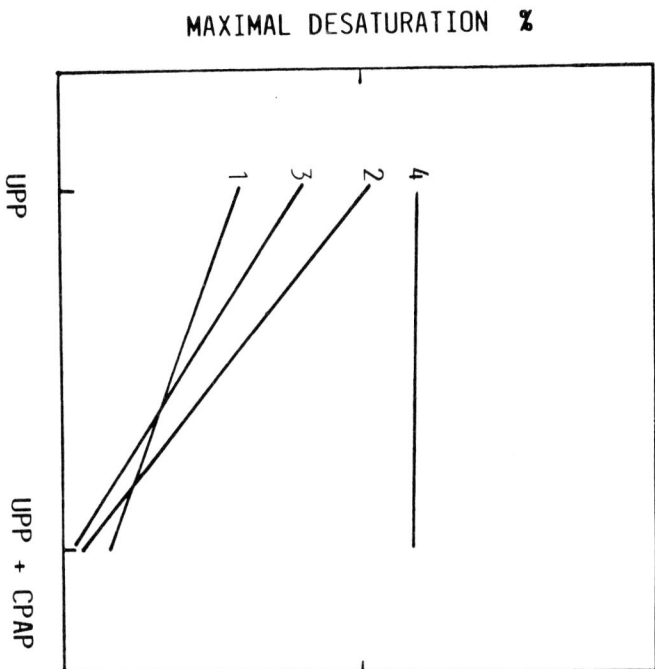

Fig III

Evolution of the maximal desaturation of oxyhemoglobin during sleep after UPP, with and without CPAP.

During NREM Sleep, apneas were abolished in three patients (N°1, 2 and 3) with a nasal pressure, of 10, 13 and 4,5 cmH20. In the patient N°4 significant reduction of the apnea index was obtained (from 63 to 14 apneas per hour) with a nasal pressure of 10 cmH20. During REM Sleep the apneas were abolished in three patients (N°2, 3 and 4) and only 7 apneas per hour were observed in the patient N° 1.

Once apneas were abolished, all subjects showed sustained sleep, which returned toward normal architecture.

A marked reduction of the sleep oxyhemoglobin desaturation was obtained in 3 patients concomittently to the reduction of apneas (Fig 3). In one patient (N° 4), in spite of reduction of apneas index, a persistant sleep oxyhemoglobin desaturation was observed ($>$ 50 % of the awake baseline of SaO2)

DISCUSSION - CONCLUSION

In spite of the anatomical changes of the oropharynx secondary to UPPP, a curative positive airway pressure delivered by nasal route can be obtained in OSAS patients.

Persisting sleep oxyhemoglobin desaturation after suppression of apneas, as seen in one of our patients has been reported after tracheostomy for OSAS (FLETCHER et al, 1985).

It is probably due to an associated chronic obstructive pulmonary disease (COPD). A COPD is present in our patient and can explain in part the persisting desaturation under CPAP in spite of apneas suppression.

BIBLIOGRAPHY

FLETCHER E.C., BROWN D.L.,
Nocturnal oxyhemoglobin desaturation following tracheostomy for obstructive sleep apnea
Am. J. Med., 1985, 79, 35-41

FUJITA S., CONWAY W., ZORICK F., ROTH T.,
Surgical correction of anatomic abnormalities in obstructive sleep apnea syndrome : uvulopalatopharyngoplasty
Otolaryngol. Head. Neck. Surg 1981, 89, 923-934

FUJITA S., CONWAY W.A., ZORICK F., SICKLESTELL J., ROEHRS T., WITTIG R., ROTH T.,
Evaluation of the effectiveness of uvulopalatopharyngoplasty
Sleep Res. 1983, 12, 248

GUILLEMINAULT C., SIMMONS F.B., MOTTA J.,
Obstructive sleep apnea syndrome and tracheostomy : long term follow up experience
Arch Intern Med. 1981, 141, 985-988

SULLIVAN C.E., ISSA F.Q., BERTHON-JONES M., EVES L.,
Reversal of obstructive sleep apnea by continuous positive pressure applied through the nares.
Lancet 1981, 1, 862-865

Surgical management of chronic snoring with obstructive sleep apnea and polysomnographic evaluation

Shiro Fujita, Robert Wittig, Frank Zorick and Thomas Roth

Henry Ford Hospital, Detroit, Michigan, USA

RESUME

Surgical treatment of obstructive sleep apnea is basically aimed at either bypassing the obstructive area by tracheostomy or eliminating the obstructive lesion in order to prevent soft tissue collapse in the upper airway during an apneic episode. Although tracheoplastic technique with advancement of skin flaps has significantly reduced undesirable side effects often associated with standard tracheostomy, other surgical alternatives are preferable to eliminate the need for tracheostomy.

Uvulopalatopharyngoplasty (UPPP) was designed to enlarge the potential oropharyngeal lumen in an attempt to reduce airway collapse during sleep. It consists of excising redundant oropharyngeal tissues from the fr-e margin of the soft palate, tonsillar pillars and uvula, preserving underlying musculature. After excision, the non-collapsible oropharyngeal space is reconstructed. This is highly effective (80-90%) in eliminating snoring and significantly reducing obstructive apnea for patients whose airway compromise is primarily in the oropharynx (Type I & IIa).

When extensive airway compromise exists (Type IIb), UPPP is performed with tracheoplasty as the first stage procedure, then followed by hypopharyngeal surgery. Hypopharyngeal surgery is divided into two categories, 1) soft tissue reduction or 2) skeletal surgery (mandibular advancement, hyoid suspension). Our recent experience indicates that CO_2 laser midline glossectomy is effective for those who have hypopharyngeal collapse in antero-posterior dimension due to retrognathia.

REFERENCES

1. Fujita S, Conway WA, Zorick F et al. "Evaluation of effectiveness of uvulopalatopharyngoplasty". Laryngoscope 95:70-74, 1985.

2. Fujita S, Woodson T, Rosner A et al. "Midline laser glossectomy as treatment for obstructive sleep apnea syndrome". (in preparation), presented at Western Section of Triological Society, January, 1987.

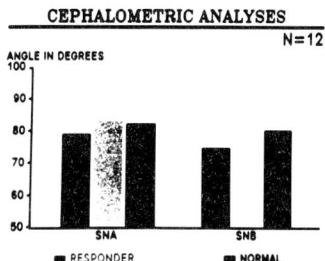

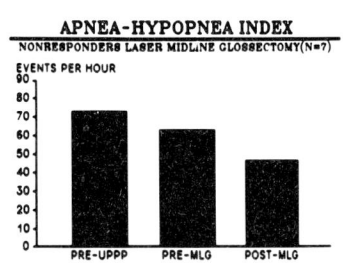

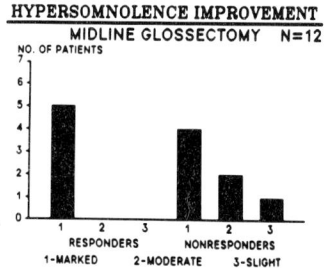

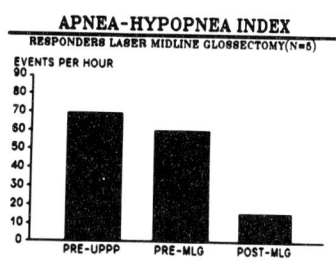

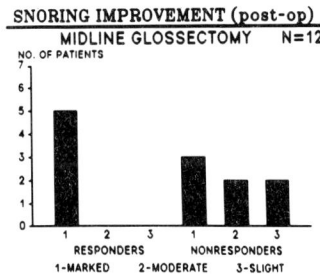

TABLE 2
SUBJECTIVE RESPONSE TO UPPP

	Improved Markedly	Moderately	Slightly	Unimproved
Snoring	56% (37) (98.5%)	38% (25)	4.5% (3)	1.5% (1)
Excessive Daytime Sleepiness	40% (26) (85%)	36% (24)	9% (6)	15% (10)

TABLE 3
NOCTURNAL RESPIRATION PARAMETERS

Parameters (N = 66)	Preoperative	Postoperative
# Apneas/hr TST*	59.2	32.1
Mean apnea duration	26.2	21.8
#SaO_2 < 85%/hr TST	65.1	27.6
Lowest SaO_2	40.9	61.3

*TST (Total Sleep Time)

TABLE 4
NOCTURNAL OXYGENATION

	Apnea Index		Oxygenation			
			#SaO_2 < 85%/hr TST*		Lowest SaO_2	
	Preop	Postop	Preop	Postop	Preop	Postop
Responders (N = 33)	58.3	9.5	77.2	20.3	46.3	68.7
Nonresponders (N = 33)	60.2	55.4	61.9	36.6	35.1	52.0

*TST (Total Sleep Time)

TABLE 5
ANATOMIC DATA

Principal Site of Airway Narrowing	Responder (N = 33)	Nonresponder (N = 33)
Oropharynx	23	5
Hypopharynx	2	0
Mixed		
(Both involved)	8	28

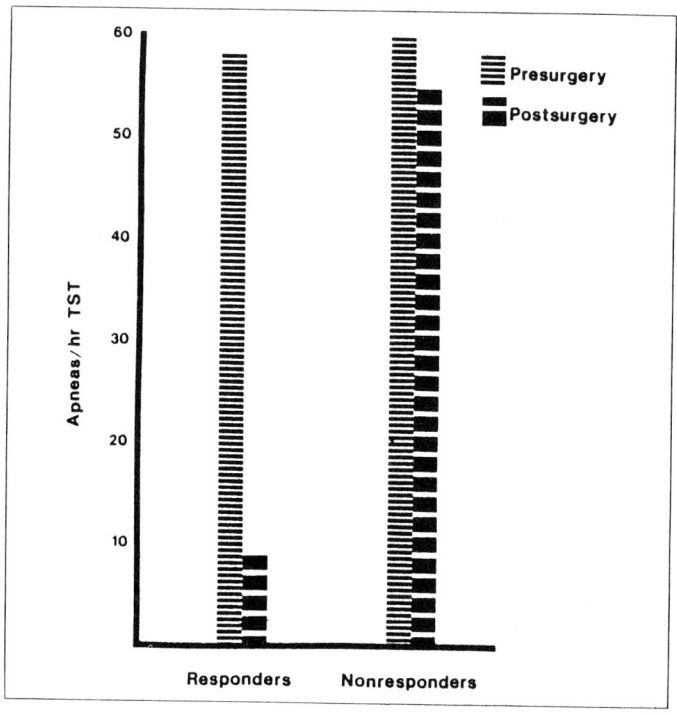

Figure 6. Apnea index for 66 patients undergoing UPPP.

RESUME

Le traitement chirurgical du syndrome d'apnée obstructive au cours du sommeil (AOS) a évolué rapidement de la trachéotomie permanente à diverses alternatives chirurgicales que les patients trouvent plus acceptables.

L'uvulopalatpharyngoplastie (UPPP) a été effective dans 50 à 60% des patients non sélectionnés souffrant de l'AOS sévere. Les échecs de l'UPPP sont causés par des obstructions ailleurs, généralement par l'effondrement hypopharyngeal. On a proposé plusieurs procédés chirurgicaux pour traiter et empêcher l'effondrement hypopharyngeal, éliminant la nécessité d'une trachéotomie permanente. Parmi ceux-ci il y a l'avancement maxillaire-mandibulaire avec ostéotomie fendue sagittale et l'ostéotomie mandibulaire glissante avec suspension hyoïde. Chacun de ces procédés a ses avantages et ses désavantages.

Récemment, nous avons développé un nouveau procédé chirurgical où il s'agit d'une glossectomie centrale à laser comme procédé alternatif afin de corriger une obstruction hypopharyngeale. Quand on combine ceci avec l'UPPP, l'effet en est excellent pour éliminer la nécessité d'une trachéotomie permanente des patients AOS ayant des rétrécissements étendus des voies respiratoires supérieures. On discutera l'indication, la techniquechirurgicale, les complications possibles, et les résultats (data polysommnographiques avant et après l'opération de l'UPPP et de la chirurgie hypopharyngeale pour AOS.

Mots Clef: uvulopalatpharyngoplastie, syndrome d'apnée obstructive au cours du sommeil, glossectomie centrale à laser, trachéoplatie

Chronic rhonchopathy. Ed. C.H. Chouard. © 1988, John Libbey Eurotext Ltd. pp.305-310.

Effectiveness of uvulopalatopharyngoplasty in snorers with sleep apnea syndrome

F. Chabolle*, B. Fleury**, B. Meyer* and J.P. Derenne**

*Service ORL, Hôpital Saint-Antoine, 75012 Paris, France
**Service de Pneumologie, Hôpital Saint-Antoine, 75012 Paris

ABSTRACT

About 23 cases of S.A.S, all having undergonne U.P.P.P the authors compared clinical and polysomnographic results at the third month after the operation. A success rate of 78 % appears, representing a 50 % decrease of mean apnea index. Authors report the absence of exact correlation between clinical and polysomnographic results. At last, Pa CO_2 et pre-operative weignt are the only criterions to hold to predict U.P.P.P results.

KEYWORDS

Oro-pharynx ; Sleep Apnea Syndrome ; Snoring ; Uvulopalatopharyngoplasty.

INTRODUCTION

Since Uvulopalatopharyngplasty (UPPP) was proposed as a treatment of obstructive Sleep Apnea Syndrome (SAS), numerous published works quoted very different results.

In spite of numerous studies using modern and performing means of investigation, exact determination of the obstructive site is still not possible, in a definite way, during pre-operative period.

Research of pre-operative criterions allowing to predict success or failure of U.P.P.P gave variable results in the field of criterion choice and of the quality of tis predictive character for the U.P.P.P result. Morover, for numerous authors there seems to exist no correlation between clinical results of U.P.P.P and those of polysomnographic parameters.

This work, realised in 23 patients suffering from S.A.S, sets out a comparison between clinical results and polysomnographic parameters results. Analysis of failures in function of various criterions allows to draw some orientations concerning the prediction of U.P.P.P success or failure.

MATERIAL

23 patients were selected : 22 men and 1 woman with extreme ages going from 34 to 71 years old. Average age is of 51 $\pm$ 8 S.M.

These patients weighed from 62 to 135 kilos with a theoretical weight percent from 117 to 225 %. Average weight was of 149 % $\pm$ 19 S.M of theoretical weight. All patients showed very invaliding snoring, associated to daytime sleepiness in 21 cases and a clinical notion of apnea in only 15 cases, some patients living alone.

Only 10 patients showed no associated pathology. Pre-operative exmination allowed to find high blood pressure in 10 cases, dyslipidemy in 6 cases, diabetis in 3 cases and allergic history in 3 other cases.

All patients had a pre-operative measure of arterial blood gazes as well as polysomnographic parameters recording.

Continuous arterial blood gazes assay showed Pa O2 going from 100 to 69,2 mmHg with mean value of 79.1 $\pm$ 9.9 S.M.

In the same way, Pa CO2 went from 35 to 49.7 mmHg with mean value of 40.7 $\pm$ 4.6 S.M. At last oxygen saturation went from 90.2 % to 97.5 % with mean value of 95.1 $\pm$ 2.0 S.M. For polysomnographic parameters recording, apnea/hour index was defined by a number of apnea higher than 10 per hour, every apnea being higher than 10 seconds.

Mean apnea/hour index was defined by the total number of apnea divided by the total duration of sleep. Average apnea index lower than 10 was considered as normal value.

In the 23 patients, average apnea/hour index spread from 21 to 87 with mean value of 52 $\pm$ 20. fir NREM sleep; apnea index went from 18 to 87 with mean value of 55 $\pm$ 21. For REM sleep, this index went from 0 to 72 with mean value of 42 $\pm$ 20.

METHODS

U.P.P.P was achieved under general anesthesia in 22 cases and under local anesthesia in 1 case. Fibroscopic intubation was necessary in 10 cases. U.P.P.P was associated to tonsillectomy in 15 cases and to nasal septoplasty in 7 cases.

Soft palate resection was achieved by passing through maximum inflexion point and then going beyond in tonsil lodges. Exeresis was finished by more or less complete resection of tonsils posterior pillars. Exeresis sides were sutured edge to edge in order not to have any cruented area at pharyngeal level, and to take off the excess of oropharyngeal mucosa.

Early operating issues of U.P.P.P were marked in two cases with hemorrhagie having demanded surgical resumption with no consequences for the patient. No case of infection or death was reported. 15 of the 23 patients had in the issues a weight losse higher than 10 % and secondary to swallowing disconfort induced by surgical gesture. This emaciation has certainly contributed in the improvement of S.A.S symptomatology.

In the examination on the third post-operative month, no permanent or disabling complication existed. Only one intermittent rhinolalia was reported in 5 cases and ceased easily after orthophonic reeducation. Occasional liquid regurgitation in forward leaning head position was described in 10 patients but completly disappeared during the following months.

At last in 6 cases, an algesic syndrome persisted under the form of pharyngeal paresthesia. No soft palate stenosis was reported during post operative period.

An other clinical and polysomnographic examination was achieved 3 months after the operation, patient being seen regularly during this period.

RESULTS

Clinical evaluation relied on using a clinical score. This score was based on the clinical analysis of 5 symptoms : snoring, apnea, night awaking, awaking asthenia and at last daytime sleepiness.

Every symptom was affected with an intensity coefficient going from symptom disappearance to its increase. All patients presented pre-operative score higher or equal to 9.

U.P.P.P clinical success was said when score was lower or equal to 5.

Evaluation of the polysomnographic recording results was achieved arbitrarily, admitting as a success a higher than 50 % decrease of average pre-operative apnea/hour index, and the patient was then said responding to U.P.P.P.

Total results in 23 patients showed clinical and polysomnographic success rate of 78 %, i.e. 18 patients, and failure rate of 22 %, i.e. 5 patients.

TABLE I

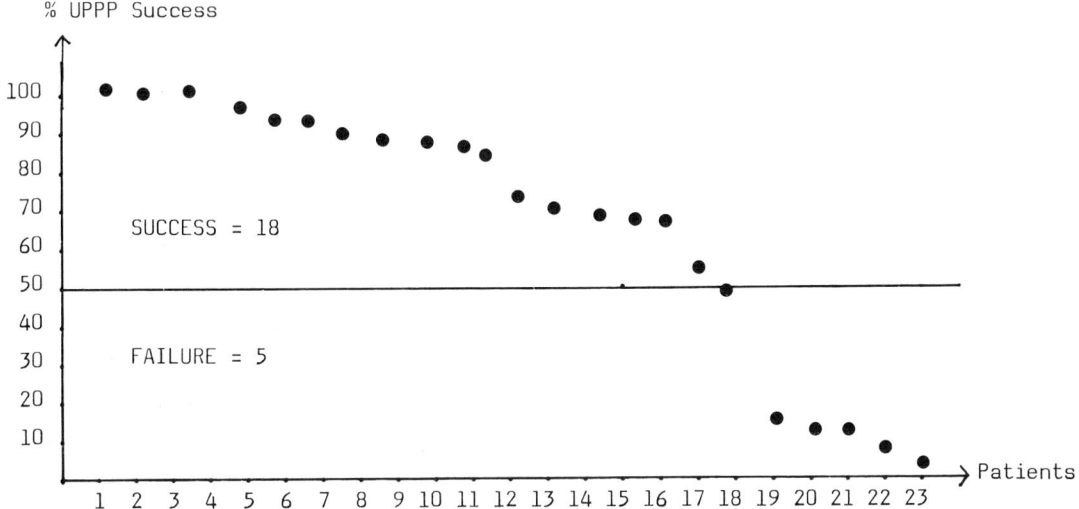

EFFECTIVENESS OF U.P.P.P ON POLYSOMNOGRAPHIC SLEEP PARAMETERS
(IMPROVEMENT % OF APNEA INDEX/HOURS)

Analysis of clinical results reveals that the 5 failures presented all a complete recovery of S.A.S symptomatology. No increase was reported. However in these 5 patients couted as clinical failure, 2 showed polysomnographic recording in favor of therapeutic success.

TABLE II

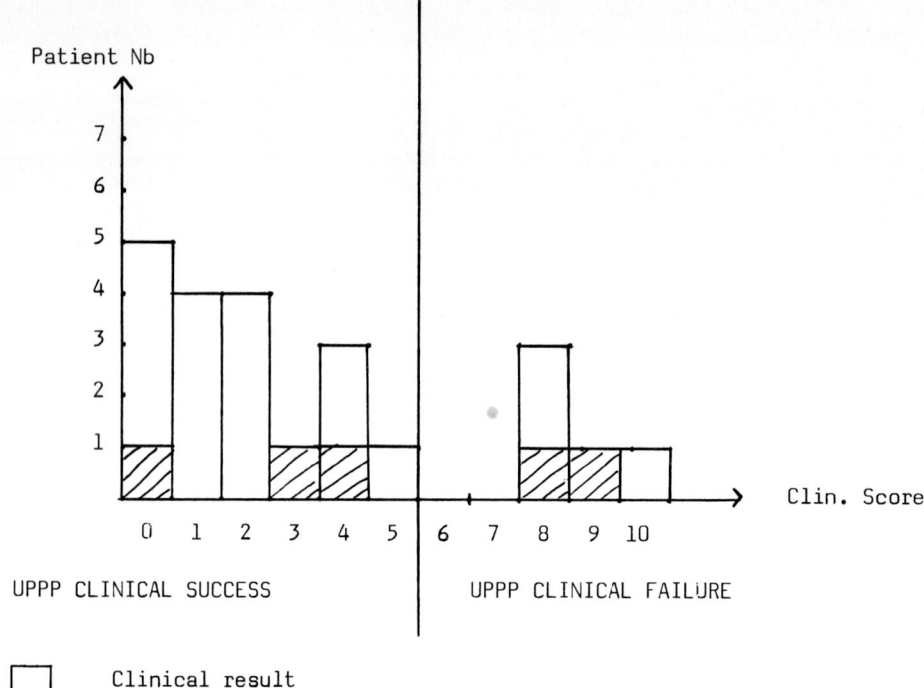

COMPARISON OF U.P.P.P CLINICAL AND POLYSOMNOGRAPHIC RESULTS

Analysis of post-operative polysomnographic recording results show that 16 patients present an improvement higher than 2/3 of their apnea index. 14 of them are considered as cured with an index lower than 10, i.e. 61 % of the patients in this study.

The 5 patients considered as polysomnographic failure are very clearly individualised v.s the patients considered as answering U.P.P.P according to polysomnographic parameters. In these 5 failures, 2 were considered as clinically cured.

TABLE III

The analysis of these 5 failures in function of patients age didn't show any distinct correlation. On the opposite, assay in function of weight quoted 4 of these patients belonging to those having highest theoretical weight in the test. But the weight of fifth patients belonged to lower limits.

In the same way, pre-operative apnea/hour index is extremely variable for these 5 patients and doesn't allow to isolate a non responding U.P.P.P group. Pre-operative analysis in function of arterial blood gazes didn't either show any signigicant difference between the 2 groups for oxygen saturation and Pa O2 as well. On the opposite, Pa CO2 in these 5 patients belongs to the 6 highest value of this study and could constitute in the future, a predicting factor fo U.P.P.P result, hypercapnia possibly making U.P.P.P failure dreadful.

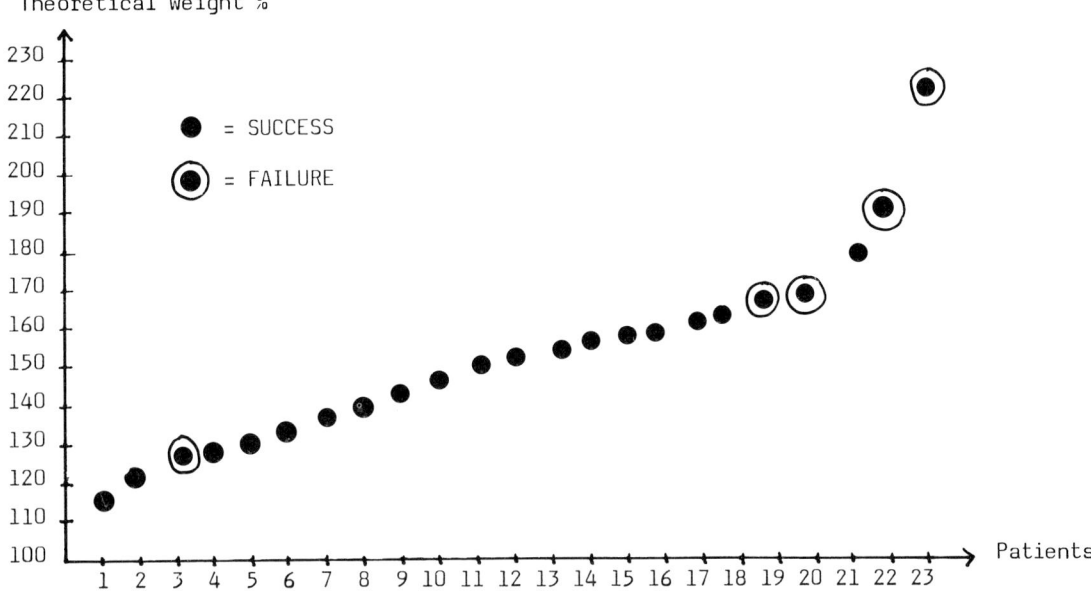

U.P.P.P FAILURE ANALYSIS IN FUNCTION OF THE WEIGHT

DISCUSSION

Clinical and polysomnographic assay in this series of 23 patients shows clear discordance between results. Thus, some patients clinically improved show non cured polysomnographic parameters. In the same way opposite situation can be found. This discordance is certainly dut to the fact that sleep is variable by its quality from on night to another. Further more, apnea/hour index is probably not completly representative of S.A.S intensity. It should then be necessary to include other criterions, especially concerning sleep organisation. This should allow better correlation between clinical and polysomnographic parameters.

Considering this work, only 2 pre-operative criterions must be held to predict U.P.P.P result : it is weight and Pa CO2.

Weight : Pre-operative weight excess higher than 160 % of theoretical weight constitutes a major failure risk of U.P.P.P.

Obesity seems then to be a pejorative criterions in U.P.P.P success. Results of this assay meet those of GUILLEMINAULT and all which quoted obesity influence in U.P.P.P failures. On the contrary, FUJITA and all would rather be in favour of U.P.P.P failure when patient get close to theoretical weight (FUJITA, 1981 ;

FUJITA, 1985).

Obesity settles the problem of a multifunctional determinism of obstructive site. Especially, numerous works demonstrated upper aerial tracts narrowing in S.A.S not only was located at soft palate lower edge but furthermore tongue base should be incriminated.

Quantification of various oro-pharyngeal structures, especially tongue volume should allow, in the next coming years, to define better the obstructive site.

Pa CO_2 : Among data defined in arterial blood gazes assay, the only pre-operative criterions allowing to predict U.P.P.P result seems to be Pa CO_2. Oxygen saturation and Pa O_2 didn't evidence any discriminative character, on the contrary of what SIMMONS and all found, using an oxygen desaturation criterious higher than 85 %. In the same way, De BERRY BOROWIECKI uses an index implicating oxygen saturation deficit.(SIMMONS, 1984 ; DEBERRY BOROWIECKI, 1985 ; WETMORE, 1986).

Pa CO_2 has never been used before as evaluation data for U.P.P.P result. However one patient in this study had a Pa CO_2 as high as the 5 failure and met therapeutic and polysomnographic success.

Weight and Pa CO_2 seem then to us, the two only pre-operative criterions to be considered in order to predict U.P.P.P result. However these criterions aren't completly reliable and today there is no dependable pre-operative mean of predicting U.P.P.P success or failure.

CONCLUSIONS

U.P.P.P consists in elementary surgery giving success answers higher than 75 % with about 60 % of S.A.S cures. This answer rate is certainly due to the important exeresis at the level of soft palate.

The 2 only pre-operative criterions to keep in order to predict U.P.P.P result are weight and Pa CO_2. These two factors aren't however completly reliable. Schematically, U.P.P.P must be proposed systematically in first intention for S.A.S therapy, as long as there doesn't exist any better method for obstructive site determination, all the more this intervention doesn't prevent other therapeutic possibilities, as tracheotomy or C.P.A.P.

REFERENCES

DEBERRY B., KUKWA, A.A. and BLANCKS. (1985) : Indications for Palatopharyngoplasty in the treatment of obstructive Sleep Apnea Syndrome. Arch. Otolaryngol. 111, 659 - 663
FUJITA, CONWAY, ZORICK. (1981) : Surgical Correction of Anatomic Abnormalities in Obstructive Sleep Apnea Syndrome : Uvulopalatopharyngoplasty. Otolaryngol. Head Neck Surg. 89, 923 - 934
FUJITA, CONWAY, SICKLESTEEL. (1985) : Evaluation of the Effectiveness of Uvulopalatopharyngoplasty. Laryngoscope 95, 70 - 74
SIMMONS, GUILLEMINAULT, SILVESTRI. (1984) : Snoring, and Some Obstructive Sleep Apnea, Can Be Cured by Oropharyngeal Surgery. Arch. Otolaryngol. 109, 502 - 507
WETMORE, SCRIMAL, SNYDERMAN, HILLER. (1986) : Post-operative evaluation of sleep apnea after uvulopalatopharyngoplasty. Laryngoscope 96, 738 - 741

Chronic rhonchopathy. Ed. C.H. Chouard. © 1988, John Libbey Eurotext Ltd. pp.311-319.

The relative importance of cranio-mandibular abnormalities in obstructive sleep apnea syndrome

M. Partinen and C. Guilleminault

Stanford University School of Medicine, Stanford, California 94305, USA

ABSTRACT

In a six-month period, 157 obstructive sleep apnea syndrome (OSAS) patients seen consecutively in clinic had cephalometric roentgenograms and polygraphic monitoring during sleep. Different variables, including cephalometric landmarks, body mass index (BMI), and polygraphic results (particularly degree of oxygen desaturation and number of abnormal breathing events) were statistically analyzed. As a rule, OSAS patients presented cranio-mandibular anatomical abnormalities and an elevated BMI. But the factors associated with a high respiratory disturbance index (RDI) and a selected oxygen desaturation index are different.

KEY WORDS

Sleep apnea, cranio-facial abnormalities, respiratory disturbance index, body mass index

INTRODUCTION

Despite the many studies published during the past 20 years on obstructive sleep apnea syndrome (OSAS), there is still significant controversy over the mechanisms involved in the development of sleep-related apneas, the long-term clinical impacts of mild to moderate OSAS, and the appropriateness of specific treatments. We investigated 157 consecutive obstructive sleep apnea patients and analyzed the cephalometric landmarks recorded on these patients. We then performed different statistical analyses to appreciate the relative role of the cranio-facial abnormalities in the development of OSAS compared with known factors such as obesity. The risk ratios for abnormal breathing during sleep and oxygen saturation drops were evaluated, taking into consideration cephalometric landmarks and other factors such as body mass index (BMI) and sleep disturbances.

SUBJECTS AND METHODS

Patient population

We saw 157 obstructive sleep apneic (OSA) patients consecutively in a sleep disorders clinic. All subjects were referred for loud snoring, excessive daytime sleepiness or disrupted nocturnal sleep. They were examined by the same investigator during a six-month period and were submitted to the same experimental protocol. Patients were included in the study if they were at least 17 years old and had a respiratory disturbance index (RDI) ≥ 10 at the diagnostic polygraphic recording. All patients were examined by the same investigator during a six-month period. None of the 157 patients meeting the above pre-selected criteria was eliminated from the study, which included 143 men with a mean age of 49.4 years and standard deviation (SD) ± 11.3 years (median 50, range 21-74), and 14 women, mean age 51.0 ± 10.4 years (median 51.5, range 32-68) (see Table 1). All had cephalometric roentgenograms and one night of polygraphic monitoring as part of the experimental protocol.

Polysomnographic recordings and definition of breathing abnormalities

The variables monitored during polygraphic recording were electroencephalogram, electro-oculogram, chin electromyogram, and electrocardiogram (modified V2 lead). Respiration was monitored by strain gauges or uncalibrated inductive respiratory plethysmography; airflow was measured by thermistors and oxygen saturation by ear oximetry (Biox^{TM}). Apnea, hypopnea, and sleep stages were scored according to standard definitions (Guilleminault et al., 1980), based upon findings obtained from respiratory, airflow, oximetric and other channels. We defined "hypopnea" as: (a) a 50 percent reduction in maximal thermistor output compared to baseline, and (b) association with a decrease of oxygen saturation to below 92 percent from a baseline of at least 94 percent, or a drop of oxygen saturation to at least 3 percent if baseline was below 90 percent. The RDI, or (apnea + hypopnea) x 60/TST, which takes into account the number of abnormal breathing events per hour of sleep, was calculated (Guilleminault et al., 1980). We also defined an oxygen desaturation index, arbitrarily considering as "significant" any desaturation below 80 percent. From the relationship of this below 80 percent level of oxygen desaturation to an apnea or hypopnea, and the number of oxygen drops below 80 percent calculated per hour of sleep, we formulated the index O_2-80-I. Sleep was scored in 30-second epochs following the international criteria of Rechtschaffen and Kales (1968). The BMI (weight x $10,000$/height^2) was calculated by the method of Khosla and Lowe (1967). (See Table 1)

Cephalometric roentgenogram studies

Lateral cephalometric roentgenograms were obtained with the Wemer cephalostatTM, using the technique of Riley et al. (1983). Tracings of the roentgenograms from all subjects were made on acetate sheets by a single investigator blind to the clinical and nocturnal polygraphic results.

The following angles in degrees and dimensions in millimeters were measured on the flat film: SNA: angle measurement from sella (S) to nasion (N) to point A (subspinale); SNB: angle measurement from sella (S) to nasion (N) to point B (supramentale); GoGn-SN: angle measurement forms by the intersection of a line passing by Go (gonion) Gn (gnathion) and by N (nasion) and S (sella); NSBa: also called cranial base flexure (angle formed by the intersection between lines drawn from nasium to sella to basion); MP-H: distance from mandibular plane (MP) to hyoid bone (H); PNS-P: distance from posterior nasal spine (PNS) to the tip of the soft palate (P), not shown in figure. The posterior airway space (PAS), defined by Riley et al. (1983) as the space behind the base of the tongue (2) and limited by soft tissues (i.e., more difficult to clearly delineate than bony landmarks), was also measured for comparative purposes. Finally, a score derived from MP-H and PAS distances was calculated. This

TABLE 1. Description of the patient population

		Men N = 143	Women N = 14	Total N = 157	p-value or X² men vs women
Age					
	mean (years)	49.4	51.0	49.5	NS
	SD	11.3	10.4	11.2	
	median	50.0	51.5	50.0	
	range	21 - 74	32 - 68	21 - 74	
BMI					
	mean (kgm⁻²)	30.5	36.4	31.0	$p < 0.001$
	SD	5.5	7.6	6.0	
	median	29.3	35.3	29.7	
	range	19.8 - 57.5	26.1 - 47.5	19.8 - 57.5	
RDI					
	mean	49.6	65.8	51.1	$p = 0.044$
	SD	27.7	34.8	28.6	
	median	44.0	62.5	47.0	
	range	10 - 130	13.5 - 125	10 - 130	
O_2-80-IND					
	mean	7.3	10.5	7.6	NS
	SD	15.5	23.8	16.3	
	median	0.0	1.5	0.0	
	range	0 - 74.7	0 - 84.4	0 - 84.4	
TST					
	mean	385.0	331.4	380.5	$p = 0.003$
	SD	61.4	55.8	62.6	
	median	391.7	342.0	385.0	
	range	130 - 552	224 - 403	130 - 552	
Treated for high blood pressure (%)		34.1	64.3	37.0	$X^2 = 3.74$*

*: almost significant; the limit of X^2 for $p < 0.05$ is 3.84.

Table 1. BMI = body mass index (kg/m²); RDI = respiratory disturbance index TST = total sleep time; O_2-80-I = desaturation index (number of desaturations below 80% per hour of sleep.

BMI = surface corporelle; RDI = index d'apnee et d'hypopnee; TST = temps total de sommeil; O_2-80-I = index du nombre de chute de la saturation en oxygene < 80%

score was based upon the variation of each measurement from normal values. For PAS, scores varied from 0 to 3, with 0 if PAS >9 mm; 1, PAS = 8-9 mm; 2, PAS = 6-7 mm; 3, PAS <6 mm. Similarly for MP-H, 0 was given for MP-H <18 mm, 1, MP-H = 18-21 mm; 2, MP-H = 22-24 mm; 3, MP-H >24 mm. Scores were summed up for each patient and varied from 0 to 6.

The normative values used to compare cephalometric roentgenogram measurements obtained on our OSAS patients were those published in textbooks and referenced articles on cephalometric landmarks and evaluation of cranio-facial anomalies (Jamieson et al., 1986; Tweed, 1946; Burstone et al., 1978; Khouw et al, 1970; Ricketts, 1961,1972; Steiner, 1959, 1962; Popovich and Thompson, 1977; MacIntosh, 1970), and from a control population of 41 subjects who were followed by orthodontists for mild to moderate malocclusion syndrome, but with no symptoms of OSAS.

Statistical analysis

Analysis of variance and Student's t tests were used for comparison between groups. Separate variance T or pooled T was used depending on the results of the Levene test for equality of variances (15). The Bonferroni criteria for significance levels were used when multiple comparisons were made (15). Mantel-Haenszel statistics, risk-ratios and corresponding 95 percent confidence limit (CL) were calculated, using the BMDP statistical program 4F (Dixon et al., 1985). Using RDI and O_2-80-I as dependent variables, we did covariate and multiple stepwise regression analyses. Independent variables were: cephalometric measurements, age, BMI, TST, stages 1, 3 and 4 NREM sleep, and REM sleep. If the kurtosis of the distribution of a variable was higher than 2, logarithmic transformation was done, and the logarithm was added to the model. We also did a factor analysis of all the above-mentioned variables.

RESULTS

Cephalometric analysis

The mean sella-nasion-point A (SNA) angle was $82.0°$ (SD 4.2, median 82) (normative data = $82°\pm2$); the difference between the patients' and normative mean SNA is nonsignificant.

The mean sella-nasion-point B (SNB) angle was $78.7°$ (± 4.4) (normative data = $80°\pm2$), nonsignificant. Females had smaller SNB (76.0 ± 4.3) than males (79.0 ± 4.3). (Pooled variance T = 2.50, p = 0.013.)

The mean NSBa, i.e., basal angle, was $128.7°\pm6.5$ with a median of $129°$ (normative data = $137\pm5.2°$), p <0.001.

The mean mandibular plane-hyoid (MP-H) distance was 26.4 ± 6.8 mm (median 26.0) (normative data = 15.4 ± 3 mm), p <0.001. The mean length of the soft palate (PNS-P) was 46.3 ± 6.8 mm (median 46.0) (normative data = 37 ± 3 mm) p <0.001. The mean PAS distance was 5.4 ± 3.3 mm (median 4.0) (normative data = 11 ± 2 mm), p <0.001.

Statistically, females and males did not differ significantly with regard to any cephalometric measurement other than SNB (see above).

This first analysis showed that 98.7 percent (155 of 157 patients) of our patient population presented at least one cranio-mandibular anatomical abnormality, and 96.8 percent (152 out of 157) had at least two cephalometric landmarks significantly different from normal. In contrast, 41 of the 49 control subjects sent for orthodontic treatment were within two standard deviations of the mean for all considered variables. We found that our population of OSAS patients, in general, had (1) a normally positioned maxilla, (2) an increase in the length of the soft palate, (3) a retroposition of the mandible with a steeper mandibular plane than expected, (4) a different cranial base flexure with a nasion-sella-basion (NSBa) angle more acute than expected (normal mean - 137 ± 5.7 degrees), and (5) a displacement of the hyoid bone to a lower position than expected (normal mean = 15.3 ± 3 mm). Retroposition of the mandible and a more acute NSBa angle reduce posterior pharynx airway space by crowding the soft tissues anchored on the skull and mandible. The patients sent to orthodontists differed in that they had a higher position of the hyoid bone, shorter soft palate, and larger NSBa angle (Jamieson et al., 1986).

Nocturnal polysomnography

1. Sleep analysis: The mean TST for the total patient population was 380.5±62.6 min. Men (385.0±61.4) slept longer than women (331.4±55.8) ($p < 0.01$). Mean total stage 1 NREM sleep percent was 42.3±20.7 (elevated compared with normative values). Mean total stages 3-4 NREM sleep percentage was 5.5±6.9 (abnormally decreased) and mean total REM sleep percent was 13.1±6.4, also decreased compared with normal values. Men (13.4±62.1) had more REM sleep than women (9.3±8.0) ($p = 0.03$), but there were nonsignificant differences between sexes for the other sleep stages.

2. Breathing abnormalities: The mean RDI was 51.1±28.6, range 10-130. The mean O_2-80-I, i.e., the number of oxygen desaturations below 80 percent per hour of sleep, was 7.6±16.2. The mean O_2-80-I of the females was 10.5±23.8, but it did not differ significantly from that of the males (7.3±15.5).

Body Mass Index (BMI)

The mean BMI (Khosla and Lowe, 1967) of the total population was 31.0±6.0 kg/m^2. The mean BMI among men was 30.5±5.5 kg/m^2, range 19.8-57.5. (Normative data in the USA for men aged 40-65 years show 26.7 percent having a BMI >27.8) (Health United States, 1985). The mean BMI among women was 36.4±7.6. (Normative data in the USA for women aged 40-65 years show 29.8 percent having a BMI >27.3) (Health United States, 1985). The difference between the male and the female group is statistically significant ($p < 0.014$).

Risk ratio for RDI and abnormal oxygen indices

Considering the findings obtained, we tried to appreciate the risk ratio (RR) for an elevated RDI, taking into account the cephalometric results. To perform this analysis, two cephalometric variables were selected, as they were significantly different to a great degree from control population MP-H, as defined by bone structure, and PAS, as delineated by soft tissue. SNB and SNBa angles indicative of a retroposition of the mandible and of an acute cranial base flexure were also considered.

The median RDI of our patient population was 47. We divided the patients into those with RDI ≤40 and those with RDI >40. Patients with RDI >40 included about two-thirds of the patient population--a very sizable group; on the other hand, when similar analysis was performed on patients with RDI cutpoint of 20, the low number of patients with RDI ≤20 clearly weakened the strength of the findings. As RDI could be influenced by BMI, we decided to adjust our analysis in relation to BMI, i.e., we considered subjects who were slim, moderately obese, or obese, and considered the risk that a high or low RDI would be noted with a smaller or greater cranio-facial anomaly. The RR for RDI, considering an SNB angle ≤78 percent (i.e., mandibular retroposition) was nonsignificant, independent of the BMI and independent of the RDI group considered (i.e., with RDI >40, <40, >20). Similarly, when NSBa angle was considered and when statistical analysis was performed on the total patient group appreciating the RR for an abnormally acute cranial base flexure in the development of elevated RDI, there was a nonsignificant trend. When the total patient population was analyzed and the BMI taken into consideration, with the patient population subdivided based on BMI, the "thin" group defined by a BMI ≤28 demonstrated near-significant results with Pearson Chi square = 4.12 ($p = 0.04$), i.e., the chance of having a higher RDI in the slim patient group was higher with an abnormal cranial base flexure. When analyses were performed considering MP-H and PAS distance expressed in millimeters, it appears that RR for high RDI was in part a function of the cephalometric abnormalities. After adjustment for BMI, when the MP-H distance was >24.4 mm, i.e., above (mean +2SD) from controls, the RR was 3.5 if RDI was >40 (95 percent confidence limit [CL] = 1.8-7.3], it was 2.4 (95 percent CL = 1.2-5.3) if the analyzed patient group had an RDI >20. (There were a small number of patients with low RDI.) Similarly, when PAS was considered, RR was 2.9 when PAS $\leq$5 mm (95 percent CL = 1.2-5.3) if RDI was >40.

When we considered O_2-80-I, RR ratios were not significantly increased with cephalometric variables.

Multiple regression analyses and statistical models

Two other statistical analyses were performed on the data obtained. After a varimax rotation, statistical analysis using rotated factor loadings and considering 16 variables, including polygraphic sleep variables (total sleep time, stage 1 and 2, etc.), oxygen desaturation, age, BMI, RDI, and cephalometric variables indicated that three dominant factors were present: (1) oxygen saturation drop factor, (2) sleep disturbance factor, and (3) MP-H and PAS cephalometric abnormalities. A stepwise multiple regression analysis and a linear multiple regression analysis were also performed to try to appreciate if a statistical model could be determined from the collected variables, with RDI as the dependent variable. And a similar exercise was also performed with O_2-80-I as the dependent variable. The analysis of covariance, with RDI as dependent variable, indicated two significant independent variables: BMI ($p < 0.001$) and MP-H distance in millimeters ($p = 0.0058$). In the multiple linear regression analysis, the percentage of Stage 1 NREM sleep ($F = 115.9$), the logarithmic transformation of BMI (kurtosis >2) ($F = 20.7$, $p < 0.001$), age and the logarithmic transformation of PAS ($F = 7.2$) were the significant variables which gave the following model: RDI = 72.5 + 0.855 S1 + 36.8 ln (BMI) + 0.49 age - 8.29 Ln (PAS). The R^2 of this model is 0.68, i.e., it explains 68 percent of the variance. Undoubtedly, the sleep disturbance indicated by the percentage of stage 1 NREM sleep is a dominant element, but PAS is in the model.

When O_2-80-I was the dependent variable, two independent variables, BMI and cranial base flexure (NSBa angle) reached significance. But the model was poor, as it explained only 19 percent of the variance. It thus appears that abnormal cephalometric measurements play a role in the definition of RDI. Compared with other variables, their importance seems to be much more limited in the definition of important, i.e., below 80 percent, oxygen saturation drops during sleep. It is obvious from the study performed on our population that obesity, indicated by BMI, is an important factor in the definition of RDI and O_2-80-I. This population is overweight. Based on epidemiological data, one expects 26.7 percent of the U.S. male population aged 40-65 years to have a BMI >27.8 (Health United States, 1985). We found that more than 50 percent of our population had a BMI >29 kg/m^2 (median 29.7). It is also clear that the factors controlling RDI and O_2-80-I are different; and BMI seems to participate differently in the respective definition of RDI and O_2-80-I: Specific analyses of the interaction between cephalometric measurements--more particularly MP-H and PAS--with BMI indicate that the risk of having a high RDI and O_2-80-I increase with BMI, but only up to a point. It seems that there is an interaction between BMI and cephalometric abnormalities, and even if it does not reach significance, it is important to note that patients with long MP-H distance (31 mm) and low to moderate BMI can have high O_2-80-I. On the other hand, it is exceptional (three patients only) to find a long MP-H distance (>26 mm) and significant obesity (BMI >38).

COMMENTS

Our patients can be subdivided into two different sub-populations. Population A has significant cranio-mandibular abnormalities with long MP-H distance and rarely reaches massive obesity before presenting with OSAS. Population B, by contrast, has fewer bony anatomical abnormalities and, as such, is "allowed" to become obese and to develop much more soft tissue fatty infiltration, as indicated by the small PAS measurement, before showing symptoms of OSAS. An inverse correlation exists between BMI and SNB; and BMI and NSBa. Patients will often combine, to a varying degree, increased BMI and abnormal cranio-mandibular findings; but considering risks and treatment issues, it appears of interest to dissociate the elements involved in the development of OSAS. 2) These two populations have different "risks": massively obese patients have, in general, greater TST and less nocturnal sleep disruption (less stage 1 sleep). The other population has a higher RDI. Not surprisingly, higher RDI is correlated with sleep disturbance factors, i.e., decrease in TST, increase in stage 1 NREM sleep, decrease in stages 3-4 NREM sleep, and decrease in REM sleep. At the extreme, these two populations have discrete disorders, and should not be mixed when physiopathogeny or therapeutic trials are considered. Even after weight loss, patients with long MP-H will still run the risk of OSAS when they have a high RDI. Patients with short MP-H distance may improve quickly with weight loss and may not need significant upper airway surgery. It is important to measure all cephalometric variables, as PAS obviously results from several factors, including fatty infiltration and cranio-mandibular abnormality.

If one considers the relationship between RDI and cephalometric measurements, the MP-H distance appears to be the most crucial. Wickwire et al. (1972), investigating the effects of experimental mandibular osteotomy on tongue position, have demonstrated that posterior displacement of the mandible has an immediate impact on the placement of the tongue and hyoid bone. Hyoid bone location results from the combined changes affecting mandible and cranial base flexure. The relative position of these bones impacts on muscle position and on oropharyngeal soft tissues, and thus determines not only location of the hyoid bone but also width of the PAS. In our statistical model, if only one anatomical variable such as SNB is considered, the degree of abnormality compared with the mean normalcy may not be sufficient to reach significance. But the association of two independent anatomical abnormalities impacting on the position of the hyoid bone and the MP-H distance results in MP-H being the only variable significantly associated with an elevated RDI.

CONCLUSION

In conclusion, our report covers the largest OSAS patient population on which multivariate analyses have been performed. It is undoubtedly a fair representation of our sleep clinic population. It indicates that weight increase above ideal body weight, a long-suspected factor, favors OSAS, but it also emphasizes the importance of cranio-facial abnormalities in OSAS. It is possible that the position of certain cranio-facial bones and their respective relationship is a significant element in the development of partial or complete obstructive apneas during sleep. In subjects with a BMI <28, weight was found to be nonsignificant for RDI definition. The degree of cranio-facial abnormality was more marked in women than in men. Women are also known to develop OSAS much less frequently than men. Our data would indicate that in order to present symptoms, women need to exhibit cranio-facial abnormality and obesity to a much greater degree than is found in men.

RESUME

157 malades avec apnées obstructives lors du sommeil vus en succession pendant 6 mois, dans une consultation d'affections liées au sommeil, ont été soumis à un protocol experimental. Céphalogrammes et enregistrements nocturnes ont été systématiquement obtenus. Tout sujet présentant un nombre d'apnées de 10 par heure de sommeil nocturne au minimum et agé de plus de 17 ans a été accepté dans l'étude. Age, degré d'obésite (poids x 10.000/taille^2), resultats polygraphiques (y compris SaO$_2$) ont été statistiquement analysés. Les malades avec apnées obstructives liées au sommeil présentent des anomalies cranio-mandibulaires. Les distances plan mandibulaire - os hyoide, espace posterieur aerien (EPA) (derrière la base de la langue), et l'angle nasion-selle turcique-basion sont souvent anormaux. Les analyses et models statistiques indiquent que le nombre d'apnées par heure de sommeil va dépendre en partie de ces anomalies, par contre elles ont moins d'importances sur la fréquence de désaturation au dessous de 80%. Un malade avec une obésite massive présente moins d'anomalies cranio-faciales, moins de perturbation de sommeil, et un temps de sommeil nocturne plus long, qu'un malade avec un taux élevé d'apnées mais non ou peu obèse. Les anomalies cranio-faciales consistent en une anomalie de la base du crane, un retrait de la mandibule, un plan mandibulaire qui forme un angle plus obtus que normalement avec la branche montante, une position basse de l'os hyoide par rapport au plan mandibulaire, et un E P A étroit. La détection de ces anomalies va permettre de guider les traitements chirurgicaux dont certains sont vouées à l'échec si l'analyse des anomalies anatomiques est mal faite.

ACKNOWLEDGMENTS

Supported by General Clinical Research Grant 00070 funded by the National Institutes of Health.

Dr. Partinen is a Fellow from Helsinki University School of Medicine and is supported by US Public Health Service International Research Fellowship 1 FO 5TW03648-01.

We would like to thank Boyd Hayes and David Cobasco for their technical help and Alison Grant for her editorial assistance.

REFERENCES

Burstone, C.J., James, R.B., Legan, H., Murphy, G.A., Norton, L.A.(1978): Cephalometrics for orthognathic surgery. J. Oral Surg. 36, 269.
Dixon, W.J., Brown, M.B., Engelman, L., Frame, J.W., Jennrich, R.I., Toporek, J.D.(1985): BMOP Statistical Software. Los Angeles: University of California Press.
Guilleminault, C., Cummiskey, J., Motta, J.(1980): Chronic obstructive airflow disease and sleep studies. Am. Rev. Respir. Dis. 122, 397-406.
Health United States (1985). Hyattsville, MD: U.S. Department of Health and Human Services, National Center for Health Statistics.
Jamieson, A., Guilleminault, C., Partinen, M., Quera-Salva, MA.(1986): Obstructive sleep apneic patients have cranio-mandibular abnormalities. Sleep 10 (in Press).
Khosla, T., Lowe, F.R.(1967): Indices of obesity derived from body weight and height. Brit. J. Prev. Soc. M. 21, 122-128.

Khouw, F.E., Proffit, W.R., White, R.P.(1970): Cephalometric evaluation of patients with dento-facial dysharmonies requiring surgical correction. Oral Surg. 42, 179.

MacIntosh, R.B.(1970): Orthodontic surgery: comments on diagnostic modalities. J. Oral Surg. 28, 249-259.

Popovich, F., Thompson, G.W.(1977): Craniofacial templates for orthodontic case analysis. Am. J. Orthod. 71, 406-420.

Rechtschaffen, A., Kales, A., eds.(1968): A Manual of Standardized Terminology, Techniques and Scoring System for Sleep Stages of Human Subjects. Los Angeles: Brain Information Service/Brain Research Institute.

Ricketts, R.M.(1961): Cephalometric analysis and synthesis. Angle Orthod. 31, 141-146.

Ricketts, R.M.(1972): The value of cephalometrics and computerized technology. Angle Orthod. 42, 179.

Riley, R., Guilleminault, C., Herran, J., Powell, N.(1983): Cephalometric analyses and flow volume loops in obstructive sleep apnea patients. Sleep 6, 304-317.

Steiner, C.C.(1959): Cephalometrics in clinical practice. Angle Orthod. 29, 18-29.

Steiner, C.C.(1962): Cephalometrics as a clinical tool. In: Vistas in Orthodontics, ed B.S.Kraus, R.A. Reidel. Philadelphia, PA: Lea and Febiger.

Tweed, C.H.(1946): The Frankfort-mandibular plane angle in orthodontic diagnosis, classification, treatment planning, and prognosis. Am. J. Orthod. Oral. Surg. 32, 175-230.

Wickwire, N.A., White, R.P., Proffit, W.R.(1972): The effect of mandibular osteotomy on tongue position. Oral Surg. 30, 184-190.

Maxillo-mandibular surgery as a treatment for obstructive sleep apnea

Christian Guilleminault, Maria Antonia Quera-Salva, Nelson B. Powell and Robert W. Riley

Stanford University School of Medicine and Head-Neck Surgery, Palo Alto, California, USA

SUMMARY

Eighteen patients with obstructive sleep apnea syndrome (OSAS) underwent maxillo-mandibular surgery. A complete control of their OSAS was noted at 6 months' follow-up recording and interview.

KEY WORDS

Obstructive sleep apnea, surgery, maxillo-mandibular, cephalometry

INTRODUCTION

Surgical approaches to obstructive sleep apnea syndrome (OSAS) have been the first means of controlling the disabling sleepiness that impairs the well-being and, at times, the life of patients. Kulho et al. (1969) are credited with performing the first tracheostomy with the intention of bypassing an obstruction that occurred during sleep in the upper airway of a very obese patient. Since then, surgical approaches have been considered as a valid treatment of OSAS. Fujita et al. (1981) initiated uvulo-palato-pharyngoplasty (UPPP) in OSAS patients sent for tracheostomy. Reviews of long-term results using nocturnal polygraphic recordings indicated successful results in about 45% of patients undergoing this procedure (Zorick et al., 1983). Investigations of the causes of failures of UPPP lead to better presurgical investigations of the subtle and often multiple anatomical upper airway abnormalities presented by OSAS patients. Jamieson et al. (1986), after reviewing 155 consecutively seen cases, concluded that 150 had at least two anatomical cranio-facial landmarks significantly different from the norms. Most commonly, their patients had a normally positioned maxilla, a retroposition of the mandible, a steep mandibular plane, a different cranial base flexure with a nasion-sella-basion angle smaller than expected, a displacement of the hyoid bone to a lower position than expected, and a significant increase in the length of the soft palate. Rojewski et al. (1984), using video-endoscopy, had already mentioned that OSAS patients presented a "disproportionate anatomy," consisting of a large base of tongue, large soft palate, shallow palatal arch, narrow mandibular arch and mandibular deficiency, and Rivlin et al. (1984) had also emphasized the overall displacement of the mandibular symphysis.

The presence of these displacements easily explained the known abnormalities of the soft tissue of the upper airway. The presence of the different levels of obstruction during sleep explained the frequent failures of UPPP in the treatment of OSAS, as only one site of obstruction may be eliminated by this surgery. Sullivan et al. (1981) proposed the use of nasal continuous positive airway pressure (CPAP) during sleep as a home treatment of OSAS. This therapeutic approach has been shown to be successful in controlling the symptoms of many OSAS patients. And several types of CPAP equipment have been offered commercially on the world market. However, several follow-up studies have indicated that compliance with this therapeutic approach was a problem; and the largest and most recent study by Nino-Murcia et al. (1987), covering 144 OSAS patients followed for a mean of five months, reconfirm these findings. From these studies on the long-term use of nasal CPAP, it appears that between 25 and 30% of patients are non-compliant for various reasons, including nocturnal rhinitis and the inconvenience of being attached, on a nightly basis, and for many years, to a machine. These difficulties lead us to investigate new upper airway surgical procedures that would be better accepted than tracheostomy, that would be aimed at correcting the abnormal anatomy noted in OSAS, and that would allow freedom from a machine during sleep.

Surgical procedure

Maxillo-mandibular and hyoid advancement is planned in two steps, with steps 1 and 2 usually performed at a 6-month interval. Step 1 consists of a combined UPPP and inferior sagittal osteotomy of the mandible, which consists of a limited osteotomy involving the genio tubercle--the anterior point of insertion of the tongue muscles; (2) a section through a submental incision of sternohyoid, stylohyoid, and omo-hyoid muscles; and (3) the suspension of the hyoid bone to the mandible, anteriorly and superiorly with fascia.

After orthodontic preparation during the interval, phase 2 consists of a maxillo-mandibular osteotomy (i.e., Lefort one osteotomy and sagittal split mandibular osteotomy), associated with a liposuction of the neck, if needed. Step 2 was initially performed under the protection of a transient tracheotomy kept in place for 3-4 weeks. Recently, for the last 25 patients submitted to this procedure (and not presented in the study due to the short follow-up period), nasal CPAP has been used immediately post-extubation, avoiding the need for tracheostomy (Powell et al., 1982).

Pre-requirements for surgical selection

The usual contraindications to non-emergency surgery related to significant medical and psychiatric problems are present.

All patients were requested to undergo polygraphic evaluation during sleep six to eight months post last upper airway surgical procedure. All patients treated consecutively during a nine-month period and who returned for follow-up are presented here.

Patient population consisted of 18 patients, 16 men and 2 women. Their mean age was 41 $\pm$ 13.5 years, range 18 to 63. Their mean BMI was 31 $\pm$ 7.4, range 19 to 41.5, again indicating a mixture of patients from the clearly underweight to the morbidly obese. The mean BMI, however, points to an overall overweight population.

METHOD OF STUDY

Each subject had (1) nocturnal polygraphic recording pre- and 6 months postsurgery, (2) evaluation of subjective symptoms pre- and postsurgery, (3) presurgical cephalometric roentgenograms and fiberopticscope evaluation, and (4) evaluation of complications during and post surgery. Four patients also had an initial trial with nasal CPAP treatment with polygraphic recording during sleep before any surgery. Comparison was made between nasal CPAP and surgical results in these cases.

Polygraphic recordings and definition of breathing abnormalities

The variables monitored during nocturnal polygraphic recording were electroencephalogram, electro-oculogram, chin electromyogram, and electrocardiogram (modified V2 lead). Respiration was monitored by uncalibrated inductive respiratory plethysmography; airflow was monitored by thermistors, and oxygen saturation by ear oximetry (Biox). Apnea, hypopnea and sleep stages were scored according to standard definitions based upon findings obtained from respiratory, airflow, oximetric and other channels. Hypopnea was defined as (a) a 50% reduction in maximal thermistor output compared with baseline and (b) association with a decrease of oxygen saturation (SaO_2) to below 92% from baseline of at least 94%, or a drop in SaO_2 of at least 3% if baseline was below 90%. The RDI or (apnea + hypopnea) x 60/total sleep time (TST) which takes into account the number of abnormal breathing events per hour of sleep was calculated.

Definition of SaO2 indices

Several indices of SaO_2 were calculated: the lowest SaO_2 during the night, the mean nocturnal SaO_2 (X SaO_2), the percentage of time during sleep spent with an SaO_2 <90% (% T<90% SaO_2), and an arbitrarily defined SaO_2 index called Oxygen-80-Index or O2-80-I. The mean nocturnal SaO_2 was calculated using the formula of Bradley et al. (1985): The highest and lowest SaO_2 of each polygraphically recorded "epoch" were measured. Because the pattern of desaturation and resaturation in OSA approximates a sine wave, the mean SaO_2 of each polygraphic epoch, i.e., 30 s, was estimated by averaging the high and low values. Mean nocturnal SaO_2 for TST was then calculated using the mean values of all epochs. To further focus on events leading to significant O2 desaturation, even if short-lived, we calculated the number of SaO_2 drops related to apnea and hypopnea $\leq$80% and, as with the RDI, calculated the number of SaO_2 drops per hour of sleep (O2-80-I). The time spent during nocturnal sleep at a SaO_2 below 90% is self-explanatory.

Indices of sleep disturbance

Several measurements of sleep disturbances have been advocated. Using Rechtschaffen and Kales' criteria (1968), sleep is scored in 30-s epochs. We decided to perform statistical analyses on the percentage of Stages 1 and 3-4 NREM sleep and REM sleep during total nocturnal sleep time. This choice is directed by the numerous publications indicating an increase in Stage 1 and disappearance of Stage 3-4 NREM sleep with repetitive sleep apneas.

Cephalometric roentgenograms

Lateral cephalometric roentgenograms were obtained with the Werner Cephalostat, using the technique reported by Riley et al. (1983). Tracings of the roentgenograms were made on an acetate sheet and the following angles in degrees, or dimensions measured in millimeters, were selected for further analyses:

SNA: angle measurement from sella (S) to nasion (N) to subspinale (deepest point--point A--on the premaxillary contour between the anterior nasal spine and the central incisor).

SNB: angle measurement from sella (S) to nasion (N) to supramentale (deepest point--point B--on the outer mandibular contour between the mandibular incisor and the pogonion. SNA and SNB (in degrees) give information on maxillary and mandibular position as it relates to cranial base.

MP-H: distance from mandibular plane to hyoid bone (in mm).

PNS (posterior nasal spine) to (P) tip of soft palate indicates (in mm) length of soft palate.

PAS: posterior airway space (in mm) defined as the space behind the base of tongue.

The information obtained was supplemented by a visual inspection of the region by fiberoptic scoping performed on a supine patient. The reference normative cephalometric measurements were those published in textbooks, referenced articles on cephalometric landmarks (Burstone et al., 1978; Khouw et al., 1970; MacIntosh, 1970; Popovich and Thompson, 1977; Tweed, 1946; Ricketts, 1961,1972; Steiner, 1959, 1962), and confirmed on our own control population (Jamieson et al, 1986).

The BMI was calculated by the method of Khosla and Lowe (1967) (weight x 10,000/height squared).

Statistical analysis

Pearson coefficient correlation was performed as an exploratory test. A Bartlett test for homogenity of variance was calculated and, depending on results ($p<0.05$), matched pair t test or Wilcoxon signed ranks test was performed.

RESULTS

Presurgery

Complaints and symptoms

All patients complained of severe, excessive daytime sleepiness and severe loud snoring at night. Frequent apneas had been noted by a spouse in all cases. In addition, 86% complained of frequent nocturnal disrupted sleep with awakenings; 46% had violent, abnormal movements during sleep; 69% had nocturia, and 71% reported heavy sweating at night; 46% had frequent headaches on awakening; 38.5% had daily morning confusion, 61.5% sleep-talked, 15.4% sleepwalked; 15.4% presented with frequent nocturnal enuresis, and 7.7% had recurrent night terrors; 20% complained of hearing loss; 40% of the population was treated pharmacologically for hypertension.

Cephalometric findings

Mean SNA = 78.1 ± 2.7 degrees, range 72-82; mean SNB = 73.7 ± 3.2 degrees, range 67-80, mean MP-H distance = 29 ± 6.4 mm, range 17-41, mean PNS-P distance = 42.6 ± 5.5 mm, range 35-52, mean PAS distance = 3.4 ± 1.2 mm, range 1.5-5.

Nocturnal polygraphy

(See Table 1) A significant sleep disturbance was seen with a very elevated percentage of Stage 1 NREM sleep, a significant decrease in percentage of Stage 3-4, and an important reduction in percentage of REM sleep. The RDI was always elevated, with lowest oxygen saturation always during REM sleep. SaO2 was seen below 80% in all patients at least once during the night. Sinus arrest in association with sleep apnea and lasting between 3 and 5 seconds was seen at least once in 3 patients. Premature ventricular complexes (PVCs) were seen at a rhythm of 1 to 2 per minute during sleep in 5 subjects. One subject had one episode of atrio-ventricular block (Mobitz type II) in association with apnea. All subjects presented the classic brady-tachyarrhythmia seen with sleep apnea.

Table 1. Maxillo-mandibular hyoid advancement: pre- and 6 months postsurgical results.

Variable	Presurgery	Postsurgery	Statistical
	X ± SD	X ± SD	significance
TST (min)	406 ± 48	397 ± 67	NS +
S1 (%)	40 ± 22.1	21 ± 13.8	p<0.002 +
S3-4 (%)	2.7 ± 3.7	7.1 ± 9.9	p<0.04 ++
REM sleep (%)	9.9 ± 3.3	13.8 ± 6.7	p<0.01 ++
Lowest O2 (%)	64.3 ± 16.5	86.5 ± 4.9	p<0.0001 ++
X SaO2 (%)	91.1 ± 3.7	94.9 ± 0.1	p<0.0001 ++
T<90% SaO2 (%)	14.5 ± 11.0	0.2 ± 0.4	p<0.0001 ++
O2-80-I	19.5 ± 24.6	0.0 0.0	p<0.007 ++
RDI	65.5 ± 20.1	8.5 ± 5.6	p<0.0001 ++

+   matched pair t test
++ Wilcoxon signed ranks test
NS nonsignificant
Other abbreviations in text

Postsurgical evaluation

Subjective report

Six months following the last surgical procedure, BMI was not significantly different from presurgery measurement, even if immediately following surgery some patients had lost weight. Subjectively, all subjects reported significant improvement of their daytime alertness, a greater energy, an appropriate handling of their daily chores, a disappearance of the frequent morning headaches, a change in mood, an impression of being "sharper," with "better memory," disappearance of snoring, abnormal movements and restless sleep. Three subjects presented some PVCs during sleep, but well below the rate of 1 to 2 per minute of the presurgery nocturnal period. The two other PVC-positive subjects had less than 50 PVCs during total sleep time. No other cardiac arrhythmias were seen.

Polygraphic variables

Polygraphic recording results are indicated in Table 1. Statistically, with the exception of a mildly decreased TST--a nonsignificant result--all other variables were highly significantly different, and the raw numbers indicated very large differences: the mean RDI was 8.5 with a range from 2 to 20. All SaO2 indices indicated a good maintenance of SaO2 (see Table 1). Presurgery, Pearson coefficient correlation had indicated significant correlation between mean SaO2 and O2-80-I (0.55), mean SaO2 and % T <90% SaO2 (0.96), O2-80-I and % T<90% SaO2 (0.87). These correlations were again found postsurgery: mean SaO2 and % T<90 SaO2 (0.54), mean SaO2 and % T<90% SaO2 (0.54), O2-80-I and % T<90% SaO2 (0.73). The postsurgical correlation coefficient between RDI and BMI was 0.46, indicating that the few persistent apneas during sleep were still seen in the most overweight patients, i.e., those with a BMI >38 (morbid obesity). Postsurgery elevated percentage of Stage 1 NREM sleep--an index of some sleep disturbance--correlated also with RDI (0.54). But the mean percentage of Stage 1 NREM sleep was highly improved statistically, compared with presurgery.

Complications of the procedure

The potential complications are not only those reported for inferior sagittal osteotomy and hyoid myotomy, but also some more specifically related to phase 2 of the procedure, and particularly the possible damage of the inferior alveloar nerve during its difficult dissection. Paradoxically, the maxillo-mandibular hyoid advancement, i.e., part 2 of the surgery, leads to less complaints of pain and significant discomfort than when UPPP is performed. Partial facial sensory paresthesia was noted up to 6 months postsurgery in 5 patients.

COMMENTS

Maxillo-mandibular-hyoid advancement gave overall very good results at 6 months' follow-up. In the 4 patients who were also treated with nasal CPAP initially but who preferred surgery as a long-term treatment, we found that very similar positive results were obtained with both procedures. It must be emphasized that if morbid obesity was seen in our maxillo-mandibular treated population (one patient weighed 185 kg at time of surgery), none had major lung disease and none was a significant CO_2 retainer, with CO_2 tension always below 44 torr during wake, seated. Maxillo-mandibular-hyoid treatment in our 18 patients was 100% successful. We know that on a short-term basis, i.e., without a 6- to 9 months' follow-up yet, or having been completed after the data analysis for this report, this 100% success has not been maintained in the following 22 subjects, as one patient of the next 22 has been a failure. However, this failure could have been avoided if the criteria to refuse this surgery to patients with significant blood gas derangement and heavy chronic alcoholism had been respected. Overall, the results seen at 6 to 9 months postsurgery are the best obtained by far with any surgical procedure, other than tracheostomy performed in our clinic over the past 10 years. This procedure does not involve the long-term problems associated with tracheostomy. However, maxillo-mandibular advancement is a procedure which requires a solid combined expertise in maxillo-facial and oto-laryngologic surgical techniques and a good presurgical analysis of the existing anatomical abnormalities.

The good results at 6 months' follow-up are also of much theoretical interest, as they clearly demonstrate that acting upon only anatomical factors located in the upper airway can completely control a severe sleep apnea syndrome, even with maintenance of significant obesity in non-CO2 retainer OSAS patients.

REFERENCES

Bradley, T.D., Martinez, D., Rutherford, R., Lue, F., Grossman, R.F., Moldofsky, H., Zamel, N., Phillipson, E.A.(1985): Physiological determinants of nocturnal arterial oxygenation in patients with obstructive sleep apnea. J. Appl. Physiol. 59, 1364-1368.

Burstone, C.J., James, R.B., Legan, H., Murphy, G.A., Norton, L.A.(1978): Cephalometrics for orthognathic surgery. J. Oral Surg. 36, 269.

Fujita, S., Conway, W., Zorick, F., Roth, T.(1981): Surgical correction of anatomic abnormalities of obstructive sleep apnea syndrome: uvulopalatopharyngoplasty. Otolaryngol. Head Neck Surg. 89, 923-934.

Jamieson, A., Guilleminault, C., Partinen, M., Quera-Salva, M.A.(1986): Obstructive sleep apneic patients have cranio-mandibular abnormalities. Sleep 9, 469-472.

Khosla, T., Lowe, F.R.(1967): Indices of obesity derived from body weight and height. Br. J. Prev. Soc. Med. 21, 122-128.

Khouw, F.E., Proffit, W.R., White, R.P.(1970): Cephalometric evaluation of patients with dento-facial dysharmonies requiring surgical correction. Oral Surg. 29, 789.

Kuhlo, W., Doll, E., Franck, M.D.(1969): Erfolgreiche behandlung eines Pickwick-syndroms durch eine dauertrachealkanule. Dtsch. Med. Wochenschr. 94, 1286-1290.

MacIntosh, R.B.(1970): Orthodontic surgery: comments on diagnostic modalities. J. Oral Surg. 28, 249-259.

Nino-Murcia, G., Crowe, C., Bliwise, D., Guilleminault, C., Dement, W.C.(1987): Sleep Res. 16, 398 (abstract).

Popovich, F., Thompson, G.W.(1977): Craniofacial templates for orthodontic case analysis. Am. J. Orthod. 71, 406-420.

Powell, N., Riley, R., Guilleminault, C.(1987): Upper airway surgery and obstructive sleep apnea: an indication for nasal CPAP. 22nd Annual Meeting of the S.E.P.C.R., proceedings and abstracts. Antwerp, June 22-26, 1987. Also Bull. Eur. Pathophysiol. Resp. (abstract), in press.

Rechtschaffen, A., Kales, A.(1968): A Manual of Standardized Terminology, Techniques and Scoring System for Sleep Stages of Human Subjects. Brain Information Service/Brain Research Institute, University of California, Los Angeles.

Ricketts, R.M.(1961): Cephalometric analysis and synthesis. Angle Orthod. 31, 141-156.

Ricketts, R.M.(1972): The value of cephalometrics and computerized technology. Angle Orthod. 42, 179.

Riley, R.W., Guilleminault, C., Herran, J., Powell, N.B.(1983): Cephalometric analysis and flow loops in obstructive sleep apnea patients. Sleep 6, 303-311.

Rivlin, J., Hoffstein, V., Kalbfleisch, J., McNicholas, W., Zamel, N., Bryan, C.(1984): Upper airway morphology in patients with idiopathic obstructive sleep apnea. Am. Rev. Respir. Dis. 129, 355-360.

Rojewski, T.E., Schuller, D.E., Clarke, R.W., Schmidt, H.S., Potts, R.E. (1984): Video-endoscopic determination of the mechanisms of obstruction in obstructive sleep apnea. Otolaryngol. Head-Neck Surg. 92, 127-131.

Steiner, C.C.(1959): Cephalometrics in clinical practice. Angle Orthod. 29, 18-29.

Steiner, C.C.(1962): Cephalometrics as a clinical tool. In Vistas in Orthodontics, eds B.S. Kraus, R.A. Reidel. Philadelphia: Lea and Febiger.

Sullivan, C.E., Berthon-Jones, M., Issa, F.G., Eves, L.(1981): Reversal of obstructive sleep apnoea by continuous positive airway pressure applied through the nares. Lancet 1, 862-865.

Tweed, C.H.(1946): The Frankfort-mandibular plane angle in orthodontic diagnosis, classification, treatment planning, and prognosis. Am. J.

Orthod. Oral Surg., 32 175-230.
Zorick, F., Roehrs, T., Conway, W., Fujita, S., Wittig, R., Roth, T.(1983): Effects of uvulopalatopharyngoplasty on the daytime sleepiness associated with sleep apnea syndrome. Bull. Eur. Pathophysiol. Resp. 19, 600-603.

Multidisciplinary approach to the diagnosis and treatment of snoring and obstructive sleep apnea

J.M. Triglia*, F. Philip-Joet**, M. Rey***, M. Cannoni* and A. Pech*

*Clinique ORL, CHU Timone, Marseille, France
**Service de Pneumologie, Hôpital Nord, Marseille, France
***Service d'Explorations Fonctionnelles du système nerveux central, Hôpital Nord, Marseille, France

RESUME

Les symptômes qui traduisent une obstruction des voies aériennes supérieures posent le problème de leur reconnaissance, le ronflement étant la manifestation la plus évidente, et de leur traitement, celui-ci devant s'appuyer sur des critères de sélection des patients et sur des critères d'appréciation de son efficacité, tant ceux-ci sont différents d'un sujet à l'autre en raison de la variabilité de l'organisation du sommeil.

Si le ronflement peut être considéré comme une simple gêne sociale, il peut être aussi le premier symptôme d'une authentique affection médicale, soit latente et découverte par les explorations polygraphiques, soit accompagnée d'un cortège de signes cliniques que l'on doit savoir rechercher.

Les auteurs insistent sur l'approche multi-disciplinaire de cette pathologie (O.R.L., pneumo-cardiologues, électrophysiologistes du sommeil). Ils sont favorables à la pratique systématique d'un enregistrement de la saturation de l'hémoglobine en oxygène sur une nuit qui permet de séparer efficacement différents groupes de ronfleurs et de leur proposer soit une chirurgie de confort (ronfleurs socialement gênants) soit une chirurgie de nécessité (ronfleurs apnéiques).

SUMMARY

The symptoms indicating an obstruction of the upper airways pose problems for recognition. Snoring is the most obvious sign. Treatment must include criteria for selection of patients as well as for an evaluation of its efficiency keeping in mind that they will differ from one patient to another given the variabilities in sleep patterns.

While snoring can be considered as a simple social problem, it can also be the first symptom of a real medical disorder, either latent or discovered by numerous clinical signs that ont must be able to recognize.

The authors wish to emphasize the multidisciplinary approach to this pathology (E.N.T., pneumo-cardiologist, sleep electro-physiologist). They are in favor of systematically carrying out a nocturnal Sa 02 recording which makes it possible to efficiently classify the different groups of snorers and thus propose them either elective surgery (socially-disturbing snorers) or necessary surgery (apneic snorers).

INTRODUCTION

The symptoms of upper airway obstruction raise 3 types of problems (9) :

- Their recognition with early diagnosis in order to avoid further complications due to chronic hypoxemia. Snoring, long a medical enigma, has thus become the most obvious manifestation of upper airway obstruction (6).

- Treatment includes making a good selection of patients in order to obtain the most favorable and permanent results. Selection criteria are based upon the results of a multidisciplinary meeting (E.N.T., pneumo-cardiologist, sleep electrophysiologist) (3, 7).

- The results are difficult to evaluate (5) as they differ from one subject to another due to the variability in sleep patterns.

The aim of this study is to emphasize the multidisciplinary approach to this pathology of upper airway obstruction which is the only way to select patients for a "personalized" therapy. The effects of uvulo-palato-pharyngoplasty were evaluated in terms of snoring, clinical signs of airway obstruction, and also sleep pattern.

MATERIAL AND METHODS

Between October 1985 and March 1987, we selected a pool of 107 patients, all of whom had come to our E.N.T. Clinic for problems of snoring.

At this time, half of these patients have undergone complete examinations and 34 (31.7 %) have been treated by uvulo-palato-pharyngoplasty :

* The patient and his family were submitted to a precise oral examination in order to note snoring characteristics as well as to define the existence of any other nocturnal signs or daytime sleepiness.

* The E.N.T. clinical examination, including a cephalometric roentgenogram, determines the amount of upper airway obstruction (2). For this, we have two classifications :

- First, anatomical (4) permitting a first selection of patients for uvulo-palato-pharyngoplasty :

. TYPE I   - Isolated oropharyngeal obstruction (normal hypopharynx)
. TYPE II   - Low palatal arch associated with an enlarged tongue
  Type IIa   - Larynx visualized with mirror
  Type IIb   - Larynx not visible.
. TYPE III   - Hypopharyngeal obstruction (hypertrophy at the base of the tongue) with normal oropharynx.

- The second classification, morphologically typical, of the oropharynx (1) subdivides approximately under 2 headings : Long thin palates, with an abnormally lower palatal arch, and secondly, thick heavy palates which are rich in fatty elements, generally congested, with numerous mucosal folds on the lateral pharyngeal walls.

* A cardio-pulmonary exam for complications due to chronic hypoxemia (arterial hypertension, arrhythmia, polyglobulia, etc...), and finally a general check-up to note obesity and endocrine problems.

* 53 patients were recorded for SaO2 (oxygen saturation) for 1 night (OHMEDA BIOX 3700). Only those with more than 10 desaturations (more than 4 %) (27 patients) were submitted to polysomnographic recording, hemoglobin saturation (Sa 02), electrocardiogram (EK6), electroencephalogram (EE6), electro-oculogram (EO6), electromyogram (EM6), nasal and oral airflow recording by thermister, and respiratory effort by strain gauge for 2 consecutive nights.

The results were analyzed hour by hour all night. The following criteria were taken into account : The number and duration of apneas with their type -central, mixed, or obstructive- ; the number and depth of saturations superior to 4 % as well as the peaks superior to 20 %, the average length of apnea and apnea index.

Three months after surgical treatment, patients were again monitered for 2 consecutive nights for comparison with the preoperative results.

* 34 patients underwent uvulo-palato-pharyngoplasty. Buccal intubation is carried out in order to determine with as much precision as possible the height of the palate to be resected, so as to avoid surgical sequelae such as velopharyngeal insufficiency. Using a blunt instrument, the soft palate is pushed against the posterior pharyngeal wall. This pusches out the section being resected for removal of the cellular-fatty tissue situated in the lowest part of the soft palate and, at the same time, conserving a maximum of pharyngo-palatal arch muscular tissue. We no longer infiltrate the tonsil and soft palate arches. Tonsillectomy is systemically performed along with half of the anterior pillar. Once the tonsillar fossa is located, resection is extended through the soft palate.

At this level, the most posterior pharyngo-staphyle muscle is conserved. A prolonged transfixion incision sectioning the uvula azygos muscle is made and care must be taken in the hemostasis of its artery. The incision is then continued toward the controlateral side, along with the tonsillectomy.

In the presence of very large lateral pharyngeal folds, causing redundant mucosa, we separate the mucosa from the muscle and, when necessary, section this lateral pharyngeal mucosa. The suspension of this lateral pharyngeal mucosa on the anterior pillar makes it possible to unpleat the pharynx and suturing is done with separate stitches using a slow absorbable thread.

RESULTS

Ages ranged from 16 to 66 years with a mean age of 45.5 years in the operated patients ; 75 % were males and 25 % were females.

Snoring was described as being very intense and always a social problem. In 38 % of the cases, it dated back many years, often to infancy. Other nocturnal signs were essentially represented by nightmares (20 %) and sudden awakening associated or not with fits of respiratory suffocation (47 %). Daytime symptoms included sleepiness (44 %), morning headache (41 %), and physical (35 %), psychic and intellectual (20 %) asthenia.

Arterial hypertension and polyglobulia were remarked in 26.5 % and 29.5 % respectively. Mean weight prior to the operation was 79.4 Kg with a range from 45 Kg to 120 Kg. Half of the patients were considered as obese or morbidly obese.

Anatomically, the oropharynx was rated as Type I in 42 % of the cases, Type IIa in 54 %, and Type IIb in 4 %. Morphologically, 40 % of the cases had long palates with a mean age of 32 years and a mean weight of 64 Kg ; 54 % of the cases had thick palates with a mean age of 52 years and a mean weight of 85 Kg.

Uvulo-palato-pharyngoplasty was proposed for 3 types of snorers :

1 - Asymptomatic snorers without apnea (14 patients) and whose SaO2 recording was completely normal.
2 - Asymptomatic snorers with sleep apnea as discovered by polysomnographic examinations (14 patients).
3 - Symptmatic snorers (6 patients) presenting clinical and biological symptoms of obstructive sleep apnea syndrome and in whom the polysomnographic exams only confirmed their existence and degree.

An analysis of these 20 polysomnographic tests produced the following data :

- 255 apneas per night (from 113 to 368) with a total duration of 1.5 hours (from 20 min. 45 sec. to 2 hr 20 mn), a mean duration of 17 sec (81 sec for the longest), and an apnea index of 44.8 apneas per hour.
- 26 peaks of Sa O2 superior to 20 % were remarked (from 0 to 80), the value of the lowest trough in relation to the base value was 29.8 % (from 8 % to 60 %) and the mean saturation value per night reached 10.3 % (from 5 % to 17.8 %).

U.P.P.P. surgical follow-ups were generally simple with a few cases of minior pain which were rapidly resolved. As for complications, we noted one case of long-term paresthesia and 2 cases of minimal velopharyngeal insufficiency which disappeared within 2 months.

DISCUSSION

Clinical

* Snoring can be strictly that. It is then merely a social problem and surgery may be performed for the comfort of the patient and his family. Of our 53 patients, 26 presented a normal Sa O2 and 14 decided to undergo U.P.P.P.

* Snoring can also be the first symptom of a real medical disorder. Two aspects must be considered :

- Relatively severe obstructive sleep apneas can exist in spite of rather insignificant symptoms. Sleep recordings reveal these apneas. We are in favor of systematically carrying out a nocturnal Sa O2 recording of any snorer who feels it necessary to come to the E.N.T. clinic. Out of our 53 patients tested, obstructive apneas were discovered in 20 and 14 decided to undergo U.P.P.P. In these cases we really encouraged the patient to have the operation and warned him of the possible risks if not operated (aggravation of sleep apneas and the appearance of cardio-pulmonary symptoms).

- Certain patients can present a multitude of clinical signs of upper airway obstruction that one should be able to remark (daytime sleepiness, abnormal nocturnal behavoir, arterial hypertension, polyglobulia...). In these cases, surgery is obsolutely indicated given the vital risks involved. Seven of our patients fell into this group and 6 of them agreed to undergo U.P.P.P.

Surgical

A good selection of patients is examined for possible U.P.P.P. contra-indication. Sooner than the standard profile radiography in both recumbent and standing positions, we prefer to practice cephalometric roentgenograms which allow for a more precise study of the cause of the symptoms, keeping in mind the ecistence of often ignored maxillo-facial problems, leading to the most effective therapy.

At present, apneic snorers are submitted to a scanner exam. While it makes it possible to analyze the pharynx stage by stage, it is sometimes difficult to define the role of the base of the tongue, the position of the mandibula and the hyoid bone.

Post-operative results

Uvulo-palato-pharyngoplasty is an excellent solution for the problem of socially disturbing snoring (70 % to 100 % improvement). As for patients with sleep apneas, the quality of the results is open to debate. Clinically, most of the patients claim to be greatly improved as witnessed by a reduction or disappearance of diurnal and nocturnal symptoms. It is for this reason that certain patients decide not to undergo a postoperative polysomnographic exam. Our preliminary results, however, suggest that the U.P.P.P. is efficient in 75 % of the cases of asymptomatic apneic snorers and in 60 % of the cases of symptomatic apneic snorers.

REFERENCES BIBLIOGRAPHIQUES

CHOUARD Ch. (1985) : La ronchopathie chronique ou ronflement. Aspects cliniques et indications thérapeutiques. Ann. Oto-Laryngol., 103, 319-327
DEJEAN Y. (1985) : Intérêt de l'examen O.R.L. dans le syndrome d'apnées au cours du sommeil. Traitement chirurgical et indications. Cahiers O.R.L., 10, 571-584
FUJITA S. (1981) : Surgical correction of anatomic abnormalities in obstructive sleep apnea syndrome : Uvulo-palato-pharyngoplasty. Otolaryngol. Head and Neck surg. 89, 923-934
FUJITA S. (1985) : Uvulo-palato-pharyngoplasty (U.P.P.P.) : A new surgical approach for treatment of obstructive sleep apnea. New dimensions in Otolaryngol. Head and neck surg., MYERS Ed., Vol. 1, Elsevier Science Publisher B.V. 193-196
FUJITA S. (1985) : Evaluation of the effectiveness of uvulo-palato-pharyngoplasty Laryngoscope, 95, 70-74
IKEMATSU T. (1985) : Clinical study of snoring for the past 30 years. New dimensions in Otolaryngol. Head and Neck Surg., MYERS Ed., Vol. 1, Elsevier Science Publishers B.V., 199-202
SIMMONS F.B. (1983) : Snoring and some obstructive sleep apnea can be cured by oropharyngeal surgery. Arch. Otolaryngol., 109, 503-507
RILEY R. (1985) : Palato-pharyngoplasty failure. Cephalometric roentgenograms and obstructive sleep apnea. Otolaryngol. Head and Neck Surg., 93, 240-244
TRIGLIA J.M. (1986) : Les apnées obstructives du sommeil chez l'adulte. Drugs and Diseases. Rapports du XIIIème congrès mondial d'O.R.L. John LIBBEY EUROTEXT Ed. Vol. 2, n° 1, 159-170

X TREATMENTS OF CHRONIC RHONCHOPATHY
Chairman: E. Lugaresi

Veloplastics in simple rhonchopathy

A.H. Morgon and F. Disant

ENT Department, Edouard Herriot Hospital, 3 place d'Arsonval, 69374 Lyon Cedex 08, France

The literature concerning soft-palate surgery for the treatment of rhonchopathy by uvulo-palato-pharyngoplasty mentions two types of possible post-operatory complications: passage of food through the nose, and nasality of voice.

A further sequel should be borne in mind: the modification of the voice subject to inadequacy of the soft palate.

This raises the following question: should a simple rhonchopathy without sleep-time apnea be thus treated at the expense of the soft palate, or should a surgical solution be sought which would reduce the symptom of snoring while preserving the functioning of the soft palate?

We are not putting uvulo-palato-pharyngoplasty in question as such, but ask whether this solution is always the right one, bearing in mind that it consists not so much in plasty as in an ectomy which alters the structure of the soft palate.

The muscles composing the soft palate fall into three groups. It is important to look at them not only from the point of view of mobility but also from that of the static state of the palate. They are arranged around the palatine aponevrosis, set in the horizontal apophyses of the palatine bones.

The inner and outer peristaphyline muscles are involved in the movement of raising the palate and also in tensing the palate in its functioning position: this is important during phonation and particularly in certain articulatory movements involved in passing from oralised to nasalised phonemes, where the palate does not revert to a full rest-position.

The pharyngo and glossostaphyline muscles involve the soft palate in two other muscle groups which operate in deglutition, phonation and respiration: these are the muscles of, on the one hand, the tongue, and, on the other, the pharynx.

Whether it be the anterior or posterior pillar muscle, the course needs to be considered, for it is in the form of an italic "S". Both of these muscles by contracting contribute to closure of palato-pharyngeal isthmus; but the glossostaphyline muscle tends to anteriorise the soft palate whereas the pharyngostaphyline muscle tends to posteriorise it.

Thus these two muscle groups situate the soft palate in a three force system : one vertical, drawing it upwards; one (glosso-staphyline) drawing it forwards; and one (pharyngostaphyline) drawing it backwards. These static components must absolutely be taken into account if surgery is to be functionally oriented.

Finally, there is the uvular azygos muscle group, which allows complete obstruction of the velopharynx during the contraction phase.

There is a criticism to be made about uvulo-palato-pharyngoplasty involving exeresis of the two soft palate ogives and affecting the anterior and posterior pillars. This exeresis cannot be performed without touching the crossed fibres, behind the palatine aponevrosis, of the two glosso and pharyngostaphyline muscles which are part of this crossover area and correspond to the fleshy, mobile and active part of the soft palate.

as in the aftermath of a badly performed tonsiplectomy, the soft palate becomes undully anteriorised : sectioning of the soft palate muscle groups abolishes the sphincter, the pharynx having become unable to play the role of sphincter alone.

In view of the anatomical and physiological data concerning the soft palate and of our long experience with congenital and acquired soft palate inadequacies in children, we have tried to strike a balande between two opposing attitudes : aiming for reduction of rhonchopathy and aiming to preserve the major functions of the soft palate.

OPERATORY PROCEDURE

- Placing of the Dott separator which replaces the intubation probe.

- A wire is pulled over the uvular mucosa.

- The wire is tensed towards the left : one centimetre incision along the right posterior pillar near where it joins the pharynx.

- Dissection of pharyngostaphyline muscle; resection after coagulation with bipolar lancet at tje upper and lower extremities of the resection.

- Likewise for the left pharyngostaphyline muscle.

- The wire is tensed in the median position so as to allow resection of the mucosa stretched by the wire; this resection is followed by dissection and resection of the azygos muscle.

- Suture of the wound left by uvula exeresis.

- Application of fibrine glue to the resection of the posterior pillar muscles.

RESULTS

For twenty six patients operated for simple snoring without sleep-time apnea, this technique :

- has never led to passage of food through the nose nor to any nasality;

- snoring ceased in six cases; it persisted, greatly reduced, in sixteen cases, but all patients were satisfied by the outcome :

- in four cases, snoring remaind unchanged;

- we shall not go into the possibility of performing this surgical operation jointly with sub-mucosal nasal resection or with tonsillectomy when the tonsils are too large.

Let us stop for a moment to consider a case such as that a youg woman who is a singing teacher : the operation abolished snoring without having any adverse effect on the voice.

From cases of congenital or acquired soft palate inadequacy, we know that persistant air-loss alters laryngeal functioning. The voice deepens. This is the begining of the cycle leading to the so-called functional lesions of the vocal cords.

It follows that snoring in those who use their voice professionally shoud be treated with great caution.

CONCLUSION

An operation which simply does away with the uvula and the immediately ajoining mucosa as well as the uvula azygos muscles and sections the posterior pillar muscle has the advantage of giving satisfactory results with respect to the symptom of snoring while preserving the functions of the soft palate : deglutition, respiration and above all phonation.

Such a procedure seems sufficient when the snoring is simple and not accompanied by sleep-time apnea.

RESUME

Le risque d'un geste chirurgical sur le voile du palais, comportant une résection importante des muscles, est de déterminer d'éventuelles séquelles soit à court terme, soit à long terme (trouble de la déglutition, rhinolabie).
En prenant en compte la physiologie du voile du palais et la disposition anatomique des muscles, en tenant compte aussi du mécanisme physio-pathologique du ronflement, il est possible de proposer un geste chirurgical qui, tout en respectant les grandes fonctions du voile du palais, permette la suppression du ronflement.

Chronic rhonchopathy. Ed. C.H. Chouard. © 1988, John Libbey Eurotext Ltd. pp.338-348.

Nocturnal respiratory obstruction and modified technique of uvulo-pharyngoplasty

Jacques Piché

Hôpital Sacré-Coeur et Cité de la Santé de Laval, 1435 boulevard St-Martin, Chomedey, Laval, Québec H73 2C6, Canada

RESUME

In this paper we have reviewed 260 cases of straightforward snorers without sleep apnea. A "bio-mechanical" model is presented so as to better understand the pathophysiology of oro-pharyngeal collapse and to attempt to regroup the many etiologies of this problem. Moreover, an important modification in the surgical technique is presented so as to reduce the morbidity associated with the surgery: a transposition flap is used to displace, in a forward manner, the implantation of the palate and create a "Z" closure of the lateral walls. The pharyngeal cicatricial contracture seems controlled and the velo-pharyngeal stenoses are avoided.

KEYWORDS

Physiopathology, aerodynamic model, etiologies, evaluation, velo-pharyngeal stenosis, modified U.P.P.P.

INTRODUCTION

As we gained knowledge about sleep pattern, its architecture and disturbances, we also learned about obstruction of the upper respiratory tracts during sleep.

New notions and a revolution in concept also, as the patients were often asymptomatic and normal in appearance on diurnal examination. Moreover, the multiple symptoms had never been united in one entity and would often be accepted as being part of a normal evolution, i.e., laughable snoring, hyperactive child, sleepy adult, the whole gamut, what.

The advent of the sleep lab allowed us to elucidate the problem: sleep brings about a muscular relaxation and, if accompanied by a disturbed airway, will favor a collapse of the oro-pharynx. When partial or complete inspiratory obstruction intervenes, it is accompanied by a multiplicity of clinical symptoms and complications.

Because of Dr. Jacques Montplaisir's sleep lab, our Montreal experience was precocious. We were brought to evaluate all the manifestations of nocturnal respiratory obstruction and our main interest focuses on snorers who do not have sleep apnea but a social and personal problem which brings them to consult.

This problem touches 25-45% of the population and will often bring about smiles and mockery. Nevertheless, the social implications are often immense: let it suffice to question these snorers on their sleep partners and we shall learn that the majority sleep alone, deserted by their partners who oblige the guilt-ridden snorer to consult.

Snoring affects males twice as frequently as females and augments with age. The obese and hypertensive are the ones most frequently affected and the mean intensity of the snoring is 35 decibels but, in some extreme cases, it can reach 85 decibels. The frequency is situated around 300 Hz. This is accompanied by few medical problems other than a high incidence of hypertension and the fact that this labile hypertension will frequently regress after surgical correction.

Today we would like to present 260 cases of snorers without apnea who were seen between 1984 and 1985. We will first describe our clinical material, after which we will present a new variation of the pharyngoplasty, a variation so as to minimize the morbidity and standardize the surgery.

PHYSIOPATHOLOGY OF THE OBSTRUCTION

In a way we have always known that a nasal obstruction or a mass projecting into the upper respiratory tract can lead to an increased resistance to respiration and, for that reason, snoring.

Nevertheless, the physiopathology of nocturnal respiratory problems in anatomically normal patients was left unexplained...

It became necessary and useful to create an aerodynamic model to as to attempt to understand the snoring process in the light of the anatomical and physiological particularities of the pharynx.

MODEL:

The pharynx behaves like a Starling resistance in a way similar to the nasal valve: two rigid air-filled cavities are united by a collapsing zone which leads to a limited air flow. During the day and in the absence of specific pathology the flow will be turbulent. The irregularity of the walls, the increase in the speed of the flow, the increase in the amount of the flow, and the decrease in the diameter of the respiratory tracts, are all factors which will favor the accentuation of this turbulence. At the same time, the energy expended to move the flow of air will be greater and the negative inspiratory pressure will have to increase to maintain the same flow. Let us see, with the help of this model, the conditions which are susceptible to modify the equilibrium of the valve:

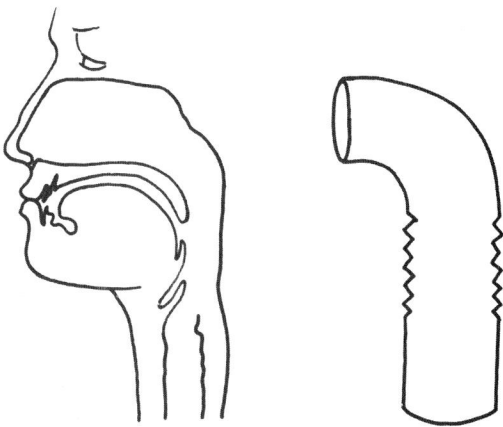

PHARYNX = RÉSISTANCE STARLING

I. Nasal Obstruction

An inspiratory effort made in the presence of an increased nasal resistance will always be associated with a more negative pharyngeal pressure and by this fact a collapse will be favored: when the sides get closer the need to maintain the same air flow creates a greater speed of flow, a greater turbulence after which the collapse accentuates. In the course of events snoring will appear and will finally be followed by apnea.

The patient will theoretically have to open his mouth to breathe and avoid apnea: studies have shown that, if during the day, buccal respiratory resistance is effectively inferior to nasal resistance, the pattern is quite different at night where the buccal resistance increases more than the nasal resistance and the nose becomes the easiest airway to breathe through.

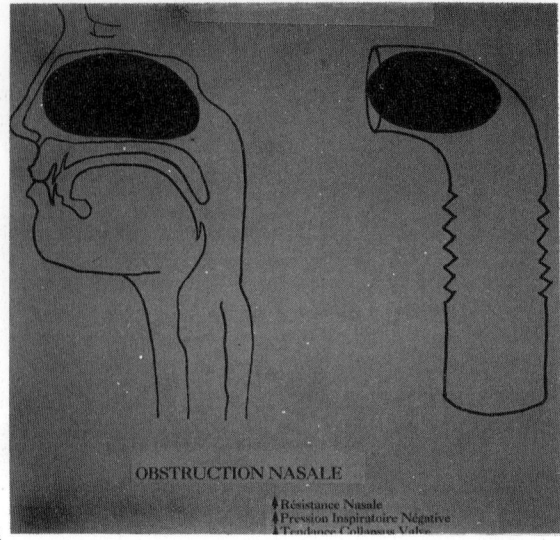

2. Presence of an Abnormal Mass of the Respiratory Airways

Knowing that any decrease in the diameter of a respiratory tube is followed by an accentuation of the speed and an increase in the negative pressure of the intraluminal pressure, and knowing also that a mass projecting into the lumen will favor turbulence, it is also evident that this mass will favor a premature collapse.

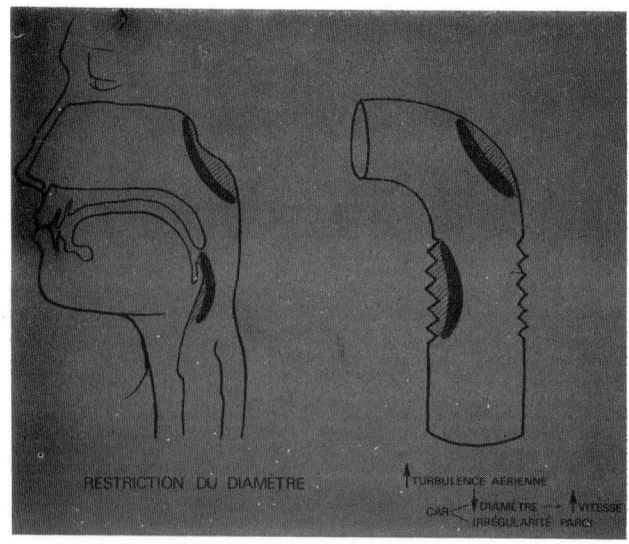

3. Decrease of the Transmural Resistance

The model and the principles already expressed speak for themselves and we easily understand that the collapse of the oro-pharynx can induce an increase in the negative intraluminal pressure and, afterwards, snoring. The genesis of the oro-pharyngeal nocturnal collapse can be explained in two ways:

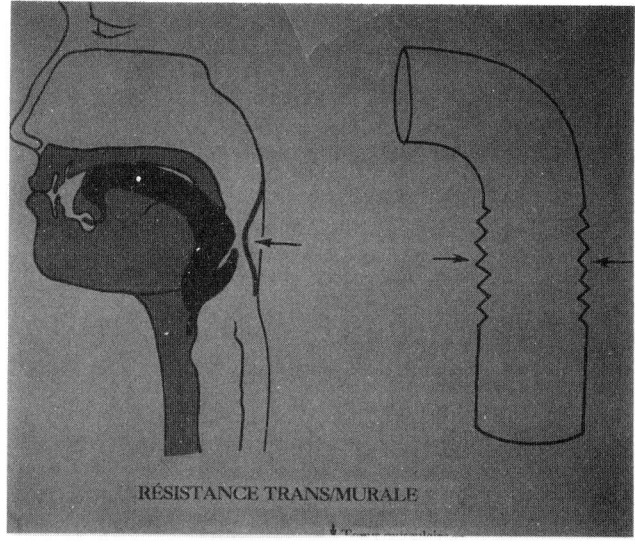

I. In the electromyographic sleep studies we observe a decrease in the tonus of the genioglossus muscles during the REM phase of sleep. The tongue and the lateral walls have a tendency to fall towards the center and it is probable that this mechanism explains why some people will snore more in the supine position when the tongue falls backwards. Moreover, studies of the phases of emergence following the periods of apnea show that the induced asphyxia will be the signal to terminate the apnea and that this event is accompanied by an increase in the registered EMG potentials of the submental muscles just before the break of the obstruction.

2. Presence of a particular pharyngeal morphotype with a relative oro-pharyngeal constriction secondary to:
    I. A palate which is longer and posterior.
    2. A very posterior insertion of the palato-pharyngeus.
    3. A large uvula.
    4. Hypertrophy of the palatine tonsils.
    5. Redundant pharyngeal mucosa.
    6. Enlarged tongue and small mandible.

CLINICAL STUDIES

We have accumulated 260 cases in a 2-year period and these patients have been seen in the ENT clinics of the Sacré-Coeur and Cité de la Santé of Laval Hospitals. The initial evaluation consisted of a standard history and physical examination with particular attention to sleep habits. When questioning about sleep habits the bed partner was usually present and in this way we had a witness to the nocturnal activities.
In all patients that consulted we attempted to elucidate 2 factors:

Clinical Experiences of Snoring

Number of Patients:		260
Sex:	Men	193
	Women	67
Age	Under 30 years	36
	From 30 to 50 years	180
	From 50 to 70 years	44
	Over 70 years	Nil
Weight:	More than normal	57

1. The site of obstruction
2. The importance of the clinical manifestation of the obstruction.

1. Site of Obstruction

As we all know, the obstruction can be situated in different anatomical areas. Moreover, it has been shown with the help of a scan that in 36-60% of cases there was a multifocal localization of narrowing. It is thus vital to attempt to identify all the factors which may cause obstruction so as to identify the cases which will not respond to treatment. To this effect, our patients underwent cephalometric studies which in all cases did not demonstrate narrowing of the posterior pharyngeal space. Four cases of micrognathia were detected but this micrognathia was not accompanied by a decrease of the posterior pharyngeal space and effectively these four patients stopped snoring after the uvulo-palato-pharyngoplasty. The majority of patients also underwent a flexible laryngoscopy in the supine position with Muller's manoeuvre so as to document more precisely the site of obstruction. This manoeuvre was not diagnostic by itself but helped to demonstrate the many foci of obstruction in certain patients. Let it suffice to mention 2 cases who presented an omega-shaped epiglottis and who continued to snore after the uvulo-palato-pharyngoplasty.

2. Importance of the Obstruction

As we all know, it is important to differentiate between straightforward snorers and those presenting snoring with sleep apnea. This differentiation has a medical and a prognostic connotation, as we know that the results of the U.P.P.P. depend on the type of snorers who we operate: indeed, in cases of simple snoring, approximately 90% of cases will respond to the U.P.P.P. whereas in cases of sleep apnea 50-60% will respond.

The patients first underwent a selection based on the importance of the diurnal and nocturnal symptoms which they presented. The doubtful cases were referred to sleep lab and the cases presenting sleep apnea in the sleep lab were excluded from this study. It is probable that a certain number of straightforward snorers included in our series could also have presented sleep apnea but because of the economic burden of having all patients studied in the sleep lab this was not done. After the evaluation all patients were given a thorough explanation on the causes of their snoring and a medical treatment was recommended so as to normalize the upper respiratory airway: stoppage of smoking, weight loss, attention to good living habits and nocturnal hygiene.

Afterwards, 110 patients underwent corrective surgery, 37 patients are on the waiting list and, in 41 cases, the patients have not yet decided to undergo the surgery.

Technique of Uvulo-Palato-Pharyngoplasty

The advent, in the last 5 years, of a new surgical technique which is not yet standardized but is used by many people, has brought about many variations according to the authors. The classical approach of uvulo-palato-pharyngo-plasty consists of a tonsillectomy, a

Clinical Experience of Uvulo-Palato-Pharyngoplasty

Number of cases:	90
Smokers:	28
Obese:	25
Anterior nasal surgery	14
-2 anterior surgeries	2
-3 anterior surgeries	1
Association of U.P.P.P. with nasal surgery:	
Diverse:	56
Cephalometry: Normal in:	90

resection of the uvula with a rim of the posterior border of the palate and variable portions of the anterior and posterior tonsillar pillars. Afterwards, sutures are placed so as to bring together the anterior and posterior surfaces of the palate and the anterior and posterior tonsillar pillars so as to displace the palate anteriorly while creating a curvilinear scar. The results of this conventional technique have been pretty good and, effectively, the worldwide analysis of the results of U.P.P.P. show that, in problems of straightforward snoring without sleep apnea, all techniques will carry a 90% success rate. Our experience in following the conventional technique is comparable to the above results but, in the course of our work, we noticed a significant incidence of patients who presented a contracture along the palato-pharyngeus: in fact, as we witnessed the immediate evolution of these patients postoperatively, many of them presented a dehiscence of the incision at the level of the tonsillar fossa. This is easy to understand: as we attempt to approximate the palato-pharyngeus to the palato-glossus with sutures, nature refuses this type of treatment, particularly when we have to deal with a structure which contracts continuously all day.

U.P.P.P. CONVENTIONAL TECHNIQUE: 25 cases

Results:
No snoring   17/23 cases
Light snoring   3/23
Same snoring   3/23
No follow-up   2/25

Velo-pharyngeal contracture

no snoring 5/23
with snoring 2/23

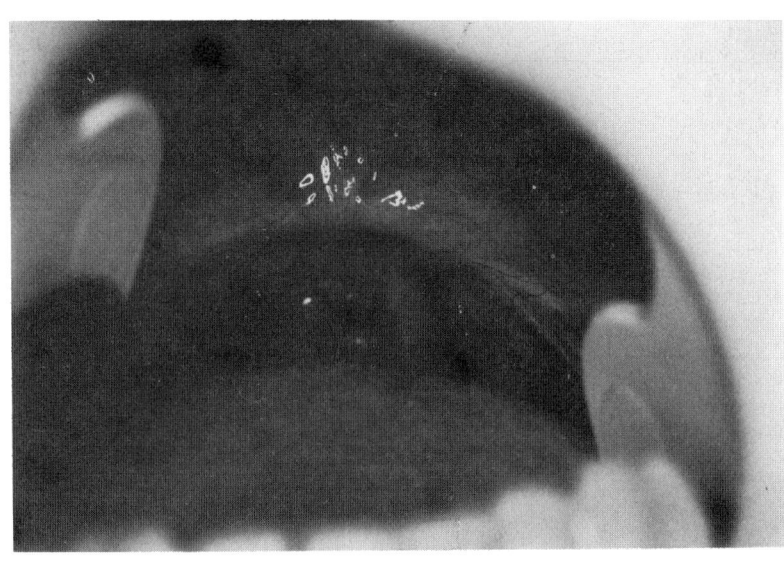

After a longer follow-up, certain patients developed a contracture along the palato-pharyngeus muscle with a tendency to velo-pharyngeal stenosis. This complication can be easily explained by study models that have been made of curvilinear skin scars studied by Dr. David Min-Chyang-Ju: in the course of the closure of a curvilinear cutaneous scar the tension effort aims at closing the hemicircle on itself and attracts it to the top.

Moreover, remembering that at the level of the palate we are dealing with a double curvilinear scar, back-to-back, and that this scar undergoes repeated extensions and retractions in the course of each deglutition, it is demonstrated that microscopic hemorrhages occur along the line of closure which, in effect, are microtraumas and this mode of closure creates extensive fibrosis. To compensate for this state, certain authors have completely resected the palato-pharyngeal muscle and attempted to meticulously suture the sectioned mucosa. Our approach was different: we were not pleased to sacrifice uselessly a muscular structure which served in the suspension of the laryngo-pharynx and larynx: we only have to think of the studies of Riley and Guilleminault, proven by cephalometric studies, which demonstrate an increase in the distance between the mandible and the hyoid in cases of sleep apnea. Theoretically, if we sacrifice the palato-pharyngeus, we may partially lose this suspension and jeopardize the improvement in this distance by fibrosis of the palato-pharyngeus.

Equally, as we began seeing patients who had stopped snoring postoperatively but who began snoring again afterwards at the same time as the onset of velo-pharyngeal stenosis this brought us to modify the technique in a more logical fashion. We have adopted a technique with section and transposition of the pillars in 65 cases and we have noticed a nearly complete absence of contracture along the palato-pharyngeus and also the absence of velo-pharyngeal stenosis.

Our goal was thus to attempt to decrease surgical morbidity, that is, to decrease postoperative pain, to decrease the percentage of dehiscence of the wound due to traction of the palato-pharyngeus, to decrease the percentage of naso-pharyngeal stenosis due to scar contracture of the palato-pharyngeus, to decrease the delayed healing of wounds and mostly to avoid the excessive shortening of the palate as advocated by certain authors so as to avoid complications of velo-pharyngeal insufficiency. Moreover, we have attempted to rationalize the approach so as to standardize the quantity of excision at the level of the palate and so as to popularize the procedure.

DESCRIPTION

1. Standard tonsillectomy
2. Transposition flaps at the level of the anterior and posterior tonsillar pillars by sectioning the palato-pharyngeus and its overlying mucosa at the level of its attachment to the soft palate. At the level of the anterior pillar we do a triangular resection of the palato-glossus with its overlying mucosa. Following this, we shift the myomucous flap anteriorly and inferiorly so as to break the tension line and so as to pediculate the line of circular fibrosis much more anteriorly, that is, at the entrance of the palato-glossus in the tongue. Finally, we minimally resect the posterior border of the palate and, the curvilinear fibrous scar being displaced anteriorly, the cicatricial contracture will form in an anterior and inferior direction and will maintain the soft palate during the night. The effect of this is to completely erase, in a majority of cases, the palato-pharyngeal projection at the level of the air column of the oro-pharynx and, in the long-term, because of the Z-plasty equivalent on the lateral walls of the oro-pharynx, to prevent the cicatricial contracture favored by continuous deglutition which can in the long-term cause velo-pharyngeal stenosis.

ANALYSIS OF RESULTS

We first noticed that the postoperative pain was decreased either due to the absence of an open wound at the level of the oro-pharynx or because of the infiltration of the greater palatine foramen and the lateral pharyngeal walls that we do with Marcaine at the end of each case. Moreover, there has been a significant decrease in dehiscence of the postoperative wound and a decrease in cases of necrosis at the level of the lateral pharyngeal wall. The most important has been the dramatic decrease in the number of velo-pharyngeal stenoses and the absence of long-term velo-pharyngeal insufficiency.

U.P.P.: Technique of Modified "Z" Plasty in 65 Cases:

Results:

No snoring	45/55
Light snoring	6/55
Same snoring	4/55
No follow-up	12/65

Velo-pharyngeal contracture: 1/55 cases without snoring

The percentage of those who responded to U.P.P.P. by a decrease in snoring was the same with both techniques. We have spent time studying those cases that did not completely respond to surgical treatment only to notice that in the majority of cases there were predisposing associated factors: in effect, 5 of 6 patients presenting a mediocre response to surgery were chronic smokers or obese people. Our impression vis-à-vis this second modified technique is that we can standardize the surgical approach, we can make a minimal resection of the lateral wall and of the soft palate while still achieving excellent results and decreasing the dangers of complications.

U.P.P.P. Failure:

Technique of Modified "Z" Plasty:

Light snoring: 6/55: 3 weight and tobacco
1 weight
1 tobacco
1 idiopathic

Same snoring: 4/55 3 idiopathic
1 weight and omega-shaped epiglottis

CONCLUSION

In all scientific fields whether medical or others, new discoveries negate or clarify the old truths and impassion those who are committed. We are now living this stimulating breakthrough in ENT and we can better understand the magnitude of the problem presented by respiratory obstruction. We have reviewed 260 cases of straightforward snorers and we have presented a surgical experience particularly regarding the pharyngoplasties. It is important to understand that surgery is not the answer to the problem of snoring and that the global approach to the patient has to be underlined: the problems of obesity, of chronic smoking,

FINAL ASPECT

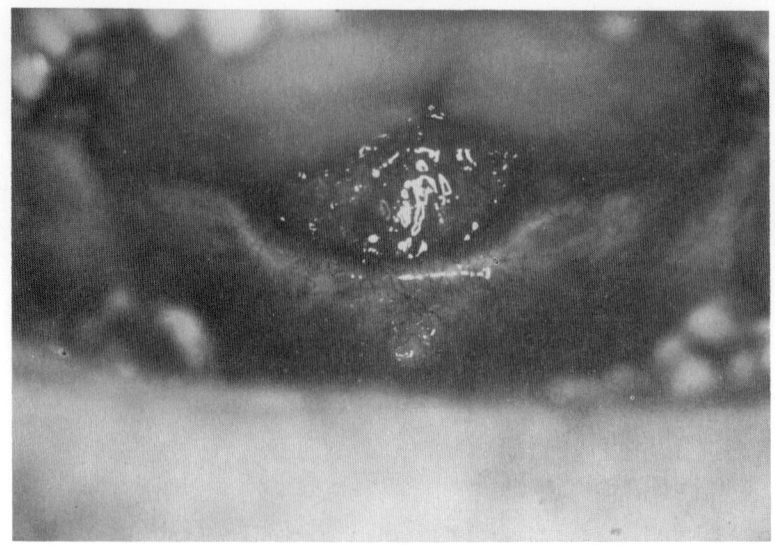

DESIRED ARCHITECTURAL MODIFICATION

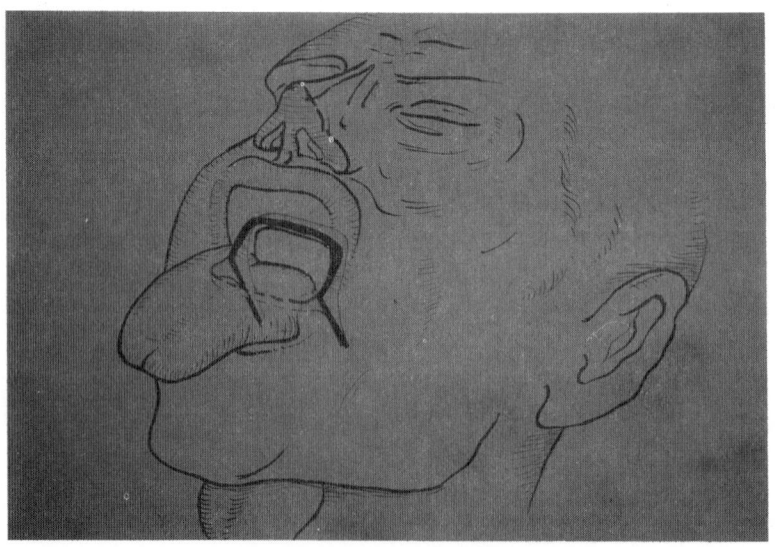

Tableau 7

1.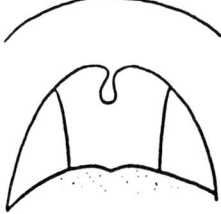
Etat post-amygdalectomie

2.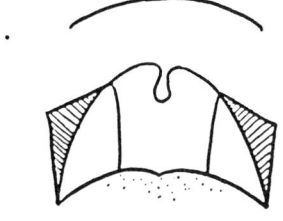
Résection d'un triangle du pilier antérieur

3.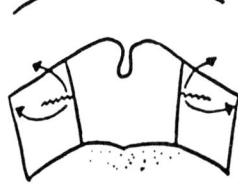
Section transversale du palato-pharyngien

4.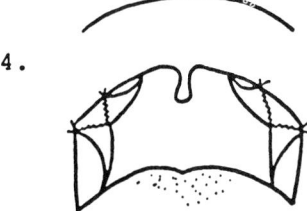
Mobilisation des lambeaux de transposition

5.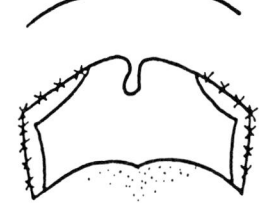
Fermeture

6.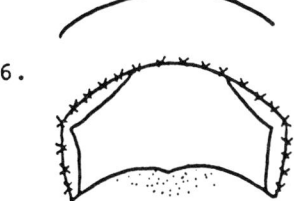
Résection luette et bordure voile palais

of sedentarism and sleep habits have to be addressed with the patient. Equally, it is important to pinpoint the multiple foci in the upper respiratory tract that can cause snoring so as to predict the long-term results of treatment.

Moreover, we have attempted to rationalize the surgical technique of pharyngoplasty so as to foresee the final surgical result and to prevent complications. Finally, a better standardization of the technique will allow a diffusion of this technique among the non-initiated and will also allow them to avoid the long-term complications and pitfalls.

RESUME

Ce papier revoit notre expérience de 260 cas de ronfleurs simples ne présentant pas d'apnée du sommeil. Un modèle bio-mécanique est présenté pour tenter de mieux comprendre la physiologie du collapsus oro-pharyngé et tenter de regrouper sous la même bannière les différentes étiologies mises en cause dans cette maladie.
De plus, une modification importante de la technique chirurgicale est introduite pour tenter de diminuer la morbidité associée à la chirurgie : par la section transversale du muscle palato-pharyngien, un lambeau de transposition est utilisé pour déplacer l'implantation du palais vers l'avant et créer une fermeture en "Z" des parois latérales.
La contracture de la cicatrice pharyngée semble contrôlée et les sténoses vélo-pharyngées sont évitées.

Snoring revealing hypothyroidism

J. Soudant, J.M. Ziza, G. Lamas, K. Boussen, B. Wechsler, M. Chic and
C. Chapelon

Service ORL et Service de Médecine Interne, Hôpital Pitie-Saltpétrière, 75013 Paris, France

SUMMARY

Snoring has become an increasing reason for consulting in the Ear-Nose-Throat departments.
Clinical examination often shows abnormalities of the uvula and pharynx which are surgically curable with uvulopharyngoplasty.
This is a case report of a patient attending for snoring with respiratory pauses as objectivated by polygraphic recording of sleep.
Hormonal therapy for hypothyroidism and snoring will be studied and the litterature shows snoring has rarely been the first complaint in hypothyroidism. This shows the different causes of sleep apnea syndrome must be borne in mind by the E.N.T. surgeons. Indeed, a surgical procedure performed in a patient with mild hypothyroidism might trigger severe decompensation of the disease.

INTRODUCTION

For the last few years, many patients have attended an E.N.T. out patient department because of snoring.
On clinical examination, abnormalities of the soft palate and pharynx have often been noted, indicating an "uvulopharyngoplasty".
However, every E.N.T. surgeon must know the other causes for snoring, particularly hypothyroid states, mainly in subclinical forms.

KEYWORDS

Sleep apnea syndrome, hypothyroidism, snoring.

MATERIAL AND METHODS

Case observation

This fifty year old male patient, originally from the West Indies, is living in France for the last twenty years.
He was complaining of snoring with the following pattern, well described by his wife : progressive deterioration with numerous respiratory pauses. The respiratory pauses may wake him up, leaving him anxious with a feeling of iminent death. There is a progressive asthenia with daytime lethargy.

Medical history

- Physical and psychological slow-down.
- Carpal Tunnel Syndrome.
- Induration and dryness of the skin difficult to see in this black man.

E.N.T. examination

- There is no abnormality of the soft palate, the pharynx and the nasal cavities.
- Mild hypertrophy of the base of the tongue, and possibly a mild induration of the pharyngeal mucosa.
The examination signs were consistent with hypothyroidism ; the diagnosis was easily confirmed by the following investigations :
- hypercholesterolemia 9mmol/l (N < 6.8mmol/l)
- increased blood levels for CPK, LDH, Aldolase, SGOT
- free T4 (radio-immuno-assay) 1.7mmol/l (9.4 < N < 2Jμmmol/l)
- TSH increased to 64 micro U/ml (0.1 < N < 4 micro U/ml)
- presence of antibodies against thyroid microsome, without anti-thyroglobulin antibodies.
Those investigations were followed by a polygraphic recording during night sleep, including :
- EEG
- electro-oculography
- EMG for tibialis anterior and chin muscles
- ECG
- study of respiratory movements and oral and nasal airflow.
This later investigation showed obstructive and mixte apneic episodes occuring with a high frequency. Indeed, patient presented during his sleep :
- 368 episodes of apnea lasting from 10 to 90 seconds (mean : 17 seconds)
- i.e 108 minutes of apnea (23,3%) during the total sleeping period.
This study showed this patient was suffering from hypothyroidism with sleep apnea syndrom.

Other investigations

- Skull xray and scan of facial bones : both were normal.
- Audiogramm : confirming the sensory hearing loss of cochlear type.
- Respiratory function test : showed mild restriction without obstruction neither hypoxia.

RESULTS

The evolution of the disease with replacement hormonal treatment has been good within three months. The clinical signs and hypothyroid biological abnormalities were back to normal. Snoring and sleep apnea have completly disappeared and sleep polygraphic recordings were normal. At the same time, respiratory function tests were back to normal. Hypoxia disappeared and CO^2 transfer test was normal.

DISCUSSION

- The course of the disease with hormonal treatment leading to diappearance of snoring and sleep apnea syndrome showed that hypothyroidism was without doubt the cause of the disorder.
- The picture of sleep apnea syndrome was typical. However, one must think from the beginning of the diagnosis of hypothyroidism.
- Sleep apnea syndrome due to hypothyroidism has been mentionned on several occasions in the litterature, but this has probably been under-estimated because it is often latent and the clinical signs are dominated by the hypothyroidism.
- Rarely sleep apnea syndrome is severe and is the primary complaint as in our case presentation. RAJAGORAL found it nine times in a series of 11 hypothyroid patient in which it was systematically looked for.
- It is more often found in obese patients.
- Other endocrine disorders might also be responsible : acromegaly and WILLI-PRADER's syndrome.
The mechanism in sleep apnea syndrome during hypothyroidism probably is multifactorial.
- In fact, apnea might be of central type with depression of central centers reflexe to hypoxia.
- There is also real apnea of obstructive type due to infiltration of upper airway and upper gastro-intestinal tract mucosa.
- This could also be due to muscular hypotony seen in the hypothyroid patient leading to the obstructive syndrome.

CONCLUSION

This case report had the goal of attracting attention to the E.N.T. surgeon for a possible cause of snoring - hypothyroidism in our case. Indeed, the E.N.T. surgeon is submitted to an increasing pressure by the patient or his relatives for curing the annoying symptom.
However, we must keep in mind the different diseases responsible for snoring. Hypothyroidism is known to be present under mild forms making a difficult diagnosis.
A possible surgical procedure in such a pathological context would be detrimentous for the endocrine disease.

RESUME

Le ronflement est devenu un motif de consultation de plus en plus fréquent dans les services O.R.L.

L'examen clinique retrouve souvent des lésions vélopharyngées accessibles à un traitement chirurgical par uvulopharyngoplastie.

Il est rapporté le cas d'un patient ayant consulté pour un ronflement avec pauses respiratoires comme l'ont montré les enregistrements polygraphiques du sommeil. Le traitement hormonal de l'hypothyroïdie a permis d'obtenir une régression du ronflement et des pauses respiratoires.

Sont ensuite étudiés les rapports entre l'hypothyroïdie et ce ronflement qui, comme on le voit dans la littérature, est très rarement révélateur de l'hypothyroïdie.

Cependant, les différentes causes de syndrome d'apnée du sommeil doivent être connues par les praticiens O.R.L. En effet, un geste chirurgical sur une hypothyroïdie fruste, comme c'est souvent le cas, pourrait être responsable d'une décompensation très grave.

BIBLIOGRAPHY

Billiard M., Besset A., Brissaud L. (1984) : Le syndrome d'apnées récurrentes au cours du sommeil. Rev. Med. Interne 5, 142-151.

Billard W., Smyk K., Crampette L., Dejean Y (1985) : Le syndrome d'apnées au cours du sommeil. Cahiers d'ORL 20, 563-569.

Dement W., Carskadon M., Richardson G. (1978) : Excessive daytime sleepness in the sleep apnea syndrome. In Sleep Apnea Syndrome, eds Guilleminault C. and Dement W.C. Alan R. Liss. Inc., New York, pp 23-46.

Findley L., Barth J., Wilhoit S. et coll (1985) : Nocturnal hypoxemia and cognitive functionning in sleep apnea patients. Am. Rev. Respir. Dis. 131, A 107.

Gastaut H., Tassinari C., Duron B. (1965) : Etude polygraphique des manifestations épisodiques (hypniques et respiratoires) diurnes et nocturnes du syndrome de Pickwick. Rev. Neurol. 112, 573-579.

Guilleminault C. (1978) : Natural history, cardiac impact and long term follow-up of sleep apnea syndrome. In Sleep Apnea Syndrome, eds Guilleminault C. and Dement W.C., Alan R. Liss. Inc., New York, pp 333-345.

Guilleminault C. (1984) : Syndrome "apnée au cours du sommeil". Presse Med. 13, 433-436.

Hall B.D., Smith D.N. (1972) : Prader-willi syndrome. J. Pediatr. 28, 686-693.

Lavie P. (1983) : Sleep apnea in industrial workers. In sleep/wake disorders natural history, epidemiology and long term evolution, eds Guilleminault C. and Lugaresi E., Raven Press, New York, pp 127-135.

Mackay D., Cooper R.A., Bradbury S. et coll (1984) : Sleep apnea in myxedemia. J. Roy Col Phy, London 18, 248-252.

Maraud L., Gin H., Brottier E., Aubertin J. (1985) : Le syndrome d'apnée du sommeil chez l'acromégale. Sem. Hôp. Paris 61, 990-993.

Miller W.P. (1982) : Cardiac arrythmias and conduction disturbances in the sleep apnea syndrome. Prevalence and significance. Am. J. Med. 73, 317-321.

Onal E., Lopata M., O'Connor T. (1982) : Pathogenesis of apneas in hypersomnia-sleep apnea syndrome. Am. Rev. Respir. Dis. 128, 167-174.

Orr W.C., Males J.L., Imes N.K. (1981) : Myxedema and obstructive sleep apnea. Am. J. Med. 70, 1061-1066.

Rajagopal K.R., Abbrecht P.H., Derderian S. S. et coll (1984) : Obstructive sleep apnea in hypothyroidism. Ann. Intern. Med. 101, 491-494.

Skatrud J., Iber C., Ewart R., Thomas G., Rasmussen H., Schultze B. (1981) : Disordered breathing during sleep in hypothyroidism. Am. Rev. Respir. Dis. 124, 325-329.

Wilson W.R., Bedeil G.N. (1960) : The pulmonary abnormalities in myxedema. J. Clinic. Invest. 39, 42-55.

Zwillich C.W., Pierson D.J., Hofeldt F.D. et coll (1975) : Ventilatory control in myxedema and hypothyroidism. N. Engl. J. Med. 292, 662-665.

Five year follow-up of daytime sleepiness and snoring after tracheostomy in patients with obstructive sleep apneas

P.S. Ledereich, M.J. Thorpy, P.B. Glovinsky, B. Burack, P. McGregor, D.L. Rozycki and A.E. Sher

Sleep-Wake Disorders Center, Montefiore Medical Center, Bronx New York 10467, USA
Albert Einstein College of Medicine, Bronx New York 10461, USA

ABSTRACT

We compared the long-term efficacy of tracheostomy vs. a variety of less definitive treatments on excessive daytime sleepiness (EDS) and snoring, the major presenting symptoms of patients with Obstructive Sleep Apnea (OSA). Patients who had undergone initial evaluation at least five years previously completed a questionnaire concerning the persistence of these symptoms. Patients who had undergone permanent tracheostomy reported less daytime sleepiness and less snoring than those treated by alternative means. The present study represents the first large scale long term follow-up of OSA patients, and provides a basis for judging the efficacy of newer treatments of OSA such as Continuous Positive Airway Pressure (CPAP) and Uvulo-palato-pharyngoplasty (UPPP).

KEYWORDS

Excessive Daytime Sleepiness, Obstructive Sleep Apnea, snoring, follow-up, tracheostomy, natural history

INTRODUCTION

Tracheostomy is regarded as being the most definitive form of therapy for patients with obstructive sleep apnea. However the possibility of surgical or post surgical complications as well as the social inconvenience of having a tracheostomy has limited its use. Many studies have shown that weight reduction can decrease the severity of obstructive sleep apnea and may lead to its resolution, however substantial weight reduction is not easy to attain and maintaining a lower body weight for a prolonged period of time is also very difficult. Although a variety of alternative treatments have been used, such as the use of respiratory stimulants including Medroxy-progesterone and Protriptyline as well as surgical alternative such as submucous resection, the efficacy of these treatments over a prolonged period has not been established.

The newer surgical therapy of uvulo-palato-pharyngoplasty (UPPP) has been shown to be effective in only to 40 to 50% of patients with obstructive sleep apnea, unless selection is made on upper pharyngeal changes, in which case the success rate can be improved to as much as 85% (Sher, et al 1985). However the long term usefulness of uvulo-palato-pharyngoplasty has not been demonstrated and it is known that some patients who initially do well following the surgery regress at a later date. It is therefore important to establish not only the natural history of untreated obstructive sleep apnea, but also the effects of the various treatment modalities. In the present study we compare the long-term efficacy of tracheostomy in reducing subjective complaints of excessive daytime sleepiness and snoring against a variety of other treatments for OSA which were available more than five years ago.

METHODS

152 patients initially seen at Montefiore Sleep Wake Disorders Center (SWDC) between the years 1977-1980 were identified as having OSA according to the following criteria: (1) An Obstructive Apnea Index of greater than five events per hour of sleep, (2) obstructive apneas comprising at least 33% of all apneic events and (3) patient age greater than twelve years. All were sent an extensive questionnaire including questions regarding their prior and current subjective assessment of daytime sleepiness and snoring. 106 patients (70%) completed the questionnaire; 18 (12%) had died since the initial evaluation, 17 (11%) refused to respond, and an additional 11 (9%) were unable to be located.

30 patients (26 M, 4 F) had a permanent tracheostomy for at least 30 months that was open at the time they answered the questionnaire. These tracheostomy patients were compared to a group of 71 patients (66 M, 5 F) who were treated by alternative treatment modalities including other surgical interventions (n=17) such as temporary tracheostomy, UPPP, tonsilectomy, submucosal resection, and respiratory stimulant medications (n=7). Other patients in this group were given recommendations for weight loss alone (n=14). However, all overweight patients were advised to attain an ideal body weight. 25 of the 71 patients were recommended to undergo tracheostomy but failed to comply. Various other treatment recommendations were made to the remaining (n=8). 5 patients who had recently commenced continuous positive airway pressure CPAP were excluded from the study.

The following table presents some features the two groups which could be influencing factors on daytime sleepiness and snoring.

	Tracheostomy(T)	Alternative(A)	p Value
Age at follow-up (years)	57.3 (SD 9.0)	56.1 (SD 12.6)	ns
Time from initial evaluation to follow up (months)	79.3 (SD 8.9)	78.1 (SD 7.5)	ns
BMI at initial evaluation (weight (kg)/height (m)2)	34.6 (SD 8.4)	31.9 (SD 7.4)	ns
BMI at follow up	33.7 (SD 7.3)	31.9 (SD 7.1)	ns
Average sleep/night (hours)	7.2 (SD 1.2)	7.2 (SD 2.0)	ns
Average duration of tracheostomy (months)	72.6 (SD 16.2)		

Questionnaire response frequencies were compared between groups using a chi-square statistic (BMDP Statistical Software).

RESULTS

Sleepiness

When asked "Do you have debilitating, uncontrollable or excessive daytime sleepiness?", 59% of the Alternative treatment group answered yes, as compared to only 24% of the Tracheostomy group ($p<.01$). However, a similar percentage of both groups (26% A, 17% T) admitted to taking unexpected daytime naps. 46% of the Alternative treatment group said they were more than or just as sleepy as when originally evaluated, in contrast to only 3% of the Tracheostomy group ($p<.001$).

Snoring

When asked if they presently snored, 58% of the Alternative treatment group said that they did, as compared to only 13% of the Tracheostomy group ($p<.001$). 54% of the Alternative treatment group stated that they snore as much or more as they had at initial evaluation, as compared to only 7% of the Tracheostomy group ($p<.001$).

35% of the Alternative treatment group reported the frequency of observed apneic pauses, or the frequency of waking up gasping for breath to be as frequent or more frequent since the initial evaluation, in contrast to only 3% of the Tracheostomy group ($p<.001$)

DISCUSSION

The results of our study demonstrate the first evaluation of a large group of patients who underwent treatment for their obstructive apnea more than 5 years previously. Alternative treatments are compared with tracheostomy and both groups were similar in terms of age at follow-up, body mass index at initial evaluation and at follow-up and the average nightly amount of sleep that they received. There were clear differences between the groups as one might expect with the tracheostomy group having less tendency for sleepiness and snoring as compared to the alternative treatment group. Most of the patients treated by means other than the tracheostomy report continuing sleepiness with the majority being as sleepy if not more so then when they were initially evaluated. Despite the presence of a tracheostomy, 24% of these patients continued to have daytime sleepiness however, only 3% of this group were just as sleepy or more sleepy then they had been originally. In addition, daytime napping was equally as frequent between both groups. The presence of significant daytime sleepiness in patients with obstructive sleep apnea after such a long period of time raises the possibility of other sleep disorders being present. Central sleep apnea, narcolepsy or idiopathic central nervous system hypersomnolence may originally have been present in conjunction with obstructive sleep apnea in some of the patients.

As one would expect, the majority of the patients with tracheostomy do not continue to snore whereas a greater percentage of patients who are treated by other means snore on a regular basis. If snoring can be used as reflecting upper airway obstruction, then the majority of these patients continue to have as much if not more upper airway obstruction despite alternative treatment recommendations. A significant percentage of patients in the alternative treatment group continue to have apneic episodes and episodes of waking up gasping for breath, whereas the symptoms were present in only 3% of the tracheostomy group. Despite having a tracheostomy some patients continue to snore, which suggests either some form of stoma obstruction may be occurring such as due to excess chin tissues in obese patients, or that some passage of air occurs through the upper airway during sleep.

Although all patients who were overweight were recommended to lose weight, the initial and final weights of both groups did not differ significantly. One might have expected that patients with tracheostomy, who are symptomatically better than those treated by alternative means, would have lost more weight, possibly because of increased activity as a result of reduced daytime sleepiness. However the tracheostomy patients as a group were not able to significantly alter their body weight.

Overall, the tracheostomy group were much more improved in terms of sleepiness and snoring compared with the patients treated by alternative means, however not all patients are "cured". The high percentage of patients treated by alternative means who continued to have as severe if not more severe symptoms is of concern, however it must be stressed that newer forms of treatment such as continuous positive nasal air pressure therapy (CPAP) are not included in this analysis. The number of patients with UPPP are not sufficient at this time to enable any assessment of the efficacy over the long term. In addition to symptomatic information objective documentation is also required. This study illustrates that evaluation of any treatment modality for OSA must take into consideration not only short term but also long term effectiveness.

Sher A.E., Thorpy M.J., Shprintzen R.J., Speilman A.J., Burack B., McGregor P.: Predictive Value of Muller Manuever in Selection of Patients for Uvulopalatopharngoplasty, Laryngoscope Vol 92 No 12 1483-1487, 1985.

RESUME

Nous avons comparé l'efficacité à long terme de la trachéostomie avec d'autres modes de traitement palliatifs de la somnolence diurne (EDS) et du ronflement, symptômes majeurs des patients atteints d'apnée obstructive du sommeil (OSA). Les patients ayant subi une première évaluation de leurs troubles au moins 5 ans auparavant, ont répondu à un questionnaire sur la persistance de ces symptômes après traitement. Les patients ayant subi une trachéostomie permanente présentent une diminution plus importante de la somnolence diurne et du ronflement que ceux qui ont eu un autre traitement.

Cette étude est la plus importante par l'étendue dans le temps et le nombre de cas, effectuée chez des patients atteints d'apnée obstructive du sommeil; et elle fournit une base de comparaison sur l'efficacité des derniers traitements de l'OSA, tels que la "pression positive continue du passage de l'air" (CPAP) et l'uvulo-palato-pharyngoplastie (UPPP)

XI. TREATMENTS OF CHRONIC RHONCHOPATHY
Chairman: J.P. Pieyre

Assessment and surgical considerations of snoring and OSA

H.B. Holden, A.D. Cheesman and B.H. Pickard

Department of Head and Neck Surgery, Charing Cross Hospital, London, UK

Definitions: We have defined apnoea as :
A period of cessation of naso-pulmonary airflow lasting 10 seconds or longer. Sleep apnoea is considered to occur if there are more than 5 periods of apnoea per hour.
Snoring or rhinocophony is considered abnormal if the patient's family are persistently and unduly disturbed.

The consequences of snoring may only be socially trivial, but could well produce serious social or marital problems, whereas OSA may lead to potentially fatal cardio-respiratory problems.

Symptoms of OSA include:
Abnormal sleep behaviour
Snoring
Alternating conscious state
Daytime fatigue
Intellect or ability change
Enuresis
Sudden death (cardiovascular or respiratory causes)

Before discussing the assessment of cases we should consider the anatomy and the possible sites of obstruction to the airflow.
Sites: Nasal, Palato-pharyngeal, Glossopharyngeal, Supraglottic.

The nasal problems are usually self-evident and can be dealt with by routine procedures, but the palate and oropharynx must be considered in more detail.
The palato-pharyngeal opening is controlled by muscles of the palate, particularly the palatopharyngeus, and the sup.constrictor. It is for this that the UPPP operation is designed.
We also find that the glosso-phonyngeal region is a secondary factorwhich may require surgical intervention in severe or recalcitrant cases of obsructive apnoea. Especially in short, stocky overweight persons who have a narrow oro-phonygeal configuration with a backward positioned tongue.

Assessment. A preliminary ENT examination is made to exclude other pathology, for example an undiagnosed vocal cord palsy.

In cases of snoring without apnoea we keep the investigations to a minimum, a sleep sound recording in the home is made (the microphone being placed 1 metre from the head). A C.T scan is taken to measure the total available airway in the palato-pharyngeal region at the level of the arch of atlas vertebra by Dr. J. McIvor.

Where there is any evidence of OSA then a full sleep laboratory assessment is carried out by the Respiratory Unit under the direction of Prof. Guz. This includes a full medical examination. Two nights sleep are assesed by Polysomnography and the following parameters measured:
1. Sleep pattern
2. Respiratory movement
3. Airflow
4. Blood gases
5. Electro-recordings (ECG; EEG; EMG; EOG)
6. C.T Scan
7. Video and Sound Recordings
8. Fibre-optic endoscopy.

Surgical techniques are discussed briefly , namely the two approaches for the UPPP operation and the mandibulo-hyoid advancement.

Discussion of results

Snoring: All our patients reported that snoring was vastly improved or eliminated. In most cases this has been independently confirmed by recordings or witness.

Daytime fatigue is very much less and activity is generally enhanced.

Periods of nocturnal apnoea are reduced, but still readily occur, although post-operative studies show better SaO_2 levels (this is probably due to O_2 being more readily and easily acquired during the respiratory phase). The possibility of a central apnoea pattern is considered an important factor.

CT Scans show a measurable improvement in airway configuration.

Complications:
Immediate problems can include pain, some bleeding, infection with oedema, nasal regurgitation of fluids. More prolonged pain does occur if the palatal muscles have been traumatized and occasionally if nasal and palatal procedures have been done together.

Later problems include continued nasal regurgitation, inability to gargle. These are usually due to some rigidity of the palatal velum, which subsides as the tissues become more supple. We ave not experienced any prolonged troubles of hypernasality or regurgitation using our present techniques.

Surgical concepts in uvulo-palato-pharyngoplasty. Complications and sequelae

Y. Zohar, Y. Finkelstein and Y. Talmi

Department of Otolaryngology, Head & Neck Surgery, Golda Medical Center, Hasharon Hospital, 7 Keren Kayemet Street, Petach Tikva 49372, Israel

ABSTRACT

Obstructive sleep apnea is a disorder involving metabolic, respiratory and sometimes neural abnormalities. Anatomical hypertrophies of the oropharyngeal lumen, collapse of the tongue-pharynx and hypotonicity of the soft palate-oropharyngeal muscles are the accepted factors in airway obstruction. This presentation reports evaluation, treatment and follow-up of 57 patients who have undergone uvulo-palato-pharyngoplasty (UPPP) since 1985. We consider that a generous resection of soft palate and tonsillar tissue is mandatory for a successful UPPP. Our modification of UPPP which obviates palatal stenosis is described and the post operative complications and sequelae are summarized. Most of the patients were relieved of the distressing and social unpleasant loud snoring, and in a large proportion reversal of clinical respiratory abnormalities was obtained after UPPP.

KEY WORDS

Soft palate, velopharyngeal incompetence, obstructive sleep apnea, uvulo-palato-pharyngoplasty.

INTRODUCTION

The primary cause of sleep apnea syndrome is in most cases unknown. Three types of sleep apnea have been described: Central, obstructive and mixed. In the so called central sleep induced apnea, involvement of the central nervous system is suspected. Peripheral or peripheral and central factors have been thought to contribute to the appearance of obstructive apnea. In the obstructive type, functional airway obstruction takes place in the upper respiratory passage. Treatment by tracheostomy kept open during sleep, reverses most of the symptoms. The exact site and mechanism of this functional airway obstruction is yet obscure. Guilleminault, Hill, Simmons and Dement (1978) have done fiber optic studies in obstructive sleep apnea (OSA). The most impressive feature found by these authors was the progressive opposition of the lateroposterior pharyngeal walls. Visual observation of the posterior tongue showed that it was not the initiator of the obstructive phenomenon. The collapse of the airway always occured at the onset of inspiration and the pharyngeal obstruction was mismatched with the respiratory cycle. On inspiration the vocal cords abducted widely, then returned to an intermediate position during expiration. The vocal cords exhibited normal inspiratory abduction despite the absence of a normal upward airflow pattern.

SUBJECTS AND METHODS

Fifty seven adult patients were examined and then operated on. The youngest patient was 29 years old, the oldest was 68 years old. Mean age of the patients was 47. Six of the 57 patients were women. All these patients complained of heavy snoring. Forty nine patients complained also of excessive day somnolence, headache and irritability. In 37 patients, members of the family vividly described the sleep disturbances which on evaluation were recognised as sleep apnea episodes. Forty eight patients including the group of 6 women, were obese. The overweight patients (48/57) had 10 to 30 kilos more than their ideal weight (Table 1). All patients underwent preoperative polysomnography. Their mean apnea index (number of apnea per sleep hour) was 60-90 (normal - 5). In forty five patients the polysomnogram revealed obstructive sleep apnea while in 12 patients a mixed sleep apnea was diagnosed with obstructive predominance. All patients were loud snorers and presented with clinical symptomatology typical of obstructive sleep apnea syndrome.

Surgical treatment

UPPP is considered today the preferred technique for many or most patients with OSA. The aim of UPPP is to increase the size of the oropharyngeal isthmus by partial resection of the soft palate without hampering the muscular function in what concerns swallowing, speech and blowing. Fifty seven patients underwent the UPPP as described by Fujita et al (1981) and Simmons et al (1983). When tonsils were present, their removal was an integral part of this procedure even if the tonsils were atrophic and were not considered having a significant contribution to the airway obstruction. Our patients underwent tonsillectomy followed by palatectomy with a margin of 1.5-2 cm. ventral (anterior) the uvula-soft palate junction. The entire thickness of the soft palate is resected including the anterior tonsillar pillar as described by Simmons et al (1983). The palatal line of excision is 1.5-2 cm wide. Our resection stops close to the thick muscular part of the palate, and includes segments of the palatopharyngeal muscle from both sides, a long segment of the muscle of uvula, and few fibers of the levator palati muscle. The posterior tonsillar pillar is pulled forward and a vertical segment of the palatopharyngeal arch is resected. Sufficient mucosa of the posterior pillar is left to approximate the anterior pillar and cover the tonsillar fossa. We stress the importance of excising by submucous dissection an appreciable amount of the palatopharyngeal muscle. In our technique we proceed to a rectangular shaped resection of the soft palate in which we try to achieve symmetrical right angled corners. In our experience, by this procedure, we avoid the stenosis of the nasopharynx which may appear when an ovoid cut is performed (Fig. 1).

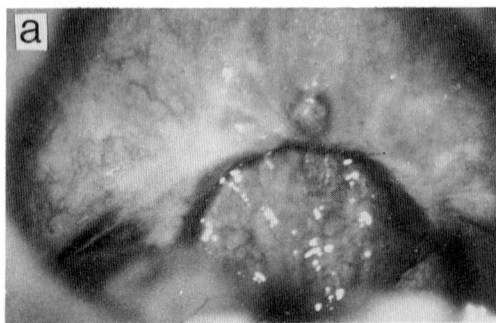
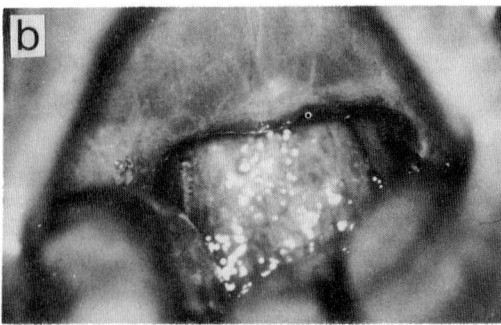

Fig. 1.a. Soft palate after UPPP with semicircular excision.
Fig. 1.b. Soft palate after UPPP with rectangular shaped excision.

It is of importance that closure of the palate, mucosa to mucosa, should be done laterally to preserve the rectangular shape of the resected palate. Four of our patients in whom nasal septal deformity and/or turbinate hypertrophy was noted underwent nasal septoplasty combined with partial resection of the inferior turbinae. None of the patients gained relief neither from snoring nor from OSA, and all were referred for UPPP. After this procedure they were relieved of snoring. The OSA was much improved in these patients. Twelve patients had surgically absent tonsils. They underwent UPPP with excision of the mucosa of the tonsillar fossa and few of the underlying muscle fibers. As described, the rest of the anterior and posterior pillars were sutured over the raw operated tonsillar fossa. It is good to remember that tension in the region of the sutures must be avoided.

RESULTS (Table 2)

Snoring was eliminated in 72% of patients. Day somnolence was eliminated in 69% and improved in another 22% of the patients. According to the family impression the apneas which were vividly described preoperatively were no more noticed in 62% of the patients, improved in 25% and unchanged in 13%. Because of economic problems and patient compliance we could not undertake a randomised post operative polysomnogram study. In twelve patients in whom a preoperative mixed sleep apnea was diagnosed by polysomnogram, the clinical signs of sleep apnea were not cured. In this group snoring was eliminated but other clinical symptoms such as day somnolence, morning tiredness, irritability and headaches, persisted. Polysomnograms done in eight of these patients revealed 10-30 episodes of apnea per hour of sleep. In four patients the polysomnogram revealed only a partial improvement.

Complications

The postoperative management is similar to that of tonsillectomy.
Pain - All fifty seven patients suffered from considerable pain 5 to 7 days after the operation. It is of interest to note that antibiotics shortened this period as shown by Telian et al (1986) and Finkelstein et al (1987).
Infection - Ten patients had mild fever for 2-3 days. A banal wound infection was observed in the region of the tonsillar bed.
Hydration - All our patients received intravenous hydration for 4-5 days because it was painful to swallow.
Bleeding - In three patients a postoperative bleeding developed. In one from the middle of the soft palate (uvular artery). In another two from the tonsillar bed.
Nasal regurgitation - All fifty seven patients had nasal regurgitation which obviated good oral hydration through the first 5-7 post operative days. All patients began to drink and swallow soft diet beginning from the 5th to 7th day. Infrequent nasal regurgitation for liquids lasted up to 6 months.
Hypernasal speech - lasted 7-14 days. Six weeks after operation none of our patients had hypernasality noticeable as to interfere with his social obligations. Teachers and lawyers returned to their previous work without disturbances.
Middle ear cleft problems - In all fifty seven patients postoperatively, retraction of both pars tensa and pars flaccida was observed and in some of the patients congestion and focal hemorrhage of the eardrums were noted. Marked negative middle ear pressure was found by tympanometry in both ears as a proof of the Eustachian tube dysfunction as shown by Finkelstein et al (1987).
Blood chemistry - In none of our patients could we find postopertive blood biochemical disturbances.

Late sequelae

Patients were periodically examined during 3-8 months after surgery.
Hypernasality - Mild hypernasality which did not cause social disturbances was permanent in four patients.
Phonetic disturbances - In seven patients there were phonetic changes in the pronounciation of the consonants "R" and "Ch" which have a special roughness in the Hebrew language.
Nasal regurgitation - On nasendoscopic examination mild regurgitation could be found in 41% of the patients. In most of the cases the patient was not aware of this subclinical sequela.

Sneezing - 47% of the operated patients suffered from uncontrollable sneezing. This disturbance can sometimes be a social disturbing phenomenon and in fact demonstrates a reduced resistance of velo-pharyngeal and lingual palatal valves.

Social and familial improvements

All patients were fully employed two to three months after surgery. The low level of confidence in their capabilities which appeared preoperative in some of our patients disappeared after the operation when they found themselves able to handle their work, while their day time fatigue and sleepiness disappeared. Domestic problems calmed down when the loud snoring which was a long lasting nightmare was eliminated. Obesity may affect the severity of the syndrome, but in our experience only few patients had improved their condition after an exhausting and substantial weight loss. It is our opinion that weight loss may not cure sleep apnea syndrome but it is an important adjuvant and is to be considered before proceeding to the UPPP.

None of our patients necessitated tracheostomy for alleviating his symptoms.

CONCLUSION

The value of all-night polysomnogram should be emphasised. Only via this evaluation can sleep apnea be documented, and tis type assessed. UPPP is perhaps not the final answer to OSA but it is today the recommended procedure for eliminating loud snoring. Post operative benefits versus the mild side effects indicate that UPPP is a valid treatment which alleviates or eliminates symptoms in more than 80% of our patients. The rectangular shaped incision and suture of the palate seems to us preferable to the ovoid classic incision which induces palatal stenosis.

Table 1. Overweight patients

Overweight	M	F
5 - 10 Kg	8	2
10 - 15 Kg	20	3
15 - 20 Kg	12	1
20 - 30 Kg	2	-
No. of patients	42	6

Table 2. Results after UPPP (57 patients)

	Eliminated	Improved	Unchanged
Snoring	72%	19%	9%
Morning tiredness	62%	25%	13%
Headache	69%	22%	9%
Day somnolence	69%	22%	9%

REFERENCES

Finkelstein Y., Talmi Y., Zohar Y., Rubel Y., Laurian N. (1987): Can uvulo-palato-pharyngoplasty be harmful to Eustachian tube function? Acta Otolaryngol (Stock). 103.

Fujita A.S., Conway W., Zorick F. et al (1981): Surgical correction of anatomic abnormalities in obstructive sleep apnea syndrome. Otolaryngol Head Neck Surg. 89, 923-934.

Guilleminault C., Hill M.W., Simmons F.B., Dement W.C. (1978): Obstructive sleep apnea: Electromyographic and Fiberoptic Studies. Experimental Neurology,

62, 48-67.
Simmons F.B., Guilleminault C., Silvestri R. (1983): Snoring and some obstructive sleep apnea can be cured by oropharyngeal surgery. <u>Arch Otolaryngol</u> 109, 503-507.
Telian S.A., Handler S.D., Baranak C.C., Wetmore R.F., Potsic W.P. (1986): The effect of antibiotic therapy on recovery after tonsillectomy in children. <u>Arch Otolaryngol. Head Neck Surg.</u> 112, 610-615.

RESUMÉ

L'apnée obstructive de sommeil est un desordre qui a des répercussions métaboliques. respiratoires et cardio-vasculaires. C'est un fait accepté que les hypertrophies anatomiques de lumen oropharyngien, le collapse de la langue, l'hypotonicité du voile du palais et des muscles oropharyngiens sont une cause de l'obstruction des voies aeriennes. Dan cet article nous reportons les observations de 57 malades, ayant subi une UPPP dans notre service depuis l'annee 1985. Nous avons utilisé une modification chirurgicale originelle de l'UPPP qui d'après notre expérience previent les stenoses du palais. La plupart de nos malades ont été libérés du ronflement qui entrainaient des problemes sociaux et familiaux. Dans une large proportion nous les avons aussi libérés des phenomènes respiratoires cliniques. Dans notre article nous voulons presenter les complications post-operatives et les sequelles tardives.

Uvulopalatopharyngoplasty sequelae and velopharyngeal valve mechanism

Y. Finkelstein, Y. Talmi and Y. Zohar

Department of Otolaryngology, Golda Medical Center, Hasharon Hospital, 7 Keren Kayemet Street, Petach Tikva 49372, Israel

ABSTRACT

Twentyseven patients undergoing uvulopalatopharyngoplasty were subjected to a comprehensive study of the velopharyngeal activities before and after surger. The patients were assessed by a peroral examination and nasendoscopy of the velopharyngeal valve during speech and non phonetic activities. New, yet unreported, findings were observed and are presented. A significant correlation was found between the postoperative course and the velopharyngeal closure patterns classified as coronal, circular, circular with passavant ridge and saggital. Our results stress the necessity of individually tailored surgical technique for each patient.

KEY WORDS

Nasendoscopy, Obstructive Sleep Apnea, Soft Palate, Uvulopalatopharyngoplasty, Uvula, Velopharyngeal valve.

INTRODUCTION

The aim of the uvulopalatopharyngoplasty (UPPP) operation is to increase the size of the oropharyngeal isthmus by partial resection of the soft palate, without hampering the active muscular action. The velopharyngeal (VP) valve integration is essential for normal speech and for non speech activities as swallowing, whistling and blowing. There are considerable variations in the size, shape and mobility of the structures forming the velopharyngeal valve (VPV). In our investigation the mechanism of VP valving in patients undergoing UPPP for Obstructive Sleep Apnea (OSAS) has been studied before and after surgery. Every patient's complaint was noted in the post operative course and correlated with a study of the readaptation capability of the VPV, in order to answer the following questions: 1) How the different closure patterns of the VPV as described by Skolnick et al (1973) influence the post operative course 2) Does the partial resection of the soft palate elicit forming a compensatory mechanism of the VPV 3) Does the partial resection of the muscularis uvulae influence the VPV mechanism?

PATIENTS AND METHODS

27 patients undergoing UPPP were included in the study (Table 1). In all of them OSAS or severe snoring were established by polysomnographic examination. None of the patients had VPV abnormality. All underwent a careful pre-and post-operative direct VPV nasendoscopy during speech and non speech activities. The endoscopic examination was performed by using the flexible Olympus ENF fiberscope type P. They were asked to produce vowels, consonants and connected speech according to a standard sample as described by Sprintzen et al (1977). The non phonetic tasks included dry swallowing, water swallowing, and forced blowing into an obstructed catheter. The patterns of valving were categorized as coronal, sagittal, circular and circular with Passavant ridge according to the classification of Skolnick et al (1973). All the patients underwent the identical surgical technique regardless of the preoperative endoscopic examination.

RESULTS AND DISCUSSION

Patients' profile and closure patterns are presented in Table 1. In the first post

Table 1. Patient profiles and post operative data

VPV closure pattern	Coronal	Circular	Circular & Passavant	Saggital	Total non coronal
No. Pat	17	4	4	2	10
F/M	4/13	/4	/4	1/1	
Age (years)/Medium range	33-56/47	51-56/53	40-66/51.5	50.5	52
Follow up (month) Medium range	3-19/11.5	3-16/10	5-13/10	7-18/12.5	10
Reflux on drinking	2 (28%)	-	-	-	-
Reflux on leaning over a tap	11 (65%)	1	-	1	2 (20%)
Inability to withold sneeze	8 (47%)	-	1	-	1 (10%)
Non specific speech alteration	3 (18%)	-	-	-	-
Alteration of uvular fricatives	7 (41%)	1	1	1	3 (30%)
Mild Hypernasal resonance	2 (12%)	-	-	-	-
Nasal escape on forced blowing	2 (12%)	-	2	-	2 (20%)

surgical week, when attempting to swallow some water all the patients of the coronal group and 6 patients from the other groups suffered from clinical nasal regurgitation. 4 patients of the coronal group and one patient of the circular group presented mild-hypernasal resonance. In all patients, on nasendoscopic examination, the velum palatum demonstrated marked edema and hypermia. The edema and sometimes the hyperemia were lateral as well as along the levator folds up to the Eustachain tubes orifices including the Torus Tubari as described by the authors (1987). On swallowing and phonation in all patients of the coronal pattern limited motion of the velum was seen, while in the other patient groups this was not observed. All patients demonstrated a positive Bubbles sign even in empty deglutition, and reflux on water deglutition. In all but two of the patients with the coronal pattern the reflux was observed in the middle third of the VPV. In these two patients resting assimetry of VPV contour was noted (Table 2) and the reflux was observed in the narrow portal side (lateral portion). In all patients of the other groups the pattern of closure mechanism remained essentially as before. On phonation all the patients of all groups presented a hesitant and restricted motion. During the first post operative 3 months, the readaptation process of the VPV was highly dynamic, and the more definite results of the operation were revealed.

In ten of the patients the VPV function became smoother and reflux of liquids disappeared within 6 or 9 post operative months. The post operative course was better in the non coronal pattern patients. During repeated nasendoscopic examinations the readaptation process of the VPV was clearly seen. The level of closure became higher and the uvular ridge received its final form. Patients' complaints are summarized in Table 1. It is seen that the long term post operative course is more problematic in the patients with the coronal pattern. The disturbances of the non phonetic tasks of the VPV were predominant while speech alterations were usually negligible. These phenomena can be explained by the basically different mechanism of function of the VPV in the phonetic and non phonetic tasks as demonstrated also by Skolnick et al (1975). During speech, the medial movement of the lateral pharyngeal waslls is located in the nasopharyngeal area generally at the level of the hard palate, while during swallowing, medial movement of entire lateral pharyngeal wall occurs. We think that this different mechanism suggests that the VPV must resist during non speech activities a higher gradient of pressure than during speech. The UPPP operation probably results in some limitation of the velar movement as well as in reduced bulk. Its contribution to the closure mechanism is affected by the operation and the resistance to the pressure gradient decreased. In the coronal pattern patients the contribution of

Table 2. Patient nasendoscopic follow up. Mild movement of a pharyngeal wall ↑. Marked movement ▲.
* VPV appearance at rest ** VPV at maximum closure A – Adenoids PPW – posterior pharyngeal wall APW – anterior pharyngeal wall

	Coronal Pattern		Circular pattern	Circular & Passavant pattern	Saggital pattern
	Preoperative	Post operative			
No change of closure pattern		6 (35%)	4 (100%)	4 (100%)	2 (100%)
Flattening of uvular ridge		10 (60%)	1 (25%)		
Increased contribution of LPW to closure	PPW ** APW	5 (30%) **			
APW PPW movement as one	PPW * APW	3 (18%) *			
Subclinical reflux of liquids in midline		10 (60%)	1 (25%)		
Assimetry of closure and reflux of liquids on ipsilatrial portal		2 (12%) * * A			
Midline Bubbles sign positive: on forced blowing		2 (12%)	3 (75%)	2 (50%)	
on /SH/		1 (6%)			

the velum to the VPV closure is obviously greater than in other groups, hence their more significant alteration of VPV mechanism. The nasendoscopic examination did not reveal any change of the pattern of VPV closure in the circular and sagittal group (Table 2). In 5 patients (30%) of the coronal group an increased contribution of the lateral pharyngeal walls to the closure was observed. Besides the gradually increased velar motion this new pattern clearly emerged as the follow up continued. The conclusion from these observations is that the lateral pharyngeal walls movement can be augmented and that it is not just the result of a postoperatively, now exposed, lateral wall movement, preoperatively disguised by the former bulk movement of the velum. This conclusion supports the idea that VPV closure can be improved by increasing the contribution of the lateral pharyngeal walls. We did not observe in any case a denovo formation of Passavant's ridge. No support can therefore be given to the concept of Passavant's ridge as a compensatory structure. The nasal reflux of liquids is a major disturbance in these patients, predominant in the coronal pattern group. Nasendoscopy revealed that the reflux is in the center of the VPV closure where the uvular ridge contacts the posterior pharyngeal wall. In 2 patients (Table 2) an assimetry of the VPV was found in rest and reflux on drinking in the middle and in the nar ow portal side was observed. An interesting observation is that in 10 patients (60%) of the coronal pattern group and one patient of the circular pattern group a mild reflux was observed in the midpoint which passed unnoticed by the patients and therefore was defined as a "subclinical reflux". 11 patients (75%) from the coronal group and 2 patients (20%) of the other groups reported a nasal reflux when bending over a sink to drink tap water. This complaint was also not noted before. From these findings and the observation on nasendoscopy of the flattening of the uvular ridge (Table 2) derives that the most important function of the muscularis uvulae is not in speech but in drinking water while bending over. In this position the naso-pharynx is at the same or at a lower level than the oropharynx contradictory to the ordinary position held while drinking. In this position the antero-posterior

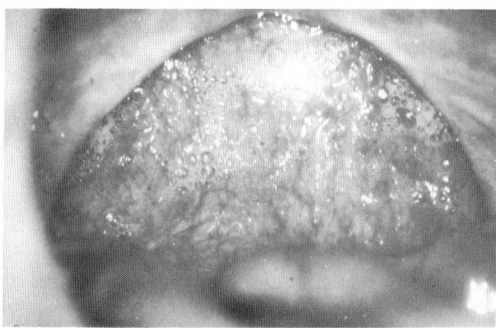 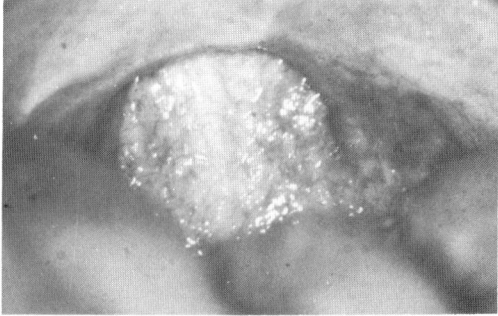

Fig. 1: A peroral appeparnace of the soft palate after UPPP. A coronal pattern (right), a circular pattern (left) were observed on nasoendoscopy.

diameter of the nasopharynx increases. 8 patients (47%) of the coronal pattern group and one of the other groups complained of an inability to withhold a sneeze. We think that this complaint can be explained by the affected Tongue-Palatal valve described by Moll (1965). In witholding a sneeze we force closed the VPV and Tongue Palate isthmus and then we gradually release them. The VPV closes the pharynx from above, and the Tongue-palatal valve which is formed mainly by the activity of the palatoglossus as shown by Fritzell (1969) located in the anterior tonsillar pillar, approximates the base of the tongue and the velum to separate the oral cavity behind the oropharynx. This valve is generally utilized during sucking activity and becomes, after the UPPP operation lateralized and tensed (Fig. 1). Three patients (18%) of the coronal group and their family reported a non specific change of their voice quality but with no possibility to define this change. Our patients' complaints can support the modern view of the VPV function according to which, the vertical aspects of closure and the tubal characteristics of VP valving influence speech. According to McWilliams and Bradely (1965) the speech appears to be less adequate as the vertical valving dimension shortens. In 7 (41%) patients of the coronal group and 3 (30%) of the other groups, uvular fricatives /r/ and /ch/ were changed to be alveolar or dental. Our findings can be explained by the characteristics of the Hebrew as a Semitic language. Before the operation the base of the bongue and the velum moved posteriorly toward the posterior pharyngeal wall and the velum rolled. After the UPPP operation the base of tongue moves anteriorly towards the palate and the /r/ became alveolar and flat. The palatine /ch/ of the Semitic language is uvular or pharyngeal and after the operation became velar as the European. Two patients of the coronal group and 2 of the other groups presented mild audible nasal escape during forced blowing. On nasendoscopic examination the Bubbles sign was positive in the midline of the VPV. In the post operative peroral examination generally the oropharynx of the coronal pattern patients is flat and larger relatively to the oropharynx and soft palate of the circular pattern patients (Fig. 1). The limitation of velar movement caused by the operation is better compensated in the circular and sagittal groups than in the coronal group. These findings with the observation of the different oropharyngeal shape between these groups support the theory that the different pattern of VP valving first described by Skolnick et al (1973) are due to anatomical variability as perhaps a different insertion of muscles.

CONCLUSION

1) The different closure patterns of the VPV are due to a variable anatomy.
2) The compensatory mechanism is less effective in coronal pattern. 3) The muscularis uvulae is important mainly in drinking. 4) Passavant's ridge is an anatomical variant rather than a compensatory mechanism. 5) The Tongue-Palatal valve is important not only for sucking but also for witholding the sneeze.
6) The dimension of VPV closure influences the speech quality. 7) It is necessary to tailor an individual surgical technique for each patient undergoing UPPP operation.

REFERENCES

Finkelstein Y., Talmi Y., Zohar Y., Rubel Y., Laurian N. (1987): Can uvulopalato-pharyngoplasty be harmful to Eustachian tube function? Acta Otolaryngol (Stockh). 103.
Fritzell B. (1969): The velopharyngeal muscles in speech. Acta Otolaryngol. Suppl. 250, 1-77.
McWilliams B.J., Bradley D.P. (1965i): Ratings of Velopharyngeal closure during blosing and speech. Cleft palate J. 2, 46-51.
Moll K.L. (1965): A cineradiographic study of velopharyngeal function in normals during various activities. Cleft palate J. 2, 112-122.
Shprintzen R.J., Rakoff S.L., Skolnick M.L., Lavorato A.S. (1977): Incongruous movements of the velum and lateral pharyngeal walls. Cleft palate J. 14, 148-157.
Skolnick M.L., McCall G.N., Barnes M. (1973): The sphinteric mechanism of velopharyngeal closure. Cleft palate J. 10, 286-305.
Skolnick M.L., Zagzebski J.A., Watkin, K.L. (1975): Two dimensional ultrasonic demonstration of lateral pharyngeal wall movement in real time - a preliminary report. Cleft palate J. 12, 299-303.

SUMMARY

In 27 patients undergoing uvulopalatopharyngoplasty a comprehensive study of the velopharyngeal activities was performed. New, yet unreported, phenomena were observed and are presented. A significant correlation was found between the postoperative course and the velopharyngeal closure patterns. Our results stress the necessity of individually tailored surgical technique for each patient.

RESUME

27 malades qui devaient subir une UPPP ont ete examines par une etude aprofondie perorale et par endoscopie nasale. Des phenomenes postoperatoires nouveaux qui n'ont pas ete observe jusqu'a maintenant, sont communiques dans notre present article. On a trouve une etroite correlation entre la symptomatologie postoperatoire et les differentes formes de fermeture de la valve velopharyngienne. Nos resultats preuvent une technique chirurgicale individuelle pour chaque malade.

Results of uvulopalatopharyngoplasty: an evaluation emphasizing preoperative selection criteria and tailoring technique of the procedure

Ph. van de Heyning, J. Claes, H. Valcke, J. de Roeck, E. Koekelkoren and J. Bru

University Clinic of Antwerp, University of Antwerp, Wilrijkstraat 10, 2520 Edegem, Belgium

ABSTRACT

Résumé.

Parmi les 75 patients se plaignant de ronflements, somnolence durant la journée et du syndrome obstructif lié au sommeil (OSAS), 34 candidats furent retenus pour UPPP sur base de 2 critères: 1. L'endoscopie nasopharyngeale avec manoeuvre de Müller montre un rétrécissement uniquement au niveau du sphincter vélo-pharyngéal, 2. absence de OSAS grave avec désaturation (SaO2) de moins de 40%. Un UPPP avec large résection et sans reconstruction de la luette fut effectué. Une classification de l'OSAS tenant compte de différents paramètres (PSG) est présentée afin d'évaluer l'UPPP. Un succès est obtenu dans 94% de ronflements, 97% de somnolence et 87% d'OSAS. Les auteurs concluent qu'une sélection per-opératoire rigoureuse forme une base solide afin de prévoir un résultat favorable de l'UPPP et ce à condition d'effectuer une résection chirurgicale importante.

Keywords.

Snoring - obstructive sleep apnea syndrome - uvulopalatopharyngoplasty - selection criteria.

INTRODUCTION

Since the first descriptive papers of obstructive sleepapnoea syndrome (OSAS) (Guilleminault, 1976) and the awareness of snoring being a social handicap, different therapeutic managements were proposed (Caldarelli et al, 1985; Moran and Orr, 1985).
A management attracting much attention is uvulopalatopharyngoplasty (UPPP), a procedure that was first introduced by Fujita et al (1981). Many investigators agreed that UPPP could cure or ameliorate snoring and OSAS. Although the UPPP procedure seemed to procure a reliable result for snoring, much less consistent benefits were noted for the OSAS varying from more than 70% success to less than 35% success. It is difficult to predict in which patients the procedure will be beneficial. (Fujita et al, 1985; Sher et al, 1985; Simmons et al, 1983; de Berry de Borrowiecki and Sassin, 1983; Cotton, 1983).
The site of obstruction, as determined by fiberendoscopy with Müller manoeuvre (Sher et al, 1985; Van de Heyning et al, 1986) or with CT scan (Crumley et al, 1987), cephalometric data (Riley et al, 1983; de Berry-Borrowiecki et al, 1985);

percentage of ideal body weight (Fujita et al, 1985) and the degree of OSAS
(Fujita et al, 1981;de Berry-Borrowiecki, 1985) were all parameters to predict
the result of UPPP.
It is clear that different variations of surgical techniques are used
(Fujita et al, 1981; Simmons et al, 1983) and some investigators stressed
the importance of the surgical technique and the extent of resection (Colman
and Rice, 1985; Kimmelman et al, 1985; Iusk, 1986).

Aim of the study.
This study investigates whether it is possible to achieve a high success rate
with UPPP concerning OSAS as well as snoring when patients are selected in a
prospective way on the presence of an obstruction at the velopharyngeal level
as determined by fiber nasopharyngoscopy and Müller manoeuvre (FNMM), and
without an extremely severe OSAS requiring a tracheotomy.

MATERIALS AND METHODS

Patients.
75 patients with complaints of snoring, excessive daytime sleepiness (EDS) and/or
OSAS were investigated by history, body indices, polysomnography with oximetry
(PSG), ENT examination, FNMM and cephalometry.
UPPP was performed on 34 of these patients, age ranging from 35 years to 70 years
(5 women and 29 men). These patients were selected on the presence of obstruction
limited to the velopharyngeal sphincter and not suffering from an extremely severe OSAS.

Site of obstruction.
The tendency of the velopharyngeal sphincter region and the hypopharynx to collapse was evaluated with FNMM, as was first described by de Berry-Borrowiecki
(1978). The patient is positioned in a lateral decubitus. After topical anaesthesia of the nose,a slender fiberoptic endoscope (Olympus BF type 3C3 Ø 2.7mm) is
introduced in one of the nostrils. The endoscope is advanced to the level of the
tongue base. With the mouth closed and the free nostril obstructed, the patient
is asked to inspire forcefully in order to create a negative pharyngeal pressure. (= Müller Manoeuvre, MM). Any tendency to collapse is noted. This MM is
repeated after positioning the fiberoptic into the rhinopharynx to evaluate uvu-
lopharyngeal collapse. The degree of obstruction at each level was recorded following Sher et al. (1985): 1 +: minimal movement of the pharyngeal cross section
towards the center; 2 ++: movement towards the center diminishing cross sectional area of the pharynx by 50%; 3 +++ movement towards the center diminishing
cross sectional area of the pharynx by 75%; 4 ++++: inwards motion obliterating
the airway.
Patients with a collapse of less than 3 + at the level of the velopharyngeal
sphincter or more than 2 + at the level of the hypopharynx, were excluded as
candidates for UPPP.

Polysomnography and OSAS.
PSG during two consecutive nights is performed. Two electro-encephalographic
derivates, electrocardiogram (ECG), electro-oculogram, electromyogram, oro-
nasal airflow, thoracic movements and percutaneous oximetry are recorded.
The patient is monitored all night by video.
Postoperative recordings were performed three months after surgery. PSG is the
only reliable method for evaluating the severity of OSAS and the result of
treatment, as surgical follow-up interviews often do not correspond with the objective data of a PSG (de Berry-Borrowiecki et al, 1985; Cotton, 1983). Many indices can be derived from a PSG such as Apnea Index, hypopnea index, lowest SaO2,
frequency and extent of SaO2 decreases, EEG sleep stages and ECG. Up to now there
is no agreement among investigators which parameter should be selected to determine the severity of OSAS and to which extent they should ameliorate in order to

define a post treatment success. Some suggest the use of a combination of several parameters (Wetmore et al, 1986).
We are reporting results of PSG in a score for the severity of OSAS:
0: the minimal requirements for OSAS are not fulfilled, i.e. a minimum of 30 episodes of apnea with a duration of at least 10 sec.; +: light OSAS in which 95% of the a-or hypopnea periods yield SaO2 of no lower than 80%; ++: moderate OSAS in which 95% of the a-or hypopnea periods yield SaO2 of no less than 60%; +++: severe OSAS in which 95% of the a- or hypopnea periods yield SaO2 of no less than 40%; ++++: extremely severe OSAS with SaO2 decreasing under recording sensibility and accompanied by life threatening arythmias. Patients with OSAS degree IIII are candidates for tracheostomy and are excluded for UPPP.

Surgical technique.
The technique of UPPP used is similar to the modification of Simmons et al. (1983) of the UPPP as first described by Fujita et al (1981). Preoperatively no sedative medication is given. The patient is intubated orally and positioned in Roosen's position. A Dingmann-gag is used. Resection includes the inferior part of the palate, the uvula and both anterior tonsillar pillars with the tonsils if they are still present. The extent of palatal resection is crucial: as much as possible has to be resected without inducing nasopharyngeal incompetence. The bulk of the levator veli palatini, the palatopharyngeal and palatoglossal muscles should remain. This is determined by gently palpating the soft palate parasagitally. It enables to determine a zone of $\pm$ 5mm where the muscular part changes into the mucosal part. The decision whether or not this zone is incorporated into the resection specimen is based on PSG and FNMM. A PSG indicating a moderate or severe OSAS and a FNMM showing total collapse of the velopharyngeal sphincter meet the requirements for a wide tailoring resection. Postoperative light microscopic examination of the specimens provided a feed back for the peroperative estimation of muscle removal. At the midline the uvular muscles are also resected by connecting the parasagittal margins of incision horizontally. Pharyngeal augmentation is achieved by pulling the posterior pillar margin forward to meet the remainders of the anterior pillar margin. This movement should lift the latero-posterior pharyngeal mucosa in a way that transverse wrinkles do not just appear. If this requirement is not met, additional palatopharyngeal muscles can be resected or anterior pillar margins. The resection should never be at the expense of posterior pharyngeal wall mucosa in the upper two thirds of the oropharynx. Otherwise a nasopharyngeal stenosis could develop postoperatively (Katsantonis et al., 1987). Mucosa to mucosa closure is achieved laterally by bites including muscle of anterior and posterior pillar and with double cross knots (poliglycon 2/0) in order to avoid tearing through.
Mucosa to mucosa sutures of the soft palate will not include submucosa or muscle (double cross knots 4/0). The uvula is not reconstructed. The first 24 hours patients are observed in intensive care units, although up to now no major problems have to be mentioned, no tracheotomy had to be performed.

RESULTS

The results of UPPP are reported in terms of snoring (table 1), excessive daytime sleepiness (table 2) and OSAS (table 3). The post-operative evaluation is done three months after UPPP.

TABLE 1.
Results of UPPP on snoring.

Number of patients	Preoperative score*	Postoperative score*	
3	++++	O	
10	++++	+	
2	++++	++	32 success = 94%
7	+++	O	
8	+++	+	
2	++	O	
2°	++++	+++	

*: O: no snoring at all in any position; +: intermittent and discrete snoring only lying on the back; ++: constant and clear snoring only lying on the back; +++: loud or constant snoring in all positions; ++++: socially unacceptable snoring (partners were not sleeping together anymore).

°: In two patients velopharyngeal snoring changed into guttural snoring in a clear and constant way.

TABLE 2.
Results of UPPP on excessive daytime sleepiness.

Number of patients°	Preoperative score*	Postoperative score*	
8	++++	O	
8	++	O	29 success = 97%
11°°	+	O	
2	+++	+	
1°°°	++	++	

* : O: no EDS; +: EDS is noted by the patient; ++: EDS is interfering with dayly activities; +++: dayly activity impossible.

° : 4 patients had no preop. EDS; °°: 3 patients noted postoperatively by their change of alertness that EDS existed preoperatively; °°°: the patient turned out postoperatively to present also narcolepsy.

TABLE 3.
Results of UPPP on OSAS.

Number of patients*	Preoperative score.	Postoperative score.	
1	+++	O	
12	++	O	26 success = 87%
10	+	O	
4	+++	+	
3	+++	++	
1	++	+	

Score: cfr. text.

* : 4 patients had no OSAS.

Complications were limited to one case who received speech therapy for rhinolalia aperta, remaining permanent to some extent. Seven additional patients experienced permanent minor velopharyngeal incompetence. Some liquid leakage through the nose existed when we asked to drink with their head upside down. One case with tendency to nasopharyngeal stenosis was noted.

DISCUSSION

A high success rate of UPPP was achieved for snoring (32/34), EDS (29/30) and OSAS (26/30). This rate is among the highest ever published. The explanation for this high success rate is the combination of the selection procedure and the extended surgical procedure. Both factors proved already to be beneficial for rather high success rates. (Kimmelman et al, 1985; Sher et al, 1985).These results demonstrated that predicting results is possible in a reasonable way. The draw back of this selection is that we have refused patients on the base of our criteria, that might have benefited from this procedure.
Severe OSAS seems to be another relatively unfavourable sign for the results of UPPP surgery, as has been reported by others (de Berry Borrowiecki, 1985). No universal way of interpreting PSG is available and the criteria used for according "success" might bias the results. It should also be noted that although patients are classified as OSAS score 0, sleep apnoea tendency may exist or remain without attaining the minimal requirements for OSAS. The subjective status of the patient underestimates clearly the nocturnal respiratory efficacy and postoperative PSG is necessary.

ABSTRACT

Out of 75 patients with complaints of snoring, daytime sleepiness (EDS) or obstructive sleep apnoea syndrom (OSAS), 34 patients were selected for uvulopalatopharyngoplasty (UPPP) on the basis of two criteria:

1. Fibronasopharyngoscopy with Müller manoeuvre shows only a narrowing on the velopharyngeal level,
2. No excessive severe OSAS with SaO2 decreases under 40%.

An extended surgical UPPP procedure was used.
A classification of OSAS is proposed to evaluate UPPP results, and that takes into account different PSG parameters.
Success rates were 94% of snoring, 97% of EDS and 87% of OSAS.
It is concluded that these pre-operative criteria form a solid basis for predicting the post-operative result, on condition that an extended procedure is used.

References.

Caldarelli, DD., Cartwright RD., Lilie K. (1985) Obstructive Sleep Apnea: variations in surgical management, Laryngoscope 95: 1070-1073.

Colman MF., Rice DH. (1985) A method of determining the correct amount of palatal resection in palatopharyngoplasty. Laryngoscope 95: 609-610

Cotton RT. (1983) Uvulopalatopharyngoplasty, Arch. Otolaryngol., 109:502

Crumley L., Stein M., Golden J., Gamsu G., Dermon S. (1987) Determination of Obstructive Site in Obstructive Sleep Apnea, Laryngoscope 97: 301-308

de Berry Borrowiecki B., Sassin JF. (1983) Surgical Treatment of Sleep Apnea, Arch. Otolaryngol. 109: 508-512.

Fujita S., Conway W., Zorick F. and Roth T. (1981), Surgical Correction of Anatomic Abnormalities in Obstructive Sleep Apnea Syndrome-Uvulopalatopharyngoplasty. Otolaryngol. Head Neck Surg. 89: 923-934

Fujita S., Conway WA., Sicklesteel JM., Wittig RM., Zorick FJ, Roehrs TA., Roth T. (1985) Evaluation of the Effectiveness of uvulopalatopharyngplasty. Laryngoscope 95: 70-74.

Guilleminault C., Tilkian A. and Dement WC., (1976) The Sleep Apnea Syndromes, Ann. Rev. Med., 27: 465-484.

Katsantonis P., Friedman WH., Krebs FJ., Walsh JK, (1987), Nasopharyngeal complications following uvulo-palatopharyngoplasty, Laryngoscope 97: 309-314

Kimmelman CP., Levine SB, Shore ET., Millman RP. (1985) Uvulopalatopharyngoplasty: A comparison of two techniques. Laryngoscope 95: 1488-1490.

Lusk P. (1986) Accurate Measurement of Soft Palate Resection during uvulopharyngopalatoplasty, Laryngoscope 96: 697-698.

Moran WB., Orr WC (1985) Diagnosis and Management of Obstructive Sleep Apnea, Arch. Otolaryngol., 111: 650-658.

Riley R., Guilleminault C., Herran J. and Powell N. (1983) Cephalometric Analysis and Flow-Volume Loops in Obstructive Sleep Apnea Patients, Raven Press, Sleep, 6(4): 303-311.

Sher KE., Thorpy MJ, Spielman AJ, Shprintzen RJ, Burack B., McGregor PA. (1985) Predictive Value of Müller Maneuver in Selection of Patients for uvulopalatopharyngoplasty. Laryngoscope 95: 1483-1486.

Van de Heyning PH., Claes J. and De Roeck J. (1986) Endoscopic Evaluation and Video Monitoring of Obstructive Sleep Apnea Syndrome, In: Endoscopy in ENT (Ed. P.A.R. Clement).

Wetmore SJ., Scrima L., Snydermand NL., Hiller FC (1986) Postoperative Evaluation of Sleep Apnea after uvulopalatopharyngoplasty. Laryngoscope 96: 738-741.

Simmons FB., Guilleminault C. and Silvestri R. (1983) Snoring, and some obstructive sleepapnea, can be cured by oropharyngeal surgery. Arch. Otolaryngol. 109: 503-507.

Clinical results in 790 cases of operated chronic rhonchopathy

C.H. Chouard, B. Meyer and F. Chabolle

Hôpital Saint-Antoine, Service ORL, 184 rue du faubourg, Saint-Antoine, 75012 Paris, France

SUMMARY

We report the results obtained by uvulopalatopharyngoplasty, in 790 cases of chronical rhonchopathy. In every case, snoring was present symptom. It was more or less associated with other symptoms of disease.

The results, generally very satisfactoring are studied according do different symptoms taking account of morphological factors which usually increase the stage of the disease. Obesity, macroglossia, retrognathy are abnormalities which decrease the rate of total recovery by means of the only surgery.

KEYWORDS :

Snoring - Clinical Results - Surgery -

Despite the fact that from June 85 to June 87, 790 cases of chronic rhonchopathy have benefited from Uvulo-Palato-Plasty (UPP), we only report there the statistical study of the clinical results we obtained in our first 210 cases between June 85 and September 86. The whole series has been operated on using always the same technic. As a consequence the results reported there may be considered as a faithful representation of our total experience.

This technic, consists in a large resection of the soft palate, the superior limits of which is delimited by the flexion of the soft palate during the pronounciation of the phonem"A". This resection has been carried out in every cases. The percentage of cases in wich this UPP has been limited to the soft palate or associated to tonsillectomy, and / or rhinoseptoplasty is described on Table 1.

These general results include also our cases of sleep apneas syndrome, the particular results of which are described in an other paper.

TABLE 1

UPP only	**50%**
UPP + tonsillectomy	**24%**
UPP + rhinoseptoplasty	**16%**
UPP + tonsillectomy + rhinoseptoplasty	**10%**

Following tables describe the clinical results and the complications on the third month of the surgery. <u>Slight</u> significates no spontaneous complaint. On the contrary <u>important</u> significates large disturbance. <u>NP</u> significates preoperatively non precised. <u>NR</u> significates our ignorance due to the fact that the patient neglected to come back on the third month or to respond to the questionnary which we sent to him.

In Table 2 snoring has been appreciated following the descriptions of the patient and / or his bed partner. Rhinolalia is considered as slight when it appears only in some special phonems encountered in spanish or arabian languages, or as important when it appears in the current conversation. Regurgitation is considered as slight when it consist in slight sensation of liquids in the posterior part of the nasal cavity in case of rapid deglutition, but whithout outside emission. It is considered as important when this outside emission appears. Paresthesia are due to the changes in the sensibility of the new pharynx and frequently need for more than 3 months to totally disappear.

TABLE 2

	IMPORTANT	SLIGHT	ABSENT	NP/NP
SNORING	5%	16%	55%	24%
RHINOLALIA	4%	9%	63%	24%
REGURGITATION	3%	10%	63%	24%
PARESTHESIA	3%	12%	61%	24%

On must underline that regurgitation and rhinolalia are also greatly improved by time. Actually our whole series of 790 cases presents only 6 cases (less than 1%) of important rhinolalia and regurgitation. But these complications are sufficiently compatible with a normal life to have led these patients to refuse the posterior palatoplasty which has been eventually proposed.

Table 3 represents the results on some clinical data. Apneas and multiple awakes during sleep have been mostly appreciated by the patient (or his bed partner) descriptions, a few of them (10%) being observed by polysomnography.

TABLE 3

	IMPORTANT		SLIGHT		ABSENT		NP/NR	
	PRE	POST	PRE	POST	PRE	POST	PRE	POST
Apneas and/or multiple awake	3%	0.5%	28%	2%	60%	73%	9%	24%
Morning headache	5%	0%	24%	1%	62%	75%	9%	24%
Morning asthenia	6%	1%	51%	3%	33%	72%	10%	24%

We had a particular attention to the daily sleepiness, specially in case of driving a car. These results are reported in Table 4.

TABLE 4

	IMPORTANT	SLIGHT	ABSENT	NP/NP
PRE General	37%	34%	20%	9%
including driving a car	9%	27%	55%	9%
POST	1%	5%	70%	24%

We tried to understand the relationship between these uncomplete improvements or failures and the existence of risks factors. The frequency of these factors is reported in Table 5.

TABLE 5

	ABSENT	SLIGHT	IMPORTANT	NP
RETROGNATH.	68%	13%	6%	
TONGUE HYPER.	65%	15%	7%	13%
NASAL PATH.	36%	24%	27%	
OBESITY	68%		20%	12%

The relation between the most important of them, obesity, and the disparition of snoring is reported in Table 6

TABLE 6

	TOTAL	NORMAL	OBESITY	NP
PRE-OPERAT.	210	68%	20%	12%
TOTAL DISAPPEAR.	55%	40%	10%	5%
SLIGHT PERSISTANCE	16%	10%	3%	3%
FAILURE	5%	2%	2%	1%
NR	24%	16%	5%	3%

On may wonder about the great number of NR patients. Are they failure or success ? The Table 7 reports the relationship between the snoring clinical results and the number of associatated risk factors. It allows to think that the members of the NR group perhaps are not all failures.

TABLE 7

	TOTAL	0 FACTOR	1 FACTORS	2 FACTORS	3 FACTORS	NP
PRE-OPER.	210	23%	45%	4%	6%	12%
SNORING DISAPPEAR.	55%	13%	25%	7%	4%	6%
SLIGHT PERSISTANCE	16%	2%	9%	2%	0,5%	2%
FAILURE	5%	0,5%	2%	1%	0,5%	0%
NR	24%	7%	9%	3%	1%	4%

Partial rejection of palate (PRP) as surgical treatment of OSAS

E. Perelló, P. Quesada, J. Pedro-Botet and A. Roca

Residencia Valle Hebrón, Barcelona, Spain

Over an amount of 550 patients of OSAS we have operated since 1975 40 patients who did not improve with the hypocaloric diet.

The surgical procedure consists in an arciform incision of the soft palate near the junction of the bony palate with the soft palate. We resect near all the oral mucosa of the soft palate and all the accessory salivary glands, and adipose tissue, and conjunctive tissue, respecting the muscles of the soft palate and the nasal mucosa. Together with this piece we resect completely the uvula. Then we suture with catgut, the border of the nasal mucosa to the incision.

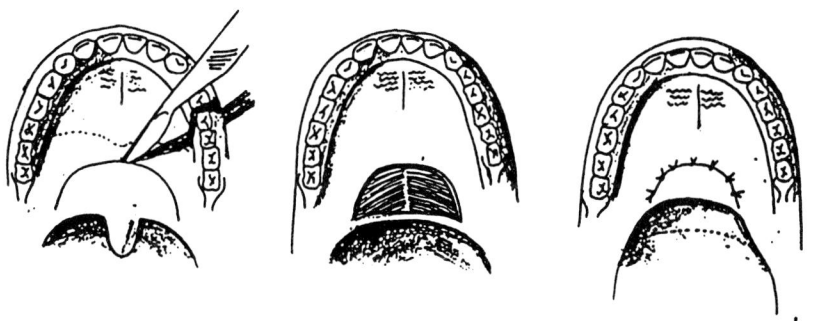

We have never had complications (as bleeding, infections, stenosis, etc.) as described with other techniques.

The snoring has disappeared in a 95% of the cases and in the other 5% it has improved.

The polygraphic studies demonstrate a healing in a 86% of the cases and a considerable improvement in the other 14%.

We prefer the name of P.R.P. instead of U.P.P.P. because the last one makes a semantic confusion with the surgical procedures for rinolalia and cleft palate.

REFERENCES :

1 - QUESADA, P., PEDRO-BOTET, J., FUENTES OTERO, J.J. y PERELLO, E. (1977) "Resección parcial del paladar blando como tratamiento del síndrome de hipersomnia y respiración periódica en los obesos". ORL Dips 5:81.

2 - QUESADA, P., PERELLO, E., PEDRO-BOTET, J. y ROCA, A. (1978) "Traitment chirurgical du syndrome de Pickwick". Comptes rendus des scéances. 75eme. Congrès de la Société Française d'O.R.L. et Patologie Cervico-Faciale. Paris. Libr. Arnette. pág. 395-399 y 61-63.

3 - QUESADA, P., PEDRO-BOTET, J., FUENTES, E. y PERELLO, E. (1979) "Resección del paladar blando como tratamiento del síndrome de hipersomnia y respiración periódica en los obesos". O.R.L. Española. 2, 119.

4 - PERELLO, E., PERELLO, J., (1980) "Intranasal Acoustic Presure in Palate Pathology". Proceedings XVIII Congress of IALP. Washington D.C. 1:237.

5 - PERELLO, E., QUESADA, P., PEDRO-BOTET, J., y ROCA, A. (1981) "Surgical treatment of the Pickwickian syndrome and allied syndromes (obstructive apnea sleep syndrome". Abstracts XII World Congress of O.R.L. Budapest. 542:123.

RESUME

Resection partielle du palais (RPP) comme traitement chirurgical du OSAS. Dr. E.Perelló, Dr. P.Quesada, Dr. J.Pedro-Botet, Dr. A.Roca. Residencia Valle Hebrón. Barcelona. Espagne.

Sur un total de 550 patients de OSAS on a opéré depuis 1975, 40 malades qui n'avaient pas amélioré avec la diete hypocalorique. L'operation consiste en une résection partielle du voile du palais de façon a l'amincir et le racourcir.

Les ronflements on disparut dans un 95% des cas, et dans l'autre 5% ils se sont amélioré.

L'étude poligraphique démontre une guérison dans un 86% des cas et dans l'autre 14% une notable amélioration.

Anesthesia for snoring surgery: methods and techniques, problems and risk factors

J.M. de Larminat, C. Boucherez, P. Brard, L. Naccache and S. Bouclier

Département d'Anesthésie, Réanimation de l'Hôpital Saint-Antoine, 184 rue du faubourg Saint-Antoine, 75012 Paris, France

SUMMARY :

Surgery for snoring was performed on 500 patients at the Saint-Antoine Hospital, either using local anesthesia or general anesthesia with intubation and carried out in such a manner as to be rapidly reversible. The main problems encountered were connected with the type of patient (often aged and/or pathological patients ; patients for whom intubation was difficult), the frequency of unforeseen prolongations of the surgery (difficult haemostasis) and/or repeated surgery (secondary bleeding) under anesthesiological conditions which were then more difficult. The potential anesthesiological risk, even greater due to these eventual problems, obviously requires great care in indicating this type of surgery.

KEYWORDS :

Anesthesia - Snoring : Surgery - Sleep Apnea Syndrome : Surgery Surgery inside of the mouth - Difficult intubation -

In the absence of sufficient bibliographical references, the methods and techniques of ANESTHESIA practiced in the ENT unit of the Saint-Antoine Hospital to allow SURGERY for SNORING (S.S.) were very largely inspired by those chosen for TONSILECTOMY in the adult (4) (6).

These two kinds of surgery, morevoer which are often associated, in fact have a common characteristic : the endobuccal operative field, near the aero-digestive junction, directly involves the respiratory aerial tract (air-way). In addition, it is susceptible to bleed immediately and/or secondarily, in a non-negligible manner. This characteristic influences, in an essential manner, the choice of the anesthesia methods and techniques.

However, there is a capital anesthesiological difference between simple tonsilectomy and surgery for snoring : rhonchopathic patients, unlike classical tonsilectomy patients, are rarely young A.S.A. class I and II subjects, but are frequently elderly patients, rather often subject to associated pathologies and/or sometimes difficult to provide intubation for.

Anesthesia for surgery for snoring is thus faced with particular problems connected not only with the operation itself but also, and mainly, with the kind of patient.

These problems also added risk factors.

It is especially the constraints which result from these problems which give anesthesia given for this kind of surgery a rather specific profile.

A - METHODS AND TECHNIQUES developed

- Isolated uvulopalatopharyngoplasty (UPPP), or associated with a tonsilectomy, can be performed using LOCAL ANESTHESIA (L. A.) or GENERAL ANESTHESIA (G. A.). It is exception for local anesthesia alone to be used to perform simultaneously a complementary septoplasty.

- The UPPP, with or without a tonsilectomy, associated to a SEPTOPLASTY, is thus performed, for the great majority of the cases, using GENERAL ANESTHESIA.

- Surgery for SLEEP APNEA, at least when it makes use of these techniques, is usually performed using GENERAL ANESTHESIA.

Whether the anesthesia is LOCAL or GENERAL :
. The CAREFUL and COMPLETE PRE-OPERATIVE, CLINICAL and PARACLINICAL EXAMINATION is the same, involving particularly and amongt other factors :

- Clinical and/or biological alterations in haemostasis, which are an absolute contra-indication for this surgery.

- Cardio-vascular, particularly coronary, disorders, notably susceptible of preventing local adrenalin infiltrations.

- Allergies, requiring appropriate pre, per and post-operative precautions (2).

- Hyperthyroid conditions, and all the concomitant complications, also, in principle, eliminating the possibility of adrenalin infiltration.

- The recent administration of I.M.A.O. drugs, which will require that the surgery be postponed for all cases.

. Immediate post-operative monitoring, in the recovery room, and secondarily, in the hospital room, must be as painstaking after LA as after GA.

. Only simple UPPP surgery, without associated tonsilectomy or septoplasty and performed using LOCAL anesthesia can allow the patients to be ambulatory, after supervision during several hours in the intensive-care awaking room.

I - LOCAL ANESTHESIA

- This is preferred, whenever possible, since it is statistically considered (1) to present a lower POTENTIAL RISK than general anesthesia (5).

Thus, for the 500 rhonchopathic patients operated on at the Saint-Antoine Hospital between May 1985 and January 1987, 367 of them, that is, 73%, received local anesthesia.

- The surgery, in this case, was performed as when simple tonsilectomy is involved (4) :

a) On a patient having received a narcotic drug last night, and, eventually, a mild premedication in the form of an intra-venous injection of an anxiolytic drug, and if possible of a vagolytic drug.

The advisibility of such a premedication can, however, be discussed :

As for dental surgery, it is desirable, in fact, for the patients to keep his TOTAL SELF CONTROL, in order to COOPERATE with the surgeon, and in order to avoid inhalation of saliva.

Moreover :

- The vagolytic drug may increase the tachycardy induced by infiltrated adrenalin, and really sometimes does increase it.

- The anxiolytic drug may induce orthostatic hypotension in a such half-sitting patient, and really sometimes does induce it.

That is why at the St. Antoine Hospital patient, in most of the cases, don't receive any more intraveinous premedication before this surgery.

b) Taking particular precautions :

in order, if necessary, to cope, under the best conditions and optimal deadlines, with any situation of distress during this endobuccal surgery, it is desirable :

- that a PERFUSION of isotonic serum connected to a peripheral venous route, having SUFFICIENT CALIBRE be installed, in order to deal with any eventuality, notably haemorrhage.

- that blood pressure as well as the electrocardioscocopic curve be monitored.

- LOCAL ANESTHESIA is given first by means of contact using VISQUOUS LIDOCAINE, then by INFILTRATION of LIDOCAINE at 1 p. 100, ADRENALIN at 0.5 p. 100,000 unless contra-indicated. For reasons of safety, no more than 0,5ml Kg-1 of this solution can be used.

— A CAPITAL POINT must be emphasised, which must influence the INDICATION FOR LOCAL ANESTHESIA :

. When the persistance, or the post-operative recurrence, of bleeding requires RENEWED SURGERY, this cannot be performed, in the great majority of the cases, except using GENERAL ANESTHESIA, in order to perform, by virtue of a larger exposure of the surgical field, a surgical haemostasis which had already been found to be difficult.

. This is why it would be unwise to perform this kind of surgery using local anesthesia SIMPLY BECAUSE of a MAJOUR COUNTER-INDICATION TO GENERAL ANESTHESIA :

> — Thus, LOCAL ANESTHESIA cannot, especially in the presence of a non-vital surgical indication, be considered here as a RECOURSE when the RISK OF GENERAL ANESTHESIA appears to be TOO MUCH IMPORTANT.

. Moreover, this is an additional reason for performing such surgery, using local anesthesia, only on patients who have been STRICTLY FASTING for at least six hours.

II - GENERAL ANESTHESIA

— This is performed in the classical manner, but responds, in particular to the following principles :

> 1) Account taken of the site of the surgery and the risk of haemorrhage, ENDOTRACHEAL INTUBATION with A CUFFED TUBE must be SYSTEMATIC.

— This intubation can be, depending on the motivated request of the operator, either ORO or NASO-TRACHEAL.

> 2) The choice of the anesthetic drugs and their administration doses, account taken of their pharmacokinetics, must have as an objective the providing of an anesthesia which is RAPIDLY REVERSIBLE in all its components.

As for all endo-buccal surgery involving the Airway and susceptible of bleeding secondarily, the observation of this principle aims at optimally ensuring the SAFETY of the patient during the post-operative hours, even if, as usually, the monitoring of this period, notably based on the freedom of the aerial tracts, is, THEORETICALLY, rigourously prescribed and organised.

In the case of punctual discontinuation of the prescribed monitoring, the persistance and especially the recurrence, after definitive awakening, of a notable decrease in vigilance, respiration and/or of the cardio-vascular system, may mask notably, during a certain time, an inhaled and ingurgitated bleeding, and thus lead to an eventually catastrophic picture.

3) The anesthesia must, obviously, be PROLONGED, and the endo-tracheal tube held in place AS LONG AS the stability of the HAEMOSTASIS does not appear to be certain.

- General anesthesia has the advantage over local anesthesia of providing the operator, by virtue of the possibility of then installing the gag, with a surgical field more largely exposed to sight and optimally accessible to surgery ; this notion largely influences the indications of general anesthesia.

B - <u>PRINCIPAL PROBLEMS encountered</u>

Although, in the MAJORITY OF THE CASES, the anesthesia and the surgery take place with no untoward effects or complication and/or in a non-pathological patient, some problems are nonetheless encountered in current practice, with notable frequency :

They are mainly as follows :

I - PROBLEMS DIRECTLY CONNECTED TO THE PATIENT :

. They are presented notably by :

1- OBESITY, which is very frequent, in the context or not of a PICKWICKIAN SYNDROME (7), with an increase in the risks and difficulties of all kinds which generally result from it : prior to operating, it would be desirable whenever possible to have the patient lose weight by prescribing an appropriate diet.

2- CARDIO-VASCULAR DISORDERS, and particularly those which are likely :

. To prevent adrenalin infiltrations.

. In addition, to increase, sometimes considerable, the risk connected to G. A.

. They are, notably :
a) ARTERIAL HYPERTENSION
of which the treatment, balance and eventual visceral repercussions must be assessed.

b) CORONAROPATHY and its eventual complications.
Thus, cases of coronaropathy, sometimes latent, must be investigated and the outcome established, using pre-operative clinical and paraclinical cardiological examinations which are as in-depth as is deemed desirable for the patient involved.

3- RESPIRATORY DISORDERS, which are often due to the use OF TOBACCO
Certainly, the surgery performed aims at improving, FOR THE FUTURE, the ventilatory condition of these patients by freeing their upper aerial tracts. However, DURING THE IMMEDIATE FOLLOW-UP, their DECOMPENSATION may be feared.

- Functional respiratory tests, not systematic but from which at least evident chronic insufficient respiratory patients should benefit, can be made thus to complete, in these cases, the pre-operative picture, by inciting greater per and especially post-operative precautions (4).

4- DIABETES
with its risks of decompensation and the numerous eventual complications, notably cardio-vascular.

5- KIDNEY DISORDERS
particularly susceptible of prolonging the elimination of the anesthetic products administered.

6- CHRONIC ALCOHOLISM
with its whole range of classical complications.

7- As for POLYGLOBULIA, frequent in snorers, and likely eventually to increase the thrombo-embolic risk, it appears to be a probably compensation mechanism of CHRONIC HYPOXIA in the rhonchopathic patient.

. THE INCIDENCE of most of these disorders likely to complicate the administration of anesthesia or even to forbid the surgery obviously increase with AGE.

However, the age of the candidates for this kind of surgery most frequently exceeds 50 years.

> Aside from the exceptional of a 12 years old child, the mean age of the patients who underwent surgery at the Saint-Antoine Hospital was 54 years, and the extremes in age ranged from 18 to 85.

II - PROBLEMS CONNECTED WITH BLEEDING

. Per-operative bleeding is rather frequently difficult to jugulate.
It may require that the ANESTHESIA BE PROLONGED, sometimes for SEVERAL HOURS, although the anesthesia had been indicated and designed as a function of a short operation.

. The recurrence of this bleeding in the post-operative hours is not exceptional, and obliges that the ANESTHESIA BE RENEWED in order to correct the haemostasis surgically.

. This difficulty in performing the haemostasis in the surgical field, when the pre-operative clinical and biological results on coagulation were normal, appears to be clearly more frequent that in the case of a classical simple tonsilectomy : It is probably due in large part, once again, to the patient, who then reveals notably the following eventual factors :

- Arterial hypertension

- Arteriosclerosis which hinders the spontaneous retractibility of the vessels

- Tissular congestion in plethoric subjects

- Muscular hypotonicity, notably around the tonsils, decreasing the passive collapsus of the damaged vessels

- As well as the difficulty in SEEING and HAVING ACCESS to the SURGICAL FIELD, especially in cases of :

. Obesity
. Macroglossia
. Small mouth orifice
. Poor adaptation of the gag to the bucco-facial morphology

. Although the haemorrhage, of the persistant oozing kind, has little chance of being cataclysmic, it can lead to a notable decrease in blood : the accessible transfusional logistic must obviously be capable of coping with such an emergency.

> The indication for surgery given the patient must take account of the fact that the anesthesia envisaged will not of necessity be brief, but eventually of a long duration and/or renewed the same day.

III - A PARTICULAR TECHNICAL DIFFICULTY : THE DIFFICULT INTUBATION of some of these patients.

- Much more often than is usual, it is found to be DIFFICULT, even IMPOSSIBLE, to expose the larynx of some rhonchopathic patients using the classical laryngoscopic technique, or at least without serious risk to the teeth, and to perform the intubation.

- This difficulty seems to be due to the PARTICULAR MORPHOLOGY of these patients, in whom the following characteristics, more or less associated, are found :

. OBESITY with SHORT NECK
. RETROGNATHISM
. MACROGLOSSIA
. SMALL MOUTH ORIFICE

- This difficulty is thus less unexpected that would initially appear, since this morphology can also play a role in favouring ronchopathy itself in the pathogeny, like some cases of sleep apnea (8).

- Besides the classical naso-tracheal "blind" intubation, which is too often random, the really adequate solution, and, moreover, the most modern, consists in performing the INTUBATION OF THESE PATIENTS via FIBROSCOPY.

. However, for reasons of SAFETY, this fibroscopic intubation can only be carried out BEFORE the induction of the anesthesia. It is in fact clear that inducing a general anesthesia WHEN A REASONABLY SUPPORTED FEAR NOT TO PERFORM INTUBATION EXISTS would be the worst kind of IMPRUDENCE : how would it be possible to avoid or limit the Mendelson Syndrom if vomiting occurred, which is always possible even in the case of a stomach which is deemed to empty.

. Yet, on another hand, despite the premedication using an anxiolytic and if possible a vagolytic drug, and despite the local contact anesthesia which accompanies fibroscopic intubation, this procedure is very disagreable for the subject who remains conscious.

. Thus, in order to preserve the comfort of a maximal number of patients and to take the minimum of risks, the candidates for C.R. were, at the end of the careful clinical examination, classifie in two categories :

1- Those - the most numerous - for whom a problem-free intubation could be envisaged : they were anesthetised, then given intubation in the classical manner.

2- Those - a large minority - for whom intubation looked as if it would be hazardous : they were systematically doomed to fibroscopic intubation before anesthesia.

. Thus :

> Out of 133 patients operated on using general anesthesia, and thus provided with intubation, 29, that is 21%, were given fibroscopic intubation at the outset.

- This fact solicits two remarks concerning good sense :

> . More than ever, it is necessary to be attentive to the STABILITY of the HAEMOSTASIS prior to removing the INTUBATION from a patient for whom intubation was difficult, or who received intubation via fibroscopy.

. It is highly desirable, for the performance of this surgery, to have a fibroscope available 24 hours a day, as surely it is occasionally necessary to re-operate during the post-operative hours ....

CONCLUSION

Of course, IN MOST OF THE CASES, local or general anesthesia for surgery for snoring does not present any insurmontable problem : thus more than 800 patients were able to benefit from such surgery at the Saint-Antoine Hospital, since May 85.

It is no less true that this surgery does have a POTENTIAL AND NON-NEGLIGIBLE ANESTHESIOLOGICAL RISK, connected to the anesthesia itself, and moveover increased by the fact that the surgical field involved the Airway.

This risk is MORE AGAIN COMPLICATED by problems frequently resulting from the PATIENT in whom the surgery for snoring is currently called upon.

Besides, unfortunately, it must be here emphasized again that local anesthesia, theorically not so dangerous than general anesthesia, cannot be a recourse for this surgery when the patient is unable to endure general anesthesia : sometimes, indeed, this intervention, performed with local anesthesia, has to be renewed some hours later with general anesthesia.

This means that the INDICATION for this surgery, certainly helpful, but far from always being indispensable, must, for each case, be weighed, and thought out, more than ever, with GOOD SENSE.

The awareness of the potential anesthetic risk taken must certainly not lead to a limitation of EXCESS to the field opened up for this new surgery, but it nonetheless appears to be of a nature to shore up REASONABLY, the growth of operative indications likely to result quite naturally in the insistence of the request, and/or in the ENTHUSIASM which may, indeed, appear to give rise to the U.P.P.P. : because of anesthesia, of course, this surgery cannot have the reputation of being potentially anodyne.

BIBLIOGRAPHIE

1 - **HATTON F, TIRET L, MAUJOL L, N'DOYE P, VOURC'H G, DESMONTS J.M., OTTENI J.C, SCHERPEREEL P**
Enquête épidémiologique sur les anesthésies.
ANN. FR. ANESTH. REANIM. 2, 331-386, 1983

2 - **HERMAN D, DRY J**
Accidents allergiques dus aux anesthésiques.
ENTRETIENS DE BICHAT. PITIE-SALPETRIERE -
THERAPEUTIQUE, 17-20, 1976

3 - **JOHNSON J. T, SANDERS M.H**
Breathing during sleep immediately after uvulopalatopharyngoplasty
Laryngoscope, 96, 1236-1238, Nov. 1986

4 - **LARMINAT (J.M. de), BOUCHEREZ C, LIENHART A, ABEN-MOHA J, CHOUARD C. H.**
L'Anesthésie locale pour l'amygdalectomie, chez l'adulte :
Intérêt, inconvénients, indications
82ème Congrès Français d'ORL - Compte-rendu des séances.
ARNETTE Ed. 404-413, 1985

5 - **LE MAT A.M.**
Les accidents de l'anesthésie locale.
Q. S. (Revue des Laboratoires Roger BELLON), 31, 86-89, 1980

6 - **LENOIR J.L.**
In : L'Anesthésie dans l'amygdalectomie, Table ronde.
REV. OTO. LARYNGOL., 95, 756-763, 1974

7 - **NEUMAN G.G, Baldwin C.C, PETRINI A.J, WISE L, WOLLMAN S.B**
Perioperative management of a 430 kilogram (946 pound) patient with Pickwickian syndrome.
Anesth. Analg. 1986 Sep : 65 (9) : 985-7.

8 - **ROA N.L, MOSS K.S**
Treacher-Collins syndrome with sleep apnea : anesthetic considerations.
Anesthesiology 1984, Jan : 60 (1) : 71-3.